New Trends and Developments in Vaccines

New Trends and Developments in Vaccines

Edited by

A. Voller

Nuffield Laboratories of Comparative Medicine, Institute of Zoology, Zoological Society of London; and

H. Friedman

Department of Microbiology, Albert Einstein Medical Center, New York

MTP

This book is based in part on an international symposium organized by ROBERT S. FIRST, INC. which is located at 405 Lexington Avenue, New York, N.Y. 10017 and Avenue Marnix 19A, 1050 Brussels, Belgium. ROBERT S. FIRST, INC. specializes in Market and Economic Research, Conferences, and Publications in all phases of the Health Care Industry.

Published by
MTP Press Limited
St Leonard's House
St Leonardgate
Lancaster, England

Softcover reprint of the hardcover 1st edition 1978

ISBN-13: 978-94-011-6632-4 e-ISBN-13: 978-94-011-6630-0
DOI: 10.1007/978-94-011-6630-0

Trowbridge & Esher

Contents

List of Contributors vii

Preface ix

1. Introduction
H. Friedman and A. Voller 1

2. New developments in vaccines
W. Hennesen 7

3. Paediatric vaccines
S. A. Plotkin 19

4. The whooping cough vaccine controversy
G. Dick 29

5. Measles vaccines
E. Norrby 55

6. Vaccines against influenza
C. Hannoun 63

7. The New York Swine Influenza Immunization Program
P. J. Imperato 71

8. Rabies vaccines
J. Crick 87

9. Rubella vaccines
C. Huygelen 103

10. Vaccination against poliomyelitis
J. Salk and D. Salk 117

11. Hepatitis viruses and vaccines
M. R. Hilleman, V. M. Villarejos, E. B. Buynak, O. L. Ittensohn, W. J. McAleer, Arlene A. McLean, W. J. Miller, P. J. Provost, A. A. Tytell and B. S. Wolanski 155

12. Developments with hepatitis B vaccines
A. J. Zuckerman 171

13. Herpesvirus vaccine development: studies of virus morphological components
S. K. Vernon, W. C. Lawrence, Carole A. Long, G. H. Cohen and B. A. Rubin 179

14. Ribosomal vaccines: a review
T. K. Eisenstein 211

15. Cholera vaccines
H. Friedman 223

16. A vaccine for the prevention of pneumococcal infections
G. Schiffman 237

17. Meningococcal vaccines
W. A. Hankins 245

18. Development of meningococcal vaccines
R. Triau 255

19. Immunization with streptococcus mutans against dental caries in Rhesus monkeys
T. Lehner, S. J. Challacombe and Jill Caldwell 275

20. Vaccination against tropical parasitic diseases
A. Voller 299

21. Notes on veterinary vaccines
A. J. Beale 311

22. Standardization and control of allergen extracts
W. D. Brighton 315

Index 321

List of Contributors

J. BEALE
Head, Biological Department,
Wellcome Research Laboratories,
Beckenham, Kent BR3 3BS

W. D. BRIGHTON
Head, Laboratory of Allergens,
National Institute for Biological Standards and Control, Hampstead, London NW3 6RB

E. B. BUYNAK
Division of Virus and Cell Biology Research, Merck Institute for Therapeutic Research, West Point, Pennsylvania 19486, USA

JILL CALDWELL
Department of Oral Immunology and Microbiology, Guy's Hospital Medical and Dental Schools, London SE1 9RT

S. J. CHALLACOMBE
Department of Oral Immunology and Microbiology, Guy's Hospital Medical and Dental Schools, London SE1 9RT

G. H. COHEN
Wyeth Laboratories Inc.,
Philadelphia, Pennsylvania 19101, USA

J. CRICK
Biochemistry Department,
Animal Virus Research Institute,
Woking, Surrey GU24 ONF

G. DICK
Regional Postgraduate Dean,
University of London Postgraduate Medical Foundation, London NW1 5HD

T. K. EISENSTEIN
Department of Microbiology and Immunology, Temple University School of Health, Health Services Center,
Philadelphia, Pennsylvania 19140, USA

H. FRIEDMAN
Head, Department of Microbiology,
Albert Einstein Medical Center,
Philadelphia, Pennsylvania 19140, USA

W. A. HANKINS
Manager, Research and Development,
Connaught Laboratories Inc.,
Swiftwater, Pennsylvania 18370, USA

C. HANNOUN
Viral Ecology Unit,
Institut Pasteur,
F-75724 Paris, France

W. HENNESSEN
Behringwerke,
D-3550 Marburg/Lahn, West Germany

M. R. HILLEMAN
Director, Division of Virus and Cell Biology Research, Merck Institute for Therapeutic Research, West Point, Pennsylvania 19486, USA

C. HUYGELEN
Director of Research,
Recherche et Industrie Therapeutique SA,
B-1330 Rixensart, Belgium

P. J. IMPERATO
First Deputy Commissioner,
New York City Department of Health,
New York, New York 10013, USA

O. L. ITTENSOHN
Division of Virus and Cell Biology Research, Merck Institute for Therapeutic Research, West Point, Pennsylvania 19486, USA

W. C. LAWRENCE
Wyeth Laboratories Inc., Philadelphia, Pennsylvania 19101, USA

T. LEHNER
Department of Oral Immunology and Microbiology, Guy's Hospital Medical and Dental Schools, London SE1 9RT

CAROLE A. LONG
Wyeth Laboratories Inc., Philadelphia, Pennsylvania 19101, USA

W. J. McALEER
Division of Virus and Cell Biology Research, Merck Institute for Therapeutic Research, West Point, Pennsylvania 19486, USA

A. A. McLEAN
Division of Virus and Cell Biology Research, Merck Institute for Therapeutic Research, West Point, Pennsylvania 19486, USA

W. J. MILLER
Division of Virus and Cell Biology Research, Merck Institute for Therapeutic Research, West Point, Pennsylvania 19486, USA

E. NORRBY
Professor and Head, Department of Virology, Karolinska Institutet, S-105–21 Stockholm, Sweden

S. A. PLOTKIN
Director of Infectious Diseases, Virus Laboratory, Joseph Stokes Jr. Research Institute, Children's Hospital, Philadelphia, Pennsylvania 19101, USA

P. J. PROVOST
Division of Virus and Cell Biology Research, Merck Institute for Therapeutic Research, West Point, Pennsylvania 19486, USA

B. A. RUBIN
Manager, Biological Products Department, Wyeth Laboratories Inc., Philadelphia, Pennsylvania 19101, USA

D. SALK
Departments of Pathology and Biochemistry, University of Washington, Seattle, Washington, USA

J. SALK
The Salk Institute, PO Box 1809, San Diego, California 92112, USA

G. SCHIFFMAN
Wyeth Laboratories Inc., Philadelphia, Pennsylvania 19101, USA

R. TRIAU
Medical Director, Institut Merieux, F-19002 Lyon, France

A. A. TYTELL
Division of Virus and Cell Biology Research, Merck Institute for Therapeutic Research, West Point, Pennsylvania 19486, USA

S. K. VERNON
Wyeth Laboratories Inc., Philadelphia, Pennsylvania 19101, USA

V. M. VILLAREJOS
Louisiana State University International Center for Medical Research and Training, San Jose, Costa Rica

A. VOLLER
Nuffield Laboratories of Comparative Medicine, Institute of Zoology, The Zoological Society of London. Regent's Park, London NW1 4RY

B. S. WOLANSKI
Division of Virus and Cell Biology Research, Merck Institute for Therapeutic Research, West Point, Pennsylvania 19486, USA

A. J. ZUCKERMAN
Professor and Head, Department of Microbiology, and WHO Collaborating Centre for Reference and Research on Viral Hepatitis, London School of Hygiene and Tropical Medicine, London WC1E 7HT

Preface

It was not too long ago that many physicians and biomedical scientists felt that the era of 'vaccines' for protecting mankind against infectious disease was coming to an end. During the 1940s and 50s the widespread use of newly developed antibiotics and antimicrobial chemotherapeutic agents suggested a new era in medicine, i.e. the control and eventual elimination of all infectious diseases, at least those caused by bacteria, by chemical means. The magic 'bullet' proposed by Paul Ehrlich in the early 1900s seemed to be the method of choice for controling infection. However, it is now quite evident that those high expectations were unwarranted. Although many acute infections, especially those caused by pyogenic cocci, have been controlled by antibiotics, it is quite evident that infectious diseases, even those caused by bacteria, still are a major problem. Thus, the old 'standby' of preventative vaccination is making a strong comeback, not only for viral but also for bacterial infections. However, except for a relatively small number of viral diseases and those bacterial diseases due to toxin elaborated by microorganisms rather than invasion and replication of the microbe *per se*, preventative vaccination still has not fulfilled the expectations of their proponents.

There has been a recent resurgence of interest concerning all aspects of vaccines, not only their preparation and administration, but also the nature and mechanism of the host immune response to the constituent microorganisms and their products. A number of recent symposia, conferences, and scientific sessions at national and international meetings have been devoted to the subject of vaccines. This volume is an outgrowth of an international meeting held in Brussels, Belgium under the sponsorship of the Robert S. First Co. At the Conference a number of presentations were made in attempts to answer some of the vital questions concerning the value of various vaccines for bacterial, viral, parasitic and fungal infections, as well as newer developments in this ares. Both fundamental and clinical aspects of vaccine development, use, and applications were discussed. A number of participants were then asked to contribute chapters to this volume. In addition other investigators actively participating in either development or use of newer vaccines for a variety of purposes were also asked to contribute to this volume. No attempt was made to cover completely every aspect of vaccines, either historical or prospectives for the future. It is anticipated that further conferences as well as publications dealing with this rapidly re-emerging area of microbial immunology and preventative medicine will, within the next few years, permit the realization of many hopes by biomedical scientists that infectious diseases can be controlled by appropriate immunological 'engineering,' i.e. administration of effective and safe vaccines.

The editors are grateful to contributors to this volume who obviously gave of their time and effort in preparing manuscripts. The editors are also grateful to the staff of MTP Press for their forebearance and assistance. We also wish to acknowledge the excellent assistant of Ms. Leony Mills, Albert Einstein Medical Center, Philadelphia, Penna. for various editorial aspects in preparing this volume.

Herman Friedman
Alister Voller
January 1978

1
Vaccines: general background and introduction

H. FRIEDMAN AND A. VOLLER

It has only been about a century since the definitive discovery that infectious diseases were caused by micro-organisms. At about the same time it was shown categorically that many of these infections could be prevented by administering properly prepared and utilized vaccines. Once such observations were accepted by the biomedical community, the pendulum swung from a general attitude of scepticism to the belief that it was necessary only to identify the appropriate micro-organism, prepare the corresponding vaccine, inject this material on to individuals and a wide variety of diseases could be prevented, ameliorated or cured.

Obviously this concept was quite simplistic, especially since the mechanism of the host–parasite relationship in terms of infectious agents was not completely understood, either at the end of the last century or even today. Vaccines *per se* are used to confer immunity by stimulating a complex series of events culminating in development of specific lymphoid cells and their products which can interact with the infectious agents. Thus the purpose of immunization is to stimulate a specific immunological response to a microbial agent or antigens, with the expectation that this will result in humoral factors (i.e., protective antibodies) in the blood or development of cell-mediated immunity. While such protection may diminish with time, sufficient residual immunity usually remains, so that the individual is expected to respond to future exposure to the same antigenic stimulus with a rapid return of the immune response, because of heightened reactivity of the antibody forming phagocytic and/or other cell classes within the immune system.

Presumably the concept of immunity to what are now known to be infectious diseases was understood by ancient civilizations many thousands of years ago, even though the cause or even nature of such diseases was not known. It is usually assumed that modern 'vaccination' began with the observations and reports of Jenner at the end of the eighteenth century that smallpox could be prevented by first 'vaccinating' individuals with cowpox, similar to the natural situation in which milkmaids acquired cowpox in nature. However, it is acknowledged that such prevention of infection by exposing individuals to attenuated infectious agents was known at least a thousand years earlier. Apparently the Chinese were aware that smallpox could be prevented by exposure to mild cases. This information appears to have been brought back to Europe by travellers and adventurers such as Marco Polo. Nevertheless, it is conceded that the modern era of vaccination began only 100 years ago. The first 'golden era' of immunology developed rapidly at the end of the last century and the beginning of the present one, when immunity was first studied in terms of mechanisms whereby individuals can be made resistant to infections by administration of certain vaccines. It is now widely recognized that, after most infectious diseases, immunity is generally acquired and that similar forms of immunity may be induced by administration of appropriately prepared 'vaccines' derived from inactivated or live micro-organisms of modified (i.e., attenuated) disease producing potential. Thus the purpose of immunization, at least in terms of infectious diseases, is to provoke a specific immunological response to a selected agent or antigen, with the expectation that this would result in humoral (i.e., antibody) protective factors in the blood. While such protection may diminish with time, sufficient residual immunity remains, so that a heightened and more rapid immune response occurs upon a subsequent exposure to the same micro-organism.

It became quite clear at the beginning of this century that cellular aspects of immunity were also involved in protection and/or defence from microbial infection. Phagocytic activity, considered to reflect mainly a non-specific phenomenon, was thought by some of the earliest immunologists to be more important than humoral immunity in protection against infectious agents. Furthermore, in many cases humoral antibody was thought to function mainly by enhancing phagocytosis by macrophages. Other cells involved in what is now considered 'classic' cell-mediated immunity may also be stimulated by infectious disease agents, and vaccines can mimic the effects of such infections. Indeed during the last few decades interest in the role of cell-mediated immunity, especially that involving specifically sensitized T-lymphocytes, has increased in almost an explosive manner in many areas of basic and applied immunology.

For those diseases in which the role and manner of the immune responses are clearly defined, methods for prevention of infection have been readily devised by developing vaccines which are generally considered safe and effective. It has been widely acknowledged that, with adequate immunization programmes, marked reduction or elimination of such previously common diseases as smallpox, measles, diphtheria, tetanus, poliomyelitis and scarlet fever can be achieved. However, many infectious diseases present special problems which have impeded development of effective vaccines. One such example is infection with *Salmonella* bacteria; the *Salmonella* group of organisms is composed of a multiplicity of antigenic variants or strains numbering hundreds. Furthermore, among the respiratory diseases, the 'cold' viruses and pneumococci present a similar problem. Recovery from infection of any one type of organism generally leaves the individual vulnerable to others.

It should be noted that antigen–antibody reactions involved in microbial infections are not well understood in most cases. The immune response to some antigens may be absent, or meagre. In addition, pathogenesis in many diseases induced by some bacteria is often poorly understood. The presence of micro-organisms or their antigen may sometimes be advantageous or part of a complex cycle in the evolution of the disease syndrome in question. In some situations the exact host relationship to the presumed offending organism may be so obscure that factors which determine infection and/or resistance remain undefined. In this regard, the role of cell-mediated immunity, as well as factors derived of T-lymphocytes and macrophages in controlling or preventing infectious diseases, (either in individuals who have been actively exposed to micro-organisms or been treated with a vaccine) is essentially unknown. Despite these problems, marked advances concerning the use of vaccines in preventing microbial infections have been made over the past few decades. It should be noted, however, that during a period of two decades or so, shortly after the development of 'chemotherapeutic' agents and antibiotics, it was felt by many that infectious diseases could be controlled chemically rather than immunologically. This obviously has not occurred. Although some of the major acute infections of man have been readily controlled by antibiotic treatment, infections are still a major problem in human medicine. It has been estimated that at least 70% of all patient visits to physicians are due to an infection. In the USA alone, it has been estimated that over 100 000 individuals die per year because of hospital-acquired infections. Thus the advantage of preventive immunization, for controlling both acute and chronic infections of man by a wide variety of micro-organisms, is once again being seriously considered.

Recent events during the last few years have focused attention on vaccines for preventing important infections. A polyvalent pneumococcal polysaccharide vaccine, based on careful isolation and identification of polysaccharides associated with certain strains of pneumococci, has recently been approved for widespread use in the USA and elsewhere. The eradication of smallpox as an infection in man has been proclaimed by world health organizations. On the other hand, an attempt to 'prevent' a suspected pandemic of influenza, i.e., the Swine Flu Programme, brought attention to the difficulties not only in developing an effective and safe vaccine for a common upper respiratory virus infection, but also the difficulties in predicting in advance which strain of virus may be prevalent in the next epidemic, and whether or not such an epidemic would indeed occur. Some of the dangers involved in vaccine administration, especially vaccines prepared from biologically active substrates such as eggs, were pointed out by the influenza virus programme in the USA. On the other hand, the tremendous success achieved in eradicating polio by means not only of a killed vaccine, but also a 'live' vaccine, has brought the scientific community and the lay public to a level of expectation which has not been realized in other areas of medicine.

Many of the advances in preparing effective vaccines have been achieved with viruses and toxic products from micro-organisms. These advances have been achieved mainly because of knowledge of the antigens involved. However, further achievements in the area of effective vaccines will also depend upon increased understanding of the immune response mechanisms and requirements for inducing effective immunity to certain micro-organisms. It is widely accepted that certain forms of antigen are more effective than others and that there are differences in the protective immune response based not only upon the antigen used, but its route and dose of administration, the immune status of the host, etc. An understanding of the antigenic nature of the micro-organism (be it a bacterium, a virus, or a protozoan) is also essential. Much knowledge must also be gained concerning many areas of microbial immunology and the host–parasite relationship. However, based on successes achieved to date with certain vaccines, it seems likely that even greater successes will be apparent in future years.

This volume is based generally on the proceedings of a conference on the topic of New Trends and Developments in Vaccines, sponsored by the Robert S. First Co. and held in Brussels, Belgium. A number of investigators who presented scientific papers were invited to review their work for this volume. In addition, other chapters were solicited from well-known bioscientists who have made major contributions in the field of vaccines. It is apparent from the presentations at the meeting and chapters submitted for this volume that most of the successful vaccines to date have been those derived from either inactivated or attenuated virus preparations. This is not surprising since the initial vaccine developed for man almost a hundred years ago was also for a virus infection, i.e., rabies. Bacterial vaccines also have been used extensively over the last half-century or so. As stated earlier, many of these vaccines, especially those developed for cholera, salmonella (i.e., typhoid fever) etc., have had only limited effectiveness. Newer types of bacterial vaccines are dependent upon identification of the protective antigen on the micro-organism. In this regard, a number of newer vaccines have been recently developed, including a pneumococcal vaccine, as well as vaccines for meningococci. However, since many of the newer developments deal with vaccines for viral infections, a number of chapters deal with such vaccines, i.e., rubella, measles, polio, influenza, hepatitis and herpes viruses. The important role of vaccines in protecting children from infectious diseases is properly emphasized. However we are made aware that the effects of vaccination (e.g. against whooping cough) are difficult to estimate and the risks have to be carefully weighed against the benefits. Developments in the area of vaccination against dental infections, as well as veterinary vaccines for parasitic diseases, and allergies are also described.

It is anticipated that much further work will be performed in the area of microbial vaccines, especially because of the serious limitations of chemotherapeutic agents not only for microbial infections but obviously also for parasitic and viral infections. This is evident from the renewed interest in the current status and prospects for improved microbial vaccines as reviewed in a number of other recent symposia, conferences and publications. It is anticipated that in the near future much more information will be available, not only concerning the basic immune response mechanism in infectious diseases, but also the mechanism whereby effective and safe microbial vaccines influence the immune response.

2
New developments in vaccines

W. HENNESSEN

Developments are based on past experience and lead to the future. With vaccines, success in the past will show what can be expected for the future. This paper tries to demonstrate what factors are to be considered for a reliable prediction for developments in vaccines. The factors studied are:

feasibility of manufacture of vaccines
quality requirements
target populations
epidemiological considerations
costs
consequences

FEASIBILITY OF MANUFACTURE OF VACCINES

It seems safe to say that, in a decade or less, it will be possible to offer vaccines against all infectious diseases caused by viruses or bacteria. Antiparasite vaccines, perhaps even certain antitumour vaccines, will also be available. Some may regard such a plain statement as sensational, some as natural progress. In figures it looks explosive (Figure 1); on this diagram the number of antigens from which the vaccines are produced is tabulated for the period from 1950 to 1985. It does not contain all the combined vaccines which can be made out of these antigens. It shows that before 1960 there were ten antigens developed for vaccine production: diphtheria; vaccinia; tetanus; rabies (?); pertussis; influenza; typhoid (?); poliomyelitis (Salk); BCG; measles (inactivated). A number of them were not yet as effective as required today.

Between 1970 and 1975 certain other vaccines were developed (see Table 1). The steep increase of antigens for vaccines will take place during the

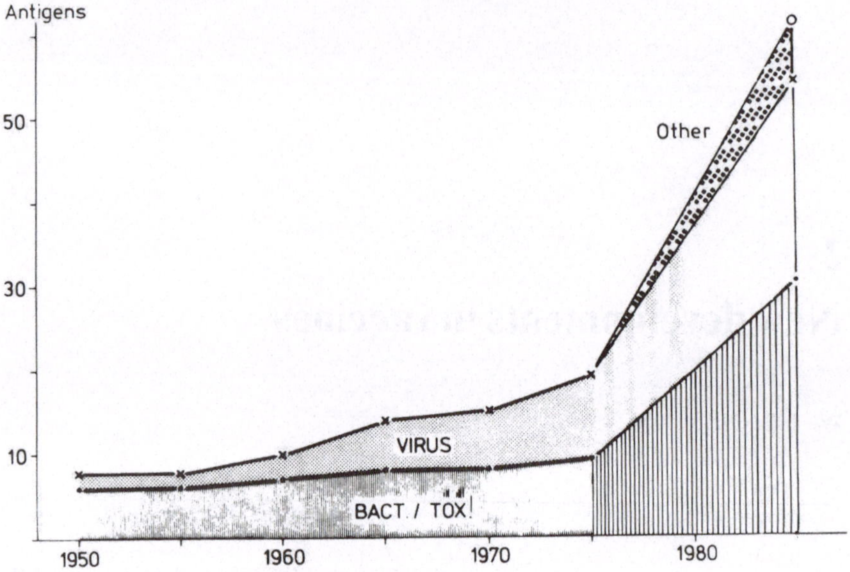

Figure 1 Human vaccines, 1950–85

Table 1 New vaccines, 1970–75

Vaccinees	*Bacteria/Toxoids*	*Virus*
Children	Meningococci A, C	Rubella Mumps Poliomyelitis HDC
Adults		Rabiės HDC

next 10–15 years. With more than double the number of antigens it will be possible to cover all infectious diseases caused by bacteria and viruses and more. These new developments are listed in Table 2. It goes without saying that, as in the past, existing vaccines will be improved, be it for better compatibility or better efficacy. Such improvements require an increasing integration of biophysical, biochemical and microbial technology into vaccine manufacture. One example may demonstrate what is meant here. Some viral vaccines (influenza-inactivated, rabies-inactivated, others to come) in routine production were only made possible by the use of centrifuges which were developed for space research. Some enthusiasts for space-labs still expect vaccine manufacture to be carried out in space to achieve more purity for the products. From what has been shown so far it is self-evident that future vaccine production, or at least the know-how, can only be found in highly industrialized areas.

Although it would go far beyond the scope of this paper to describe just

Table 2 New vaccines – expected development after 1976

Vaccinees	*Bacteria/Toxoids*	*Virus*	*Other*
Children	Meningococci B Meningococci A + B Polyv. pneumococci *H. influenza* Caries Trachoma	Herpes simplex 1 + 2 Cytomegalo Varicella/Zoster Rota	
Adults	Bact. enterotoxoids Pseudomonas Cholera-toxoids Gonococci Syphilis	Influenza, inactivated Influenza, live, att. Resp. syncytial Parainfluenza 1 – 3 Hepatitis A + B	Parasites Tumour

parts of the progress of vaccine manufacture, one development should be mentioned here. It has been proved that the virus particle – the virion – is in fact a complicated machinery for the production of protein. The reproduction of its own protein involves the multiplication of billions and billions of new virus particles. It is not the function of this machine to cause disease; disease is only the result. The essential parts for the reproductive function are known, as are the facilities to stop the machine. Among the inactivated virus vaccines the most advanced are already used under the definition of subunit vaccines. They are directed against the essential parts of the virion, not against the whole virus machinery. This is the case today for influenza virus vaccines; it has been used for measles vaccines and it will be used in due time for even better rabies or herpes vaccines.

QUALITY REQUIREMENTS

Throughout the world, vaccines are under a special, mainly national, control. The reasons for this are partly explained in Table 3. Here, some of the differences between drugs and vaccines are listed. National, supranational and

Table 3 Comparison of nature of drugs and vaccines

	Drugs	*Vaccines*
Origin	Mineral denaturated	Biological Live
Medical use	Treatment individual	Prophylaxis group
Action obvious to physician	Yes	No
Manufacturer	Pharmacist	Biologist
Quality control	Pharmacist	Biologist
Measure of active substances	Weight Chemical reaction	Biolog. reference animal experiment
Efficacy	Short	(Live) long

international requirements agree that for such sophisticated test systems only the most experienced, best-equipped institutions are in a position to perform such a control. As an example, the control of live polio vaccine is given in Figure 2. Only after all these tests are performed is it possible to define a given suspension of poliomyelitis virus as a vaccine. It will be mentioned later that national and international organizations who sponsor vaccination programmes regard quality as the condition for success of their campaigns.

As far as manufacturing is concerned, control of vaccines at present and in the foreseeable future with all its complexity is only conceivable where biology meets the highest possible standards. It should be kept in mind that

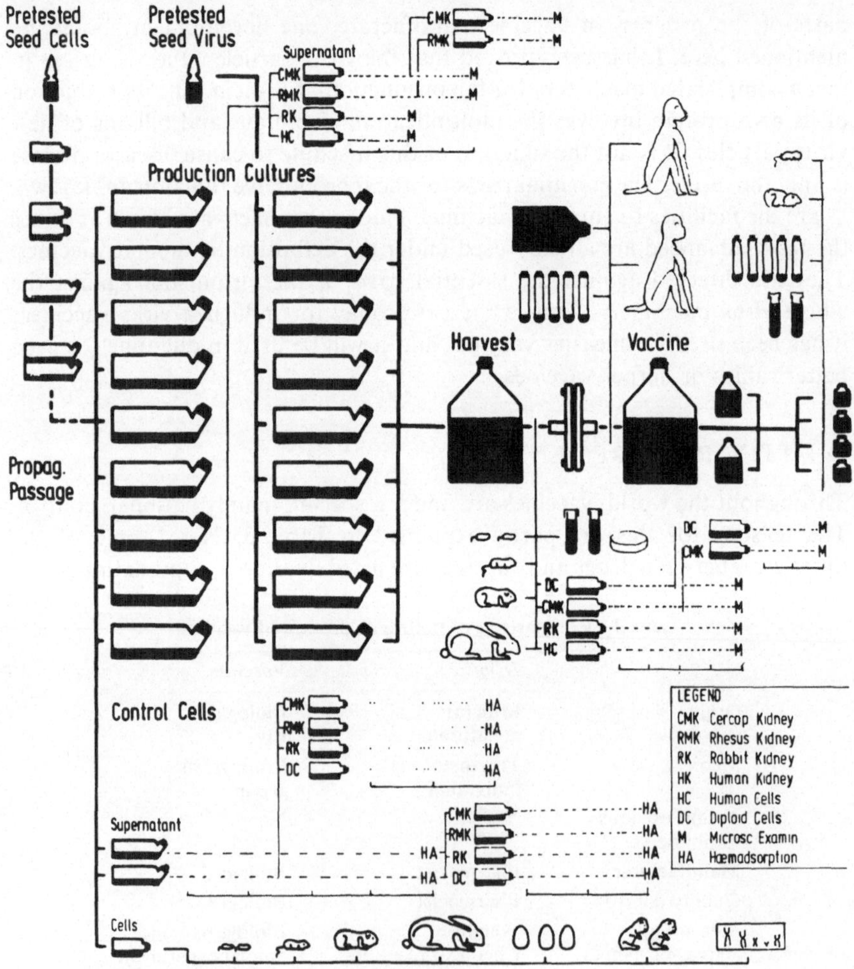

Figure 2 Control of live oral poliomyelitis vaccine (from human diploid cells)

quality control is far from being satisfactory for all vaccines. It received general attention in the mid-1950s with the arrival of virus vaccines such as poliomyelitis (inactivated) when safety and efficacy became of vital importance. The older vaccines – the classical ones – will have to be improved quickly, both for safety and efficacy, because in the years to come it will be better appreciated that an unsafe or poorly tolerated vaccine is a danger, and an inefficient vaccine is a nuisance.

TARGET POPULATIONS

The highest standards of living or civilization on this globe are found in Western Europe, North America and some communities in close contact with the nations of these areas. Infant mortality is regarded as one of the parameters of such standards. It is useful to analyse what developments took place in the industrialized parts of the world from the past to the present, in the context of vaccines.

A comparison of the mortality rates recorded in West Germany for 1910 and 1967 reflects our development. The general mortality in 1910 (Figure 3) shows a high death-rate in early childhood; by 1967 this was eliminated. The cause of such an elimination is not a reduction of heart diseases (Figure 4), nor a reduction of malignancies (Figure 5), but is exclusively a reduction of deaths due to infectious diseases (Figure 6), predominantly in childhood. As proof that vaccination was the decisive factor certain infectious diseases

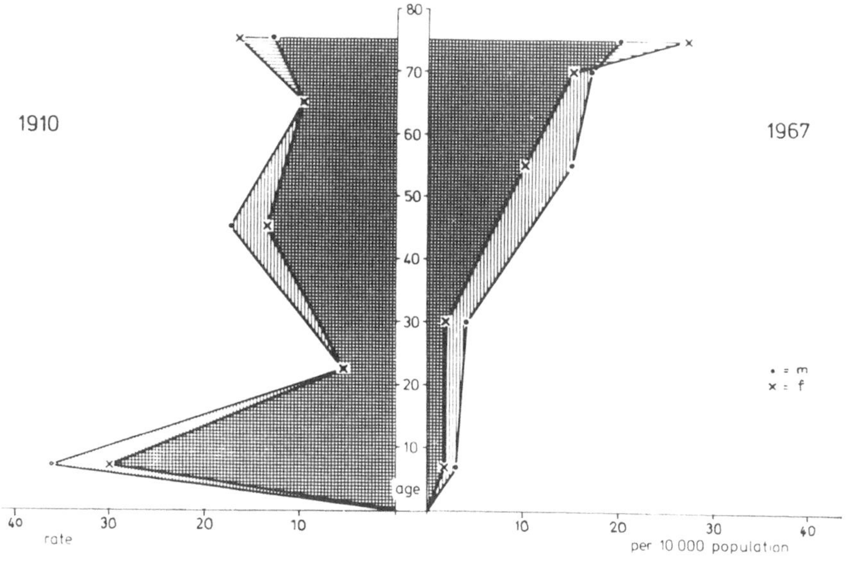

Figure 3 Age distribution of mortality in 1910 and 1967 for the Federal Republic of Germany: total

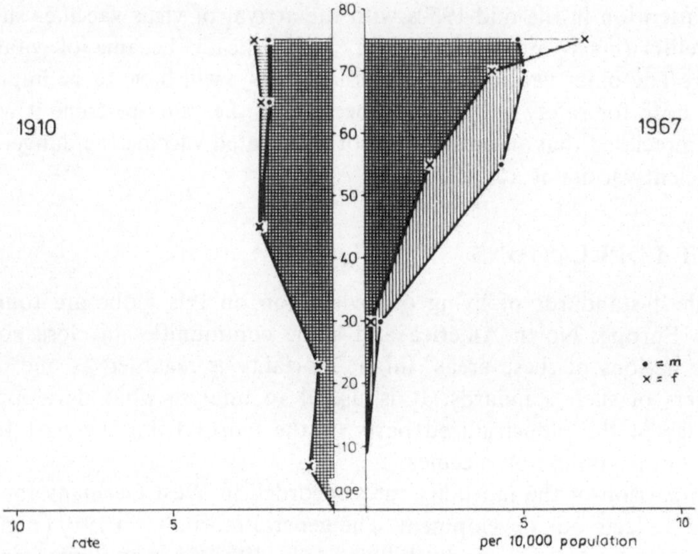

Figure 4 Age distribution of mortality in 1910 and 1967 for the Federal Republic of Germany: heart and circulation

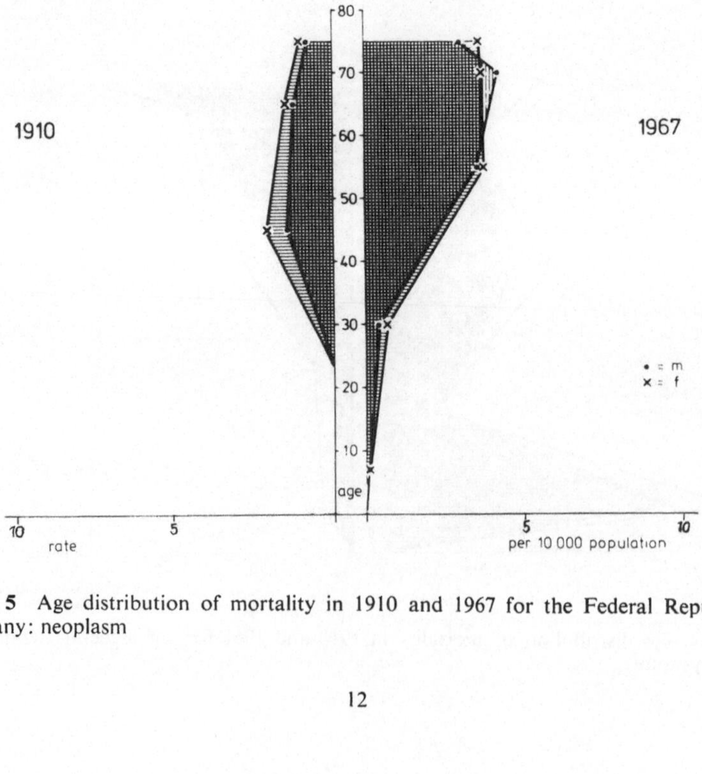

Figure 5 Age distribution of mortality in 1910 and 1967 for the Federal Republic of Germany: neoplasm

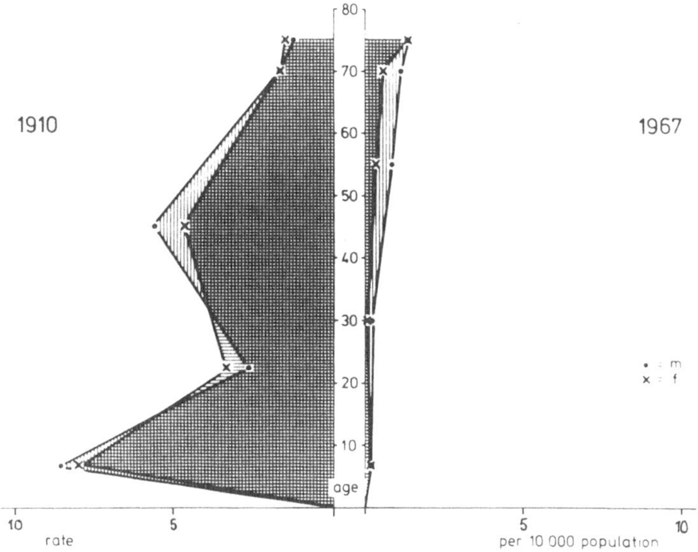

Figure 6 Age distribution of mortality in 1910 and 1967 for the Federal Republic of Germany: infectious diseases

in the same country were compared. Figure 7 demonstrates that infections for which there is excellent treatment but no vaccination (such as scarlet fever, infectious enteritis or meningitis) do not disappear. While those diseases for which there is no treatment (e.g. poliomyelitis or diphtheria) are close to eradication because of vaccination.

If the developing parts of the world wish to reach the standard of living of the industrialized nations, they will have to follow the lines drawn by our fathers and grandfathers in medicine. The smallpox eradication programme has proved already that they can achieve success similar to that reached in Europe, when smallpox vaccination was introduced in the last century, Figure 8 shows the dramatic effect such a programme had on the incidence of smallpox on a European population. The nations which we call the third world must first introduce paediatric vaccines. The order of vaccines will depend on the logistics in the country. Vaccines easy to ship into remote places should be among the first. They are smallpox and DPT (diphtheria, pertussis, tetanus). Live vaccines (polio, measles, BCG) require a more complicated system for transport and application (cooling). As soon as they are sufficiently potent, safe and easy to transport and administer, typhoid vaccines will find large populations in need of protection. The vaccines mentioned above will, when properly used, reduce the big killing diseases of children in the nations concerned and finally in the whole world. Billions of doses of first-quality products will be needed. Once started, vaccination programmes can hardly be discontinued. Vaccines do not destroy the infectious agents, nor do they eradicate the infectious agents;

but they do eradicate disease, enabling vaccinated populations to live with such agents, just as we have for decades.

It was stated before that the production of even a limited number of highest quality vaccines in enormous quantities, will require the most advanced biotechnology. This means they will have to be produced in industrialized countries. Manufacture of the vaccines will be one thing and a service system for the administration and application will have to be developed too. The example of the WHO'S successful struggle against smallpox in the world is extremely instructive from the point of view of what is needed in such a fight. Excellent smallpox vaccines have been produced since World War II, but it was not before the early 1960s that a commercial manufacturer

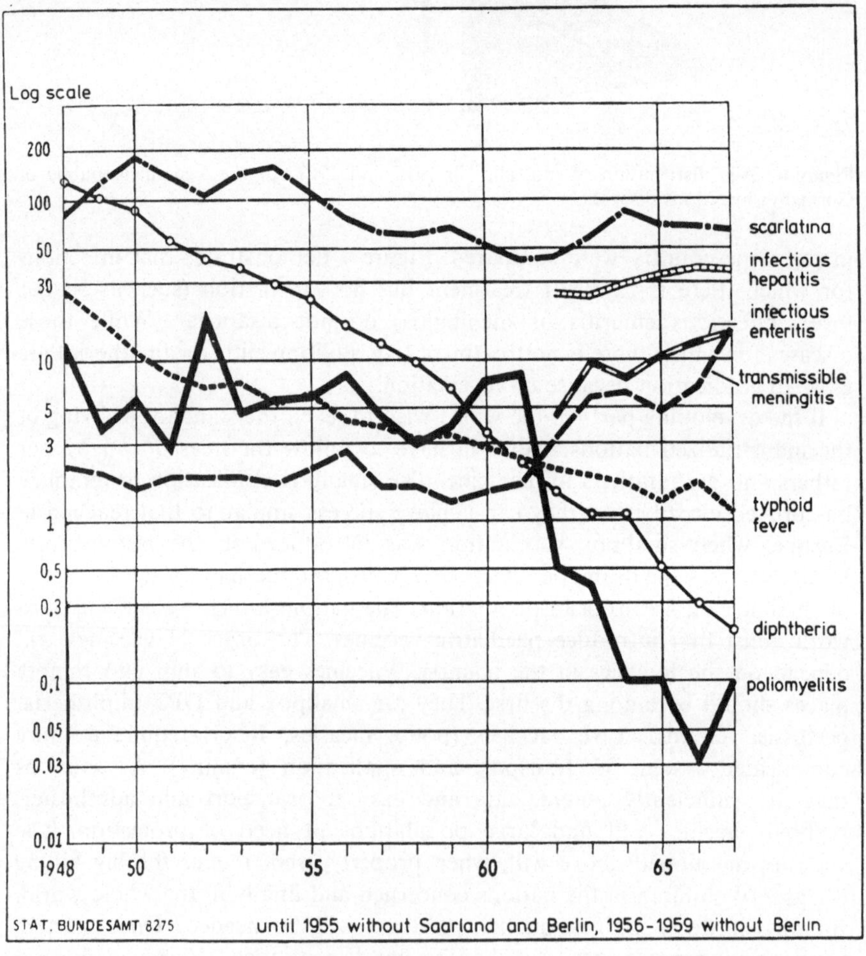

Figure 7 Development of selected diseases subject to compulsory notification (cases per 100 000 population)

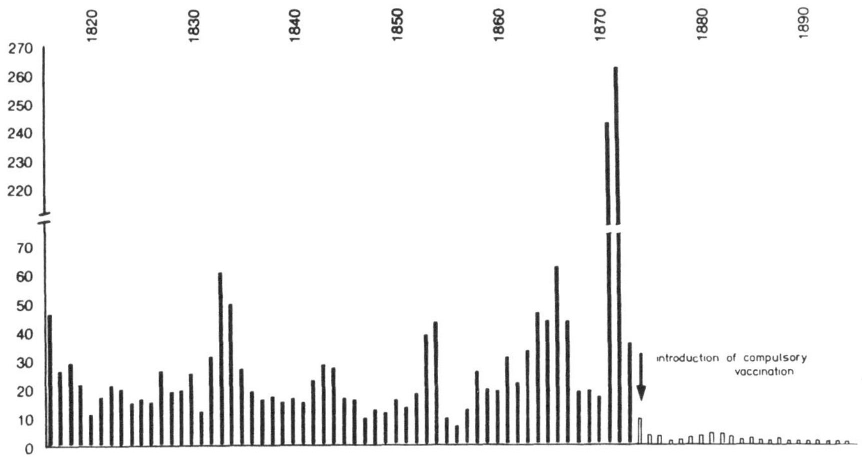

Figure 8 Smallpox mortality 1816–94 in the Federal Republic of Germany

in the USA developed the bifurcated needle. That very modest piece of metal enabled the WHO to start their eradication programme, because vaccines could now be administered under all conceivable conditions to a large number of people. As soon as anything comparable can be developed for BCG the world can fight tuberculosis successfully.

EPIDEMIOLOGICAL CONSIDERATIONS

Epidemiology is one of the disciplines of medicine which drew the largest advantage from the work of the League of Nations and later the World Health Organization. In fact, it was epidemics and pandemics which called for international cooperation first. The knowledge of the incidence and the spread of disease on this earth is, therefore, well founded and relatively dependable. The big childhood killers are recognized in all parts of the world, the causative agents are known and the immunological approaches are in the hands of the experts. It did not come as a surprise that the most important killing diseases in the non-industrialized world are very similar, if not identical, to the most important diseases we knew from 100 years ago. They are tuberculosis, typhoid, diphtheria, pertussis, tetanus and measles to mention only the most prominent ones. Some more will show up during the course of industrialization, when the age of infection will rise from early infancy to childhood. Such is the case already for poliomyelitis and meningococcal meningitis. Salmonellosis will soon follow. Natural immunity, which is achieved by very early infection that either leaves a baby immune or dead, will no longer occur for the majority of children when their respective countries become industrialized nations.

The diseases mentioned before could be reduced with the vaccines we already have. To epidemiologists it is no surprise that there is no tropical or exotic disease among the causes of high mortality. However, if the incidence of the world's most common diseases is reduced, then the need for special vaccines arises. When infants survive their early months and years due to vaccination, then it will be necessary to use those vaccines under development to protect against parasites and other transmissible agents prevalent among adolescents. Medicine will go on manipulating epidemiology in the world by prevention of transmissible diseases. The final results will be permanent programmes for vaccination for all ages. They will shift from large campaigns, sponsored by governments or other organizations, to individual immunizations given by single doctors.

COSTS

So far, this paper has described vaccines which are already available, as well as vaccines which are under development for use in the near future. On several occasions it has been stressed that either the quality will have to be improved, or the control extended. Stability and ease of application will deserve more attention than before. As previously mentioned, this requires the highest possible skill and technology. In the near future all these factors will lead to an increase in costs. These costs may, in part, be compensated by the rationalization effect of large-scale production. Manufacturers of vaccines have already experienced the consequences of the development of cost escalation. Such consequences resulted predominantly in many companies totally giving up vaccine production or in maintaining production for only the more profitable ones. If development and production costs continue to rise while, at the same time, the rich and the poor nations demand increasing amounts of vaccines, then the problem becomes one of financing active prophylaxis.

Vaccines in the present and in the future will have to be produced for both the 'haves' and the 'have-nots'. They will have to be of equal quality, although not everyone can buy such quality. The cost situation will force western manufacturers to consider the financial situation of the vaccines. Can vaccines be produced as profitably as drugs under a system which gives a return on invested capital? Is a system conceivable in which vaccines would be regarded as a service contribution from the western pharmaceutical industry to all mankind, thus helping to develop nations in need of it? Could such a system be regarded as the key to subsequent development of markets, which would never have come into existence without such early help? Can vaccination be regarded as number one item in development aid? Would the face of the pharmaceutical industry look less grim to the 'have-nots' than it seems today, if it took up this challenge and responsibility?

CONSEQUENCES

The various aspects of vaccines discussed above may be regarded as part of the painting of a philanthropical, unrealistic optimist. The claim is that infant mortality from infectious diseases could be reduced to near zero with the vaccines we already have in hand. This claim neglects one of the most urgent problems of mankind: the population explosion. Such an explosion may occur for a time, but shortly thereafter people will realize that the majority of their children survive. The number of children will then be reduced because the necessity for many children, as old-age insurance, will not exist any more. In Europe, too, many children were regarded as insurance for ageing couples. As soon as infant mortality was reduced, the birth-rate decreased.

While such thoughts sound fantastic, they are the rationale behind the WHO'S expanded programme of vaccination. Are they more fantastic than what was achieved in the last 100 years in the developed parts of the world? Industry and preventative medicine among others have made the western world the most envied part of the globe. Why could our achievements not also be applied to other nations?

Bibliography

Vaccination Against Communicable Disease (1973). 45th International IABS Symposium, Monaco. Symp. Series immunobiol. Standard, **22**, (Basel: S. Korgen).

Hennessen, W. Developments in Vaccines for prophylactic use. *Zbl. Bakt. Hyg.*, I. Abt. Orig. B, **163**, 55.

3
Paediatric vaccines

S. A. PLOTKIN

INTRODUCTION

Although much of what I have to say will be covered in greater depth by those writing on specific vaccines, it is appropriate that children be a primary preoccupation of vaccinators – for prevention of disease in them represents the best hope of preventive medicine in general.

This discussion will comprise some of the past, some of the present, and hopefully, some of the future.

In the United States, as shown in Table 1, five vaccines are in routine paediatric use. It therefore would be appropriate to begin by discussing these routine preparations. The routine vaccination schedule is given in Table 2.

Table 1 Vaccines routinely used in children in the USA

Diphtheria–Pertussis–Tetanus
Oral polio
Measles
Mumps
Rubella

Table 2 Routine vaccination schedule (USA)

3 months	DTP and TOPV
4 months	DTP and TOPV
5 months	DTP and TOPV
15 months	Measles, mumps, rubella
18 months	DTP and TOPV
4–6 years	DTP and TOPV
14–16 years	Td

DTP = Diphtheria–tetanus-polio
TOPV = Trivalent oral polio vaccine
Td = Tetanus and low-dose diphtheria

DTP

A triple vaccine against diphtheria, tetanus, and pertussis is widely used. In diphtheria and tetanus we have almost perfect vaccines. These two substances are inactivated forms of the toxins that cause the respective diseases. Complete immunization, which is three injections in infancy followed by one booster, provides probably lifetime protection against disease. Booster immunizations may be given later in life if necessary. The third component of DTP, pertussis (whooping cough) is not nearly so ideal.

In contrast to diphtheria and tetanus toxoids, pertusiss vaccine is a relatively crude preparation that contains the majority of the bacteria's constituents, most of which are probably not relevant to the induction of immunity to the disease. The reason for this vaccine being impure is that the antigenic component of the bacterium responsible for clinical immunity has not yet been positively identified.

In the United States, morbidity and mortality due to pertussis rapidly declined after increased use of pertussis vaccine in the 1940s and its official standardization in 1949, although the disease persists as a significant contributor to infant mortality in developing countries.

In the USA and in the UK it appears that current vaccine is capable of reducing total pertussis incidence considerably. In our own experience in Philadelphia, a large metropolitan city, pertussis is diagnosed only five to ten times a year, and in 1973 in the USA only five deaths due to pertussis were reported. Yet the effectiveness of the vaccine appears to be only partial.

Data from Manchester, England, and Bernalillo, New Mexico, show that during epidemics the vaccine is only about 60% effective (Table 3). It may be, therefore, that part of the reduction of pertussis in certain countries is due to improvements in living standards.

Table 3 Pertussis in Bernalillo, New Mexico

Immunization status of group	*Group size*	*Pertussis cases*		
		Symptomatic	*Subclinical*	*Total*
Good	276	7 (2.5%)	19 (6.9%)	26 (9.4%)
Bad	248	15 (6.0%)	9 (3.7%)	24 (9.7%)

Good pertussis vaccines *can* be made by extraction of types 1, 2, and 3 protective antigens from pertussis organisms. But there is still clearly a need to improve antigenicity by identifying and purifying the agglutinogens.

Unfortunately, toxic substances are extracted to some degree along with protective substances. Reaction rates are difficult to assess since reactions are seldom reported by physicians.

Reactions to pertussis vaccine consist of screaming fits, shock symptoms and neurological reactions including convulsions. Estimates of incidence vary from 1 in 3000 to 1 in 50 000. American experience suggests that the latter figure is more realistic. Since a crude mouse weight-gain test is the only measure of toxicity for vaccine lots, it is difficult to standardize pertussis vaccines.

Pertussis vaccine is currently prepared by Lilly Labs, in the USA, by an extraction procedure which destroys the whole bacterial cells. The extracted vaccine, which is combined with alum for enhancement of antigenicity, appears to be improved, as regards safety, over whole-cell vaccine.

Pertussis vaccines adsorbed on to aluminum compounds elicit fewer adverse reactions and are thought to provide better and longer protection. Unfortunately, at the present time attempts to improve immunogenicity and reduce reactivity of pertussis vaccines by purification or extraction can only be evaluated by difficult field studies in humans.

POLIOMYELITIS

Polio vaccines have almost eradicated the disease from developed countries. This result has been achieved by two completely different methods. In Holland, Sweden, and Finland, killed Salk-type vaccine has been used; whereas in large areas of the world, including the USA, oral Sabin-type polio vaccine has been widely employed. There is still disagreement as to which should be used. In favour of killed vaccine is its safety factor, if properly manufactured and tested. In favour of live vaccine is its protection against infection of the throat and intestines by polio virus, and the ease of its administration.

Infection by polio virus can be halted at one or both of two stages: intestinal or viraemic, as shown in Table 4. Polio virus invades the gastrointestinal

Table 4 Protection against polio

Vaccine	*Antibody*	*Virus spread*
		Saliva or faeces
Live	→Local (IgA)→	↓
	↘	Intestines
Killed	→Blood (IgG)→	↓
		Blood
		↓
		Brain

tract if there are no local antibodies such as are induced by previous live virus immunization or natural infection. If virus multiplies in the throat and intestine it can spread throughout the body via the blood; but the presence of antibodies in the blood produced by *either* killed or live vaccine prevents that process.

A major problem with live polio vaccine has been the tendency for reversion of the vaccine virus to virulence. Of the three types of polio virus, type 3 has the greatest tendency to reversion. The clinical result is paralysis *caused* by the vaccine. Fortunately, the risk of this is low, and becomes even lower if only children under 18 years of age are vaccinated. A more stable type 3 strain is needed, and several candidates are available; it seems unlikely, however, that an effort will be made to verify their safety and efficacy.

It is important to note that in most countries the live polio vaccine employed is trivalent—that is, containing all three types. Multiple doses (three or four) are given, not because of the need for boosters, but because each of the three types must 'take' (multiply in the intestines) and it may require three to four administrations to insure successful 'takes'.

A major problem in polio vaccination today is the vaccination of children in tropical areas. Killed vaccine is too expensive for these countries, and seroconversion after live vaccine is very poor. The reasons for this poor seroconversion in tropical areas are not understood, and a method for achieving the same success there as achieved in temperate countries is badly needed. Part of the answer to the problem in tropical areas may lie in the administration of vaccine to newborn infants.

MEASLES

Measles has been a devastating disease in the past, particularly in the poorly nourished. But even in middle-class children it causes encephalitis, pneumonia, otitis, and breakdown of tuberculous foci in the lungs. There is therefore no doubt that vaccination against measles is necessary. Three facets of this living attenuated vaccine which must be considered are: reactions, age of immunization and persistence of immunity.

The problem of febrile and other reactions has been solved by further attenuating the original vaccine, and it is these further attenuated strains that are largely in use today.

The choice of age at immunization is based on two factors: (1) the interference produced by maternal antibodies passively transmitted to the infant through the placenta; and (2) the age-specific attack rate of measles. With respect to the former, interference may persist up to 15 months of age. With respect to the latter, in some communities the measles attack rate is high *under* a year of age. Thus if vaccination is practised at 15 months of age, as is now done in the USA, some measles may occur in infants under that age. If vaccination is practised before that time there will be some failures of immunization, these unvaccinated infants will soon become susceptible, and reimmunization will be necessary. In certain regions of the world, including the inner cities of the USA, the latter scheme may be preferable.

During the last years there has been a resurgence of measles epidemics in the USA, with many cases occurring in older children. Whereas the reasons for these epidemics are complex, including failure to immunize sufficient numbers of children and immunization of some before the age of 1 year, there are data which suggest that primary vaccine failure or loss of immunity are involved. Consequently, it may become prudent to revaccinate against measles at about the 10th birthday. So far this policy has not been adopted, but may be in the future.

MUMPS

Mumps is a ubiquitous infection and the single most common cause of viral meningitis. This fact, along with the unusual but important cases of sterility following mumps infection of the testis in adult men, are sufficient reasons to vaccinate against the disease. A live attenuated mumps vaccine has been developed and so far data indicate permanent immunity from this subclinical infection. The vaccine should be given at age 1 year or at 15 months with other vaccines.

RUBELLA

In the case of rubella the object is not to protect against the disease itself, which is mild, but against the teratogenic effects of the virus which are exerted when a pregnant woman is infected. Several strains of live attenuated virus are used throughout the world, all given subcutaneously, although one of them (RA 27/3) can be given intranasally with some theoretical advantage.

Perhaps the chief question about rubella vaccine is the time of administration. In the USA a policy of administering rubella vaccine at 15 months of age together with mumps and measles has been adopted. My own preference is for the plan used in Europe, which is to vaccinate girls about 12 years old. This plan avoids unnecessary vaccination of boys, focuses on a specific target group, allows time for girls to acquire natural immunity and reduces the interval between vaccination and the age of child-bearing. The success of either American or European policy will depend on the eradication of congenital rubella syndrome, which if accomplished would reduce the toll of congenital heart disease, cataracts and deafness.

BACTERIAL VACCINES

Having covered the routine vaccines of today, I turn to a group of potential and actual vaccines against bacterial infections of childhood. Four groups of organisms cause the common serious infections of childhood: streptococci, pneumococci, meningococci, and *Haemophilus influenzae*. The diseases they cause are listed in Table 5. Vaccination against streptococci is not now feasible. Meningococci occur in a number of different antigenic groups, but most strains belong to groups A, B or C. Recently it has been possible to isolate and purify the cell-wall polysaccharide of meningococcal groups A and C and to prepare potent vaccines. These vaccines have been used in epidemic situations, notably in Brazil, Finland, and in American military recruits, with striking success.

Table 5 Major bacterial pathogens of childhood

Organism	*Diseases*
Streptococci	Pharyngitis (rheumatic fever; glomerulonephritis)
Pneumococci	Pneumonia Otitis Meningitis
H. influenzae	Meningitis Croup
Meningococci	Meningitis

In areas of the world where meningococcal meningitis is frequent vaccination of children may be considered, whereas elsewhere meningococcal vaccine does not appear to be warranted, at least until a group B vaccine is also available. There are 86 pneumococcal capsular types, although certain ones can be singled out as the cause of most pneumococcal infections. Half of the cases of pneumococcal pneumonia are caused by six types, and three-quarters by twelve types. Vaccines containing twelve or fourteen types have been tested in the USA and in South Africa with results indicating about 75% effectiveness in reducing severe bacteraemic pneumonia in adults. The types that frequently cause infections in childhood include some that also cause disease in adults, and some that are different. The reduction of pneumococcal disease in childhood would be extremely valuable. Many children have episodes of pneumococcal bacteraemias early in childhood, and in one study 80% of children had at least one episode of otitis during the first year of life, of which about one-third was caused by pneumococci.

Lastly, in *H. influenzae* we have a problem of major proportions. In the USA, *H. influenzae* is the first cause of bacterial meningitis, with one child in every *1000* becoming subject to the disease before his 5th birthday; 10% will die and 30% will have neurological damage. Croup and other serious infections are also caused by this organism. Here again it is possible to prepare a vaccine consisting of capsular material from type B organisms, which cause 90% of the serious infections.

The fly in the ointment of application of bacterial vaccines in children is this: infants less than 2 years do not respond well to polysaccharide antigens (Table 6). Evidently, the immune system is still maturing in infancy with respect to these antigens. Although the bacterial vaccines might still have value in older children, unquestionably a major desideratum is that some way be found to immunize infants.

Table 6 Relation of age to antibody response of children inoculated with *H. influenzae* type B capsular polysaccharide

Age of vaccines (months)	*Number responding*
5–12	4/18 (22%)
13–24	27/39 (69%)
25–36	24/27 (89%)

BCG vaccine against tuberculosis (TB) is an effective preventative, and in some countries is inoculated at about age 12. As TB becomes less common, as it is in the USA, the need for BCG diminishes.

RESPIRATORY VIRUS VACCINES

Unlike adults in whom many viruses cause acute respiratory disease, children are affected severely by a small number of viruses, listed in Table 7 with the respiratory disease-states they produce.

Table 7 Respiratory viruses of childhood

Virus	*Clinical manifestation*
Respiratory syncytial	Bronchiolitis
Parainfluenza (1, 2, 3)	Pneumonia, croup
Adenoviruses	Pneumonia, pharyngitis
Influenza A and B	Influenza, pneumonia, croup

Respiratory syncytial virus causes more deaths than any other virus of childhood. It acts by causing symptoms like asthma, and in small infants these symptoms are dangerous. Some work has been done both with killed and live virus vaccines, but progress has not been dramatic owing to deficiencies in our knowledge of the factors that produce immunity, and in particular the possibility that disease may occur *because* of the presence of antibodies. Not much work has been done on parainfluenza virus vaccines.

In the case of adenoviruses, vaccines against types 4, 7 and 21 have been developed for adults, and these have been dramatically successful in preventing pneumonia when tested in soldiers. The technology exists or could be developed without much difficulty for manufacture of vaccine against types 1, 2, 3 and 5, which are important in young children. For example, in the USSR, live adenovirus vaccines have been given to children combined with bovine serum inhibitor. The inhibitor is destroyed by gastric acid and the virus released in the intestine. At present the development of paediatric adenovirus vaccines is being delayed by theoretical concerns about oncogenicity which I will not digress upon.

Influenza A and B vaccines, although widely used in adults, have not been advised in children because of the lesser risk of fatal disease and higher reaction rates.

In my opinion, if influenza vaccines could be prepared that would be effective and sufficiently well tolerated by children, then they should be used in them. My basis for so thinking is that, during an influenza A epidemic, much time is lost from school and much morbidity is caused by persistent cough, croup, and pneumonia. Moreover, children appear to be the reservoir for influenza.

Influenza B is followed in some cases by a fatal disease called Reye's Syndrome that occurs only in children. During an epidemic of influenza B, mass vaccination of children might decrease the incidence of Reye's Syndrome.

In reference to influenza vaccines, one should mention the older Russian work and more recent work accomplished in Belgium and in Great Britain, in which strains of influenza have been developed which can be given by the intranasal route. This route has, to recommend itself, the induction of local antibody which may have considerable importance in protection. Problems of reactions in children will have to be solved, however. Killed influenza vaccine should be given without question to children with chronic diseases, particularly cardiorespiratory.

VARICELLA

Chickenpox, the last common childhood disease, is the subject of current attempts in Japan and in the USA to develop a live virus vaccine. The results with the Japanese vaccine have been thus far encouraging.

CYTOMEGALOVIRUS

In considering rubella vaccine, I mentioned that the object of vaccination is to prevent infection of the fetus. Another experimental live virus vaccine

Table 8 Incidence of certain causes of neonatal sepsis syndrome (per 1000 cases)

Bacterial	1.0–3.5
Cytomegalovirus	5–20
Rubella	0.25–5
Toxoplasma	0.75–1.3
Herpes virus	0.03–0.3
Syphilis	0.1–0.2

under development is one against an agent called cytomegalovirus. This virus, as shown in Table 8, commonly infects fetuses—in fact, it is the most common congenital infection. The infant born with intra-uterine infection suffers brain damage 10–30% of the time. Thus, considerable mental retardation might be prevented by an effective vaccine against cytomegalovirus. Such a vaccine would be applied in late childhood, just before puberty.

SUMMARY

In summary, vaccination against diphtheria, tetanus, pertussis, polio, measles, mumps, and rubella has made fantastic reductions in morbidity and mortality from infectious disease in children. Our next efforts must be focused on bacterial vaccines, on respiratory viruses, and on cytomegalovirus and varicella.

4
The whooping cough vaccine controversy

G. DICK

Every vaccine introduced for routine use has been associated with a certain amount of opposition. The medical and lay opposition to smallpox vaccine was vociferous and the propaganda against its introduction included pamphlets, lampoons and caricatures. In the case of diphtheria toxoid, in spite of the successful use of toxoid products in Europe and North America and the repeated recommendations of the then Ministry of Health, the British public and medical profession resisted the introduction of diphtheria toxoid in the 1930s when there were approximately 50 000–60 000 notifications of diphtheria with approximately 3000 deaths every year. The objections to these vaccines were based essentially on fear of their giving rise to complications – in both cases greatly exaggerated.

In contrast, when whooping cough vaccine was introduced in 1957, there appears to have been little concern about any possible side-effects and its general acceptance, without any continuing surveillance of efficacy or safety, was presumably related to the complete acceptance of the conclusion of the trials of whooping cough vaccines which had been carried out by the Medical Research Council for about the previous ten years[1–4]. Indeed, it appears that any untoward effects that may have occurred with whooping cough vaccine tended to have been minimized or disregarded for fear of upsetting the use of a vaccine against a disease which, in the late 1950s, was giving rise to approximately 30 000–90 000 annual notifications, and also of bringing the use of diphtheria vaccine, which had been so successful, into disrepute.

NATURAL HISTORY

The disease

Whooping cough is spread from person to person by close personal contact. It is generally accepted that there is no passive immunity in young infants born to immune mothers[5]. Preston[6] does not accept this and states that the levels of pertussis agglutinins in infants' sera are directly related to those in the mothers' sera, but that the mothers' sera rarely contain detectable amounts of antibody to pertussis antigen 3, which Preston has considered important – but this is not universally accepted.

Although the severity, complications and rate of sequelae from whooping cough appear to have been declining in recent years in the United Kingdom, in other parts of Europe and in North America, this impression does not seem to be borne out by the fact that in the United Kingdom for the past 20 or so years, the ratio of deaths to notifications has remained fairly constant at about one death per 1000 notifications. This raises the whole question as to what is notified as whooping cough. How much of the notified disease is due to *Bordetella pertussis* and indeed how much 'whooping cough' is due to infections with viruses or a mixture of viruses and *B. pertussis*. A very valuable study was recently made in Toronto by Islur, Anglin and Middleton[7] investigating the severity of whooping cough. A useful retrospective study of whooping cough was made in the United Kingdom by the British Society for the Study of Infection[8], but neither that study nor the one by Miller and Fletcher[9] has in my opinion given an accurate picture of the disease in the United Kingdom at present. The latter study was also a retrospective one, based on recall by general practitioners and on hospital notes. Severity was 'judged' from the symptoms recorded and the subsequent course of the disease. (It should be remembered in making such arbitrary judgements that whooping cough is one of the few diseases which very often increases in severity for about 2 weeks from the date of onset.) Many of the so-called 'complications' described by Miller and Fletcher would be considered by many clinicians as features of the normal pattern of the disease, and this may explain their complication rate of 78% in the hospital admissions compared with 17% in the study of Islur *et al.*[7]. In Miller and Fletcher's report *B. pertussis* was isolated from only 31% of the 555 patients from whom a pernasal swab or cough plate was taken and no viruses were recorded as having been isolated or looked for: this is to be compared with an isolation of *B. pertussis* in 87% of patients in the Canadian study and virus isolations from one-fifth of the patients with bacteriologically positive swabs and one-fifth of patients with negative swabs. In the Canadian study there were no deaths; in the British study there were ten deaths. Three of these deaths were in premature infants, one in a so-called 'post-mature' infant, and one occurred 9 months after the attack of whooping cough, one was (?) due to gastroenteritis and one was a cot death.

I do not believe the picture presented by Miller and Fletcher presents the true picture of whooping cough in the UK today, and a careful study similar to that of the Canadians is urgently required. Furthermore, their 'judgement' whether or not an infant or child was admitted to hospital for medical or social reasons is poorly defined. The pressures on general practitioners to seek admission to hospital for infants and children are numerous and varied depending on many conditions. One would hazard a guess that the admissions for small babies might have been largely for medical reasons. It would have been interesting to compare the numbers of infants and children admitted in the same period with a diagnosis of bronchitis and pneumonia, and in what proportion of the patients whooping cough had contributed to these causes of death.

Whooping cough may still be a serious disease in certain communities but to many general practitioners in England it is 'a disease with a cough which takes longer to clear up than the "usual" type of respiratory infection of infants and children, which often occurs at night, and is sometimes associated with vomiting', but accurate diagnosis depends on bacteriological confirmation. The failure of the British Society for the Study of Infection[8] to present any bacteriological confirmation of the cases in their retrospective study greatly reduces the value of their report, and it is hoped that they will now do a prospective study.

Notifications

The extent of notifications of a relatively common disease varies widely and is dependent on a number of factors. What influences, for example, have outbreaks of cytomegalovirus or other virus infections on the notification rates of whooping cough? In general, notifications represent the overall annual pattern of a disease called 'whooping cough', whatever it really is.

Whooping cough has only been notifiable in England and Wales since 1940 (Figures 1 and 2) and there have been wide fluctuations in the numbers of cases notified which are difficult to explain. The increase of notifications in 1941 has been said to have been influenced by the dispersal of mothers and children from the cities at the beginning of the Second World War and the consequent increase in contact between infected and susceptible children[10]. At that time the number of births in England and Wales was the lowest it had ever been in the twentieth century. The peaks of whooping cough notifications in the early 1950s have been attributed to the high postwar birth rates[10]. These explanations appear unconvincing and inconsistent. It is well known that 'Notification is notoriously erratic among general practitioners as a whole, worse perhaps in many hospitals, and exasperatingly inconsistent even for many an individual doctor, depending on how busy he may be or when he converts his rough notes to official records'[11]. I do not know how much better the situation is today. Obviously there are many factors which influence notification and, for example, it was suggested, in a study of measles[12], that the number of children who were notified as having measles might be related in some way with the 1948 increase in the notification fee from 1*s*. to 2*s*. 6*d*.[12]. Certainly, the Isle of Wight notifications of measles at that time showed a parallel rise with increasing fees.

So with whooping cough, motivation, interest, awareness, fashion, publicity, etc. all influence notification, but the overall picture has to be looked at. Recently there has been a 'dramatic' increase of yellow cards (notifying adverse drug reactions) submitted to the Committee on Safety in Medicines[13] and the actual number of yellow card reports submitted in the first 6 months of 1977 was more than twice the equivalent number of those submitted in

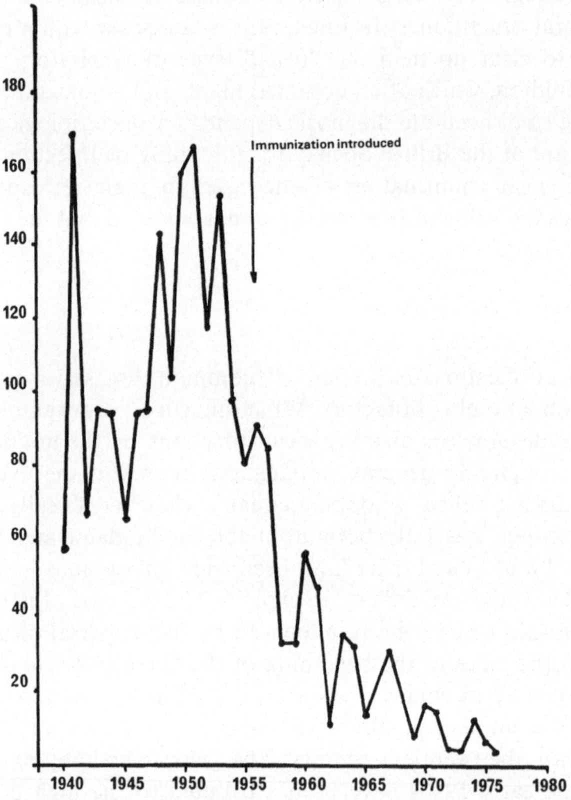

Figure 1 Notifications of whooping cough; England and Wales

1976, and more than all the cards submitted in the whole of 1975. But this no more means an epidemic of drug reactions than an increased number of notifications of whooping cough in 1977/78 will necessarily mean an increased incidence of that disease.

When one looks at the weekly or quarterly notifications of whooping cough over the years it will be seen that there has been a series of peaks followed by troughs of about 3 years' duration. (Figures 3 and 4.) A peak is expected in 1977/78, but if this is greater than that of 1974/75, as has been said, it does not necessarily mean that there is an increase in whooping cough as has been predicted by the Joint Committee[10].

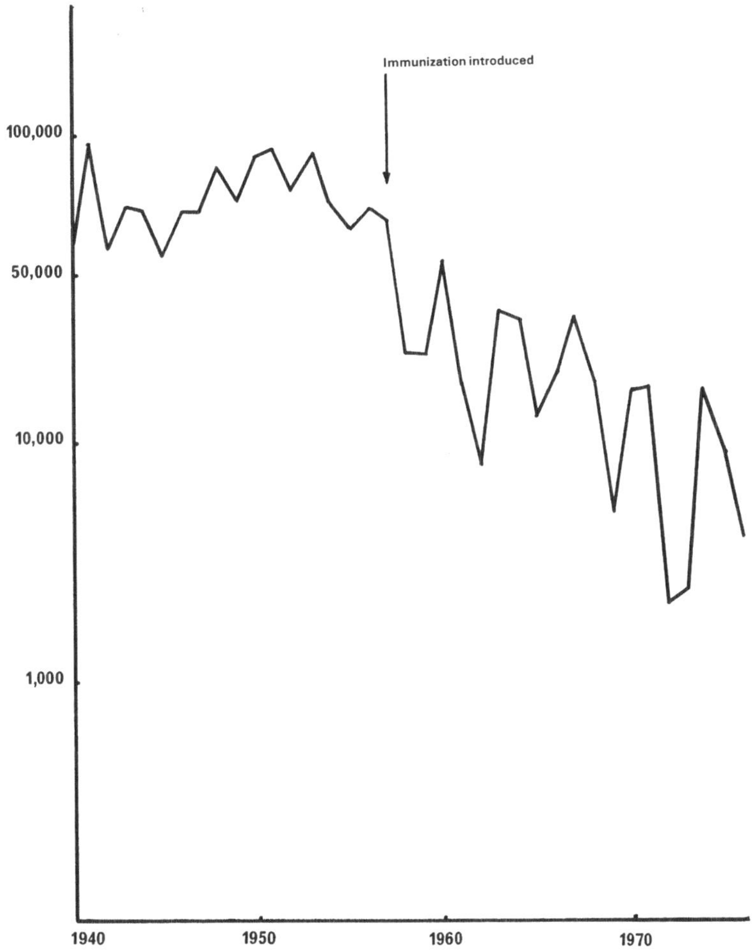

Figure 2 Notifications of whooping cough; England and Wales (log. scale)

Deaths

It is well known that infant mortality rates vary inversely with standards of hygiene and are influenced by standards of medical care, and the least equivocal indicator of community health is probably death. While mortality figures are in general a crude index of health care, nevertheless they correlate well with morbidity rates and are probably less liable to be influenced by the various factors which produce fluctuations in notifications of morbidity.

As with other infectious diseases there has in general been a steady decline in the number of whooping cough deaths reported in England and Wales since registration of deaths was started in 1836. In the early years of the nineteenth century measles and whooping cough together began to replace smallpox as the principal killing disease of infants and children. The record of mortality from measles and whooping cough diseases in children is shown in Figure 5. From 1851 to 1880 the trend of mortality from whooping cough showed little change; then it began to decline somewhat earlier than did measles and then fell below measles at the beginning of this century, until 1921–25 when measles and whooping cough exchanged their places of importance. Whooping cough deaths per million of population are shown

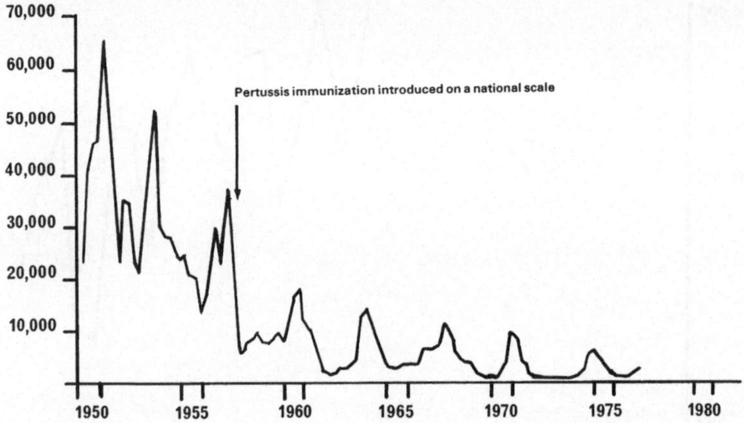

Figure 3 Quarterly notification of whooping cough; England and Wales

arithmetically in Figures 6a and 6b and on logarithmic paper in Figure 7, indicating the proportional fall. Deaths per million children under 15 years are presented in Figure 8.

In recent years the average annual number of deaths has fallen from 1205 in 1940–44 to 262 in 1950–54 and about 34 and 12 respectively in the first five years of the 1960s and 1970s. The number of deaths per 1000 notifications has been as follows:

1940–44	12.5	1960–64	1.1
1945–49	7.4	1965–69	1.0
1950–54	1.9	1970–74	1.0
1955–59	1.0		

At first sight it might be suggested that the drop in notifications and case fatality in the late 1940s was a consequence of the introduction of antibiotics; but when one looks at the proportional fall in notifications and deaths from whooping cough and scarlet fever in relation to the introduction of antibiotics (Figures 9–11) such a suggestion does not sound very convincing.

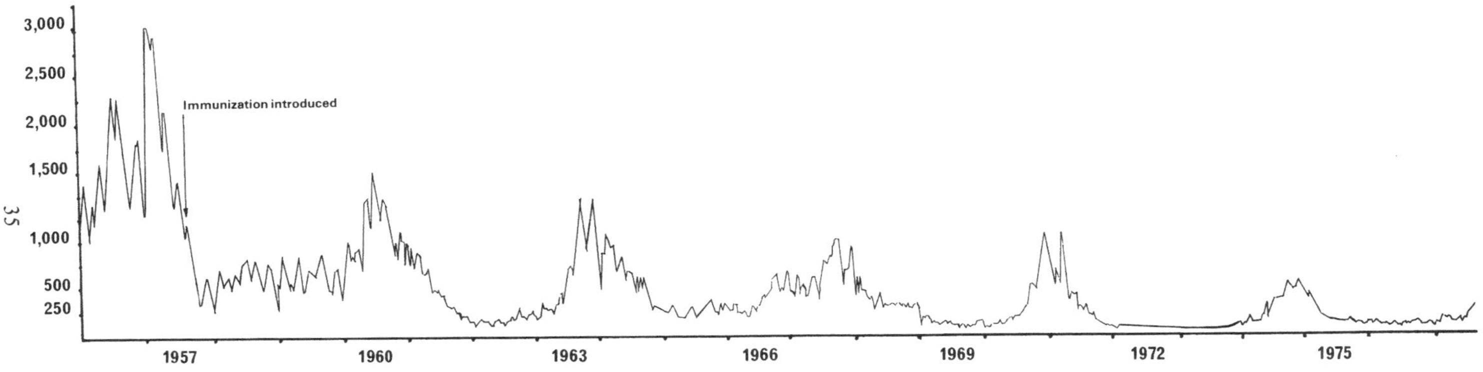

Figure 4 Weekly notifications of whooping cough; England and Wales

WHOOPING COUGH VACCINE

Effect of vaccine

When vaccine was introduced for routine use on a national scale in 1957 the number of notified cases in England and Wales declined (Figures 1 and 2) but this decline was not comparable with what had been observed following the introduction of diphtheria or of poliovirus vaccine. The drop in the number of whooping cough notifications continued until 1962 (8343 notifications) and then the number increased again and since then has continued

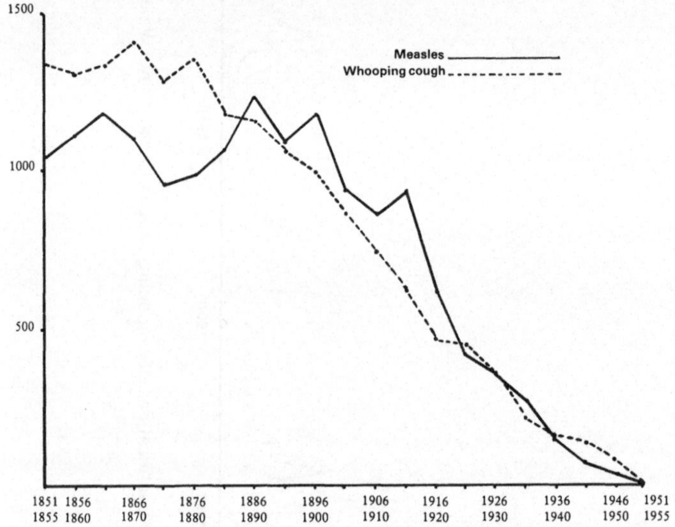

Figure 5 Deaths from measles and whooping cough; England and Wales

to fluctuate. The weekly and quarterly notification data show curves of decreasing size (Figures 3 and 4) not obviously influenced by the routine introduction of vaccine in 1957. Similarly there is no clear evidence that the reduction in deaths was markedly affected by routine vaccination (Figures 6–9).

Vaccine trials

Although it had been shown in the USA in the 1930s that it was possible to prepare a vaccine which gave a protection rate of about 60% against whooping cough in family contacts and about 90% in those exposed to infection at school[14] the early British trials were unable to show any protective effect of British vaccine[15]. Further extensive trials carried out by the Medical Research

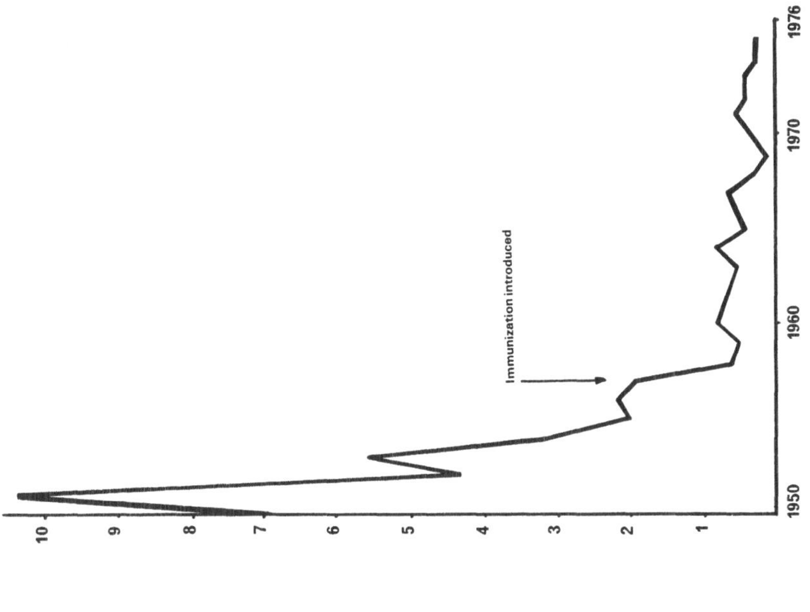

Figure 6b Whooping cough deaths per million population; England and Wales, 1950–75

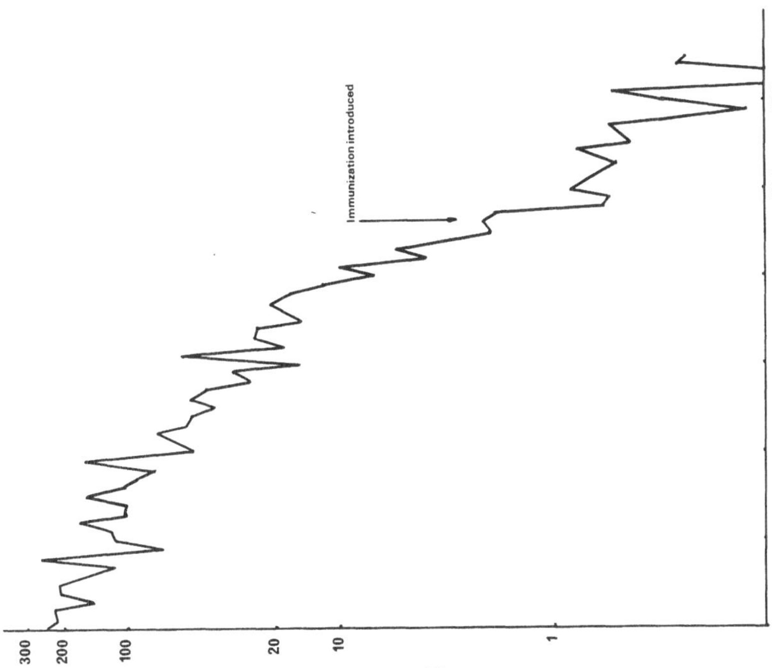

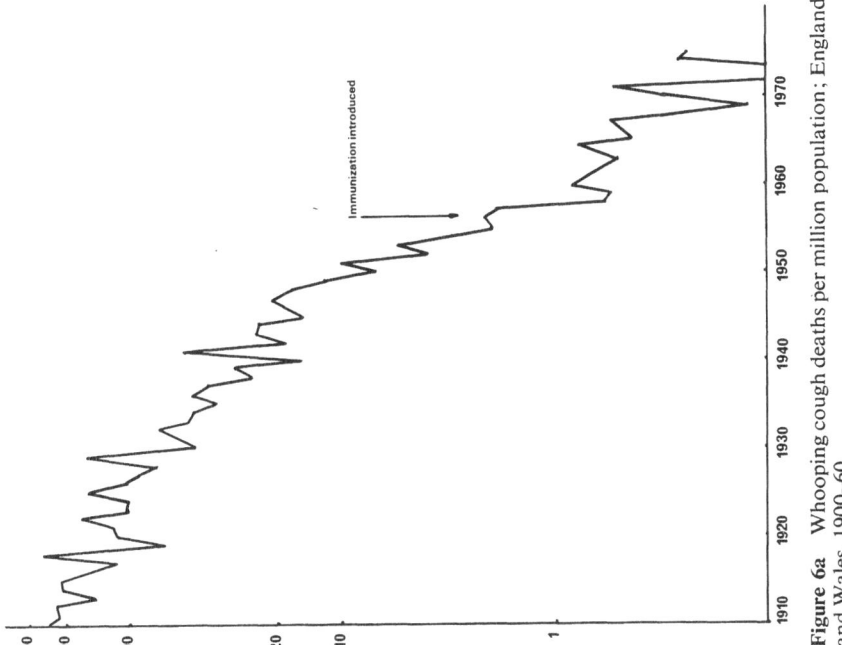

Figure 6a Whooping cough deaths per million population; England and Wales, 1900–60

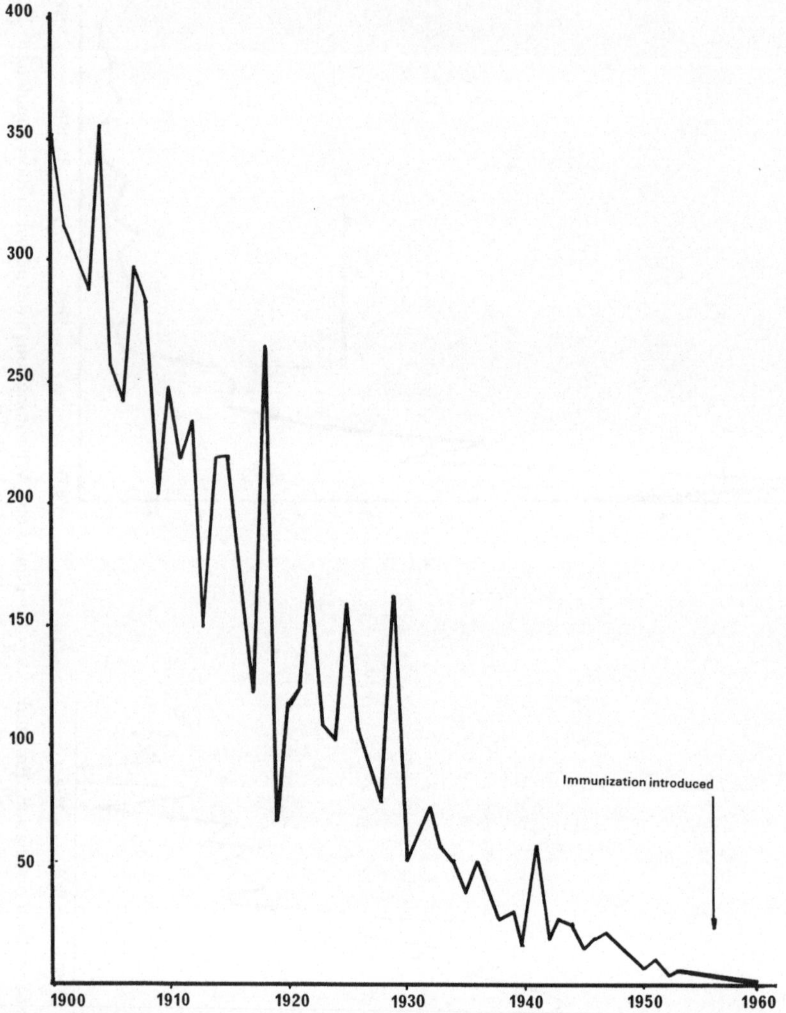

Figure 7 Whooping cough deaths per million population; England and Wales (log. scale)

Council between 1946 and 1954[1–4] showed that although there were considerable variations in the protective efficacy of whooping cough vaccines, vaccines could be made in England which could give a 90% protection against family exposure to infection. At the same time, although small numbers of cases of convulsions[1–4] were reported in each of the MRC trials, no serious complications or untoward reactions to these vaccines were recorded. The stage was thus set for the introduction of whooping cough vaccine as a routine procedure on a national scale; but there was the problem of preparing vaccines of uniform acceptability and efficacy.

Standardization of vaccine

Unfortunately, there is as yet no precise method of identifying or measuring the antigen in whooping cough vaccine which produces protection against infection by *B. pertussis* and secondly, although the agglutinins which develop following immunization tend to reflect the protective efficacy of the vaccine, there is no precise *in vitro* test which will do so.

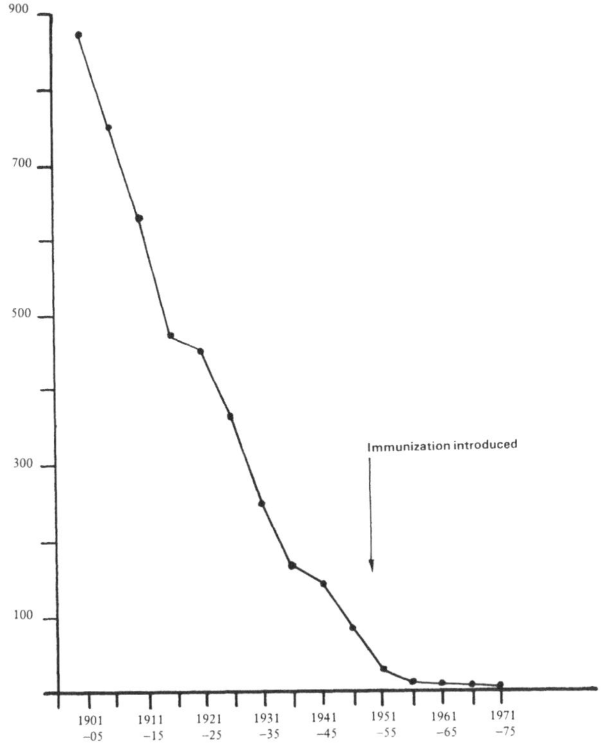

Figure 8 Whooping cough deaths per million children under 15 years; England and Wales

In order to try to standardize the potency of whooping cough vaccines a test in mice was developed which was based on the intracerebral challenge of immunized mice and a British Reference Vaccine was established in 1957 as one giving 80% protection against home exposure.

So whooping cough vaccines were introduced nationally in the UK in 1957 with the hope that they would produce the consistent type of efficacy which had apparently been achieved in North America.

Untoward reactions to vaccine

Although no serious reactions had been recorded in any of the MRC trials,

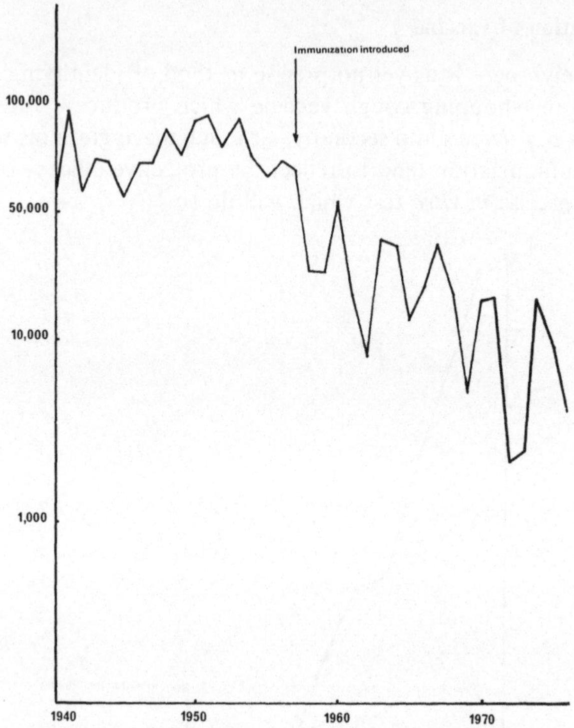

Figure 9 Notifications of whooping cough; England and Wales (log. scale)

soon after the introduction of vaccine for routine use Hopper[16] of Northumberland reported a significant number of illnesses in immunized children following inoculation of either plain pertussis vaccine or triple antigen (diphtheria, tetanus and pertussis). He noted that in an 18-month period when 1700 children had received a course of three injections at child welfare centres, forty of them became sufficiently upset for their parents to inform a health visitor, or a clinic or family doctor about the occurrence. The illnesses which he reported in these forty children were:

generalized rash	4
swollen painful arm	1
malaise	7
persistent uncontrollable screaming	10
persistent vomiting	14
collapse	4

Little or no attention seems to have been paid at the time to these observations, and indeed it appears that *no effort was made to carry out any continuing surveillance of the safety or efficacy of whooping cough vaccine after its introduction in 1957.* At about the time of Hopper's investigations, my colleagues

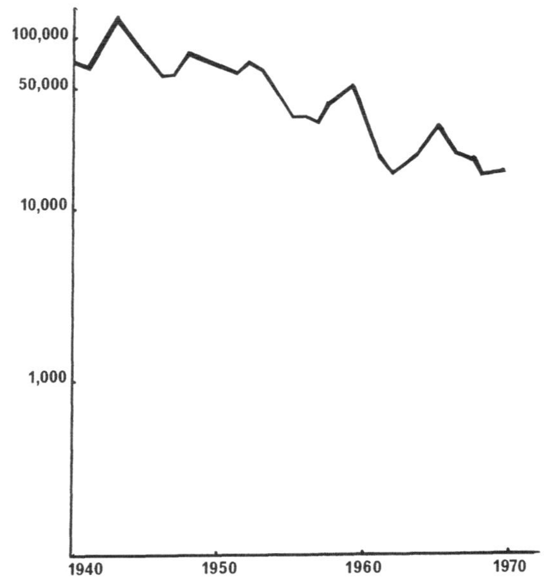

Figure 10 Notifications of scarlet fever and streptococcal sore throat; England and Wales (log. scale)

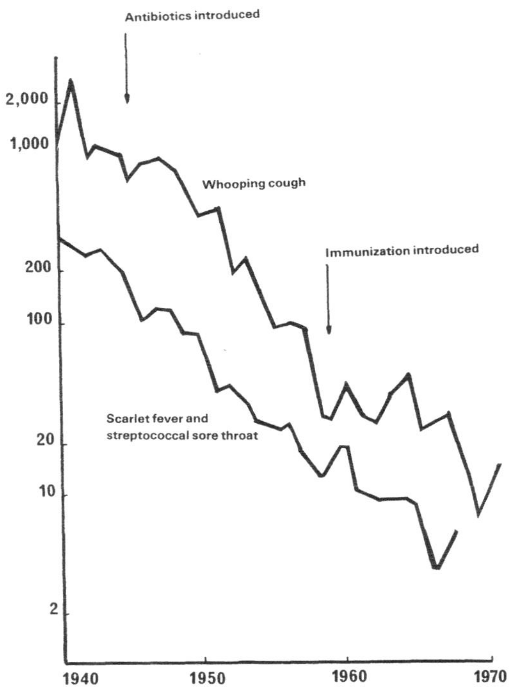

Figure 11 Deaths from whooping cough and scarlet fever; England and Wales (log. scale)

and I[17] were developing a quadruple vaccine consisting of poliomyelitis, diphtheria, tetanus and pertussis components. After the completion of our laboratory studies and trials of this vaccine, it was made available for routine use in the UK. Shortly after its general introduction we heard of a number of untoward reactions associated with its use, and subsequent investigations of commercially available quadruple vaccine and of the triple antigen (Dip/Tet/Pert)[18] confirmed Hopper's observations for Haire *et al.* found not only that there were reactions associated with the new quadruple vaccine but that reactions were not uncommonly associated with commercially available triple antigen prepared in the UK.

In one of the studies which was done at that time we compared the reactions of two commercially available Dip/Tet/Pert vaccines in two groups of sixty infants of similar age and sex. The results, which are summarized in Table 1, showed not only that the reactions following the injection of some commercially available vaccines were more frequent than was generally believed or admitted but also that there were some serious reactions – the so-called *major reactions* which consisted of persistent high-pitched screaming or collapse (see Haire *et al.*[18]).

Table 1 Comparison of percentage of vaccinees showing reactions following first doses of Dip/Tet/Pert A and Dip/Tet/Pert B

Reaction	*A*	*B*
Fretful	73	32
Flushed and feverish	18	9
Painful arm	45	12
Swollen arm	20	4
Major reactions	6.6	1.6
No reported action	18	54

These observations were made on two groups of sixty infants of similar age and sex.

All vaccines give rise to some reactions, and many babies show some malaise, a slight rise in temperature and some tenderness at the site of injection about 2–4 h after the injection of pertussis-containing vaccines which is accepted as normal. In one study in the Netherlands it was found that about one-third of the vaccinees had more serious reactions with high temperatures lasting for a longer period, frequently combined with a swelling and marked redness at the site of the injection[19]. But we were more concerned with the persistent screaming and collapse which we and Hopper and now others have observed[19] and which we had classified as *major* reactions. There is no indication as to whether these reactions are central or peripheral in origin.

The assessment of complications associated with vaccines is not easy, and in order to establish a relationship between any untoward event and the inoculation of a vaccine, the event must present a fairly consistent and characteristic clinical picture with a reasonably clear time-relationship to the inoculation, and preferably there should be laboratory evidence implicating the causal agent. The latter is not available with whooping cough vaccine. As far as persistent screaming and collapse are concerned it seems reasonable to assume from the data of Hopper[16], Haire *et al.*[18] and Hannik[19], that these *major reactions* are associated with the inoculation of pertussis-containing vaccines. They do not appear to have been observed following the inoculation of other vaccines, nor does the type of screaming or the collapse picture which has been described with whooping cough vaccines[18] seem to have been observed in children given no vaccine.

In addition to screaming and collapse, convulsions and encephalopathy have been described as being associated with whooping cough vaccine. To establish a relationship between whooping cough vaccine and the onset of convulsions and encephalopathy is much more difficult. As far as convulsions are concerned, convulsions as 'febrile convulsions' or 'first fits' occur not infrequently in the first two years of life[20–22] which is the time when whooping cough vaccine is most commonly given. Any convulsion following whooping cough vaccine could thus be a chance event, and could wrongly be attributed to the vaccine.

Encephalopathy or other serious neurological complications following whooping cough vaccination have been recorded by several individuals[19,23–31], but to establish an association between the event and the vaccine is again not easy. The problem is usually made more difficult because the evaluation of the illness and the evidence has usually been made in retrospect.

In trying to obtain accurate data on neurological complications to immunization there is the additional problem of the actual reporting of such complications. A good example of under-reporting of neurological complications was recently given by Roden[32] who pointed out that 'About six months before the national campaign for vaccination against measles was launched the Committee on Safety of Drugs [as it was then] drew the attention of doctors to the importance of reporting adverse reactions to vaccines and other immunological agents, including hyperpyrexia, meningism, prolonged drowsiness and convulsions. A subsequent analysis of the reports received showed an incidence of convulsions of a little over 19/100 000 after measles vaccination of children under the age of two years, in contrast to an incidence of 19/10 000 observed in the Medical Research Council's clinical trial.'

No doctor likes to report a serious untoward event such as encephalopathy which has followed an immunization procedure which he may unwittingly have caused by recommending the inoculation of a particular vaccine. The available reported information on the frequency of serious neurological complications of all types following whooping cough vaccine are variable, and estimates of their frequency have varied from no cases of encephalopathy in about 19 000 children who were followed up in the MRC trials of 1948 and 1957 in the United Kingdom[2–4] to four or five serious neurological illnesses in 215 000 children inoculated in Sweden in 1955–58 (Malmgren *et al.*[26], reviewing the data of Strøm[24]) which gives a rate of 1:50 000 and three cases of 'destructive encephalopathy' between 1959 and 1965 in 516 276 children in Strøm's second series in Sweden[25]. A guess of 1:10 000 to 1: 50 000 which was based on unconfirmed data from various sources using vaccines which were available in the UK prior to 1968 was made by Dick[33]. This guess is very similar to the estimates arrived at by Malmgren *et al.*[26] and Strøm[25] for the vaccines used in Sweden in the 1960s. Hannik[19] has recorded cases of encephalopathy associated with quadruple vaccine in the Netherlands, but it is not possible to calculate the frequency.

No serious neurological complications have been reported in a study which began in January 1975 and is as yet incomplete and unpublished[34], in 80 000 children in the North West Thames Region who had recently received a primary dose of triple vaccine. The number so far studied is too small to make it possible to draw any sensible conclusion. All of the above studies except that of Pollock[34] were essentially retrospective.

From personal experience of trying to evaluate retrospectively neurological complications allegedly associated with the administration of whooping cough vaccine, perhaps less than 20% of them merit serious consideration because of inaccurate diagnosis (see also Stephenson[35] and Ounsted[36]) and of the onset of an event in time which could in no way be rationally associated with immunization.

In investigations of vaccine reactions of any kind, the method employed in collecting the information is all-important. Thus in the study of Haire *et al.*[18] the homes of the babies who had been immunized at various clinics were visited, on the day after the inoculation, by a health visitor who asked one question: 'How is baby?' and this was followed by further interrogation and by a visit from a physician as required. This method was followed by Hannik[19] in the Netherlands and similarly Hopper[16] arranged visits by health visitors to all those who failed to complete the course of injections. In contrast the unpublished data on reactions to the current vaccines by the Public Health Laboratory Service[34] has been based on the *reporting* by physicians of any instance of severe reactions. The deficiency of such reports, has already been discussed.

In considering the reactions which follow immunization, it is quite wrong to assume that vaccines manufactured at different times with different compositions will give the same reaction rates. Thus some of the data of Haire *et al.*[18] related to vaccines of which some were subsequently found to have contained as many as 29×10^9 organisms/ml[37] and some of it related to reactions following quadruple vaccine as were some of the reactions reported by Hannik[19]; there is, however, no reason to suppose that anything other than the pertussis component was responsible.

It is worth noting that in one of our studies (Haire *et al.*[18]) it was found that with quadruple vaccine the reactions were about twenty times more frequent in infants less than 6 months of age compared with older children. It may be seen (Table 2) that twenty-four infants had 'major' reactions (collapse or screaming, etc.); twenty-three of these appeared after 498 inoculations in infants less than 6 months of age, but only one occurred after 471 inoculations in older infants. This observation of age in relation to reactions has not been confirmed by Pollock[38].

Table 2 Comparison of percentage of reactions to first doses of quadruple vaccine in infants under and over 6 months of age

Type of reaction	*471 Infants over 6 months of age* (%)	*498 Infants under 6 months of age* (%)
Major	0.2	4.6
Minor	48	62
None	52	33

$\chi^2 = 49.3$ DR = 2 $P > 0.001$

It is relevant to note that increasing the number of organisms in the dose of a *B. pertussis* vaccine increases the frequency of reactions[15,39], and it is therefore not surprising that we found that a decrease in the size of the infants receiving a particular vaccine increased the number of reactions observed. There may be other factors involved which could explain the discrepancy of the results of Pollock[38] and our data, but the size of the infants in relation to the number of organisms injected would seem likely to be important.

Many of those who were Medical Officers of Health in the UK prior to the reorganization of the National Health Service, will recall that there was until the end of the 1960s no central organization to which reports of untoward vaccine reactions could be made, for it was not until the Medicine Act of 1968 that the Committee on Safety of Drugs (CSD) was given the duty of monitoring adverse reactions to all drugs, *including vaccines*. The deficiency of reporting to the CSD, now called the Committee on Safety of Medicines (CSM), is again well known and 'In spite of what has been done to improve the rate of reporting of adverse reactions by doctors, there is still thought to be under-reporting'[40]. (The system of reporting to the CSM is only intended as an early warning system, and is not set up to record all adverse reactions.)

In the United Kingdom in the 1960s Medical Officers of Health usually got to know about adverse reactions to whooping cough vaccine, and the usual response to what they considered an unacceptable number of adverse reactions would be to change their supplier of the vaccine. There is, as far as I see, no national monitoring of adverse reactions to all vaccines at present. In discussing this problem Wilson[41] stated: 'a large number of accidents – I suspect the majority – have never been reported in print, either through fear of compensation claims, or of giving a weapon to the anti-vaccinationists, or for some other reason.'

There actually was some concern about pertussis-containing vaccines at the periphery in the 1960s, and indeed at one point the Research Committee the then Society of Medical Officers of Health agreed to a study which I tried to set up in England in 1967 in which a comparison was to be made of the reactions following triple antigen (Dip/Tet/Pert) and a Dip/Tet vaccine with adjuvant. This was discouraged, and was never carried out. There seemed to be no central recognition at that time that there might be a problem with whooping cough vaccine, and no official attention seemed to be paid to any adverse reactions until the Association of Parents of Vaccine-Damaged Children which was founded in 1973 brought the issue to the notice of the public and of the politicians.

In addition to the study of adverse effects of vaccine which is being undertaken by Pollock[34] a second prospective study (The National Encephalopathy Study) has been set up in the UK in order to try to obtain exact knowledge on the incidence of severe neurological sequelae following immunization with pertussis-containing vaccines. This study, which is being carried out by Professor D. L. Miller and the staff of the Department of Community Medicine of the Middlesex Hospital Medical School, got under way towards the end of 1976 and is intended to investigate the diagnosis and vaccine history of all children of 2 months to 3 years of age who have been admitted to hospitals throughout the UK with various neurological syndromes[10].

THE CONTROVERSY

The controversy could be said to have become a public one in 1970, when it was questioned whether the community effect of the vaccine outweighed the damage which it might be doing[33]. There was at that time a general disappointment that the vaccine introduced in 1957 had not been more effective, for in spite of relatively good acceptance of vaccines in many areas there was still a considerable amount of whooping cough in England, Wales and Scotland (see Figures). Secondly, following the trials of quadruple vaccine in Belfast the potency of the available vaccines was called into question[37]. Although, as noted, a British Reference Vaccine had been approved in 1957, when an International standard was established in 1964[42], it was found that British vaccine contained only half the recommended number of four International Units per dose[43]. So it looked as if much of the British vaccine used in the early 1960s may have been of low potency; but secondly it also appeared that the number of *B. pertussis* in some vaccines greatly exceeded the recommended number of organisms[37] which according to the WHO standard should not exceed 20×10^9 per dose. (As has been said, it is generally agreed that an increased number of organisms is associated with increased toxicity.) The potency of British vaccine is said to have been adjusted from

1967 onwards. Because of the concern about the efficacy of the vaccine available in the early 1960s the Public Health Laboratory Service (PHLS) initiated a field study in 1966 which showed that at that time the attack rate of whooping cough in unvaccinated home contacts was 67% compared with 56% in fully vaccinated children, and it was estimated that the protective effect of some of the vaccine current at that time was less than 20%[44]. So perhaps there was some justification for the concern of the Belfast group about the community effect of the vaccine.

As noted, the potency of British vaccine has been increased and, in addition, all current British vaccines contain antigen type 3 and also a mineral adjuvant.

There is no adequate evidence that the lack of the type 3 antigen in earlier British vaccines had rendered it relatively impotent as suggested by Preston[45,46]. Preston and Stanbridge[47] have recently indicated that they had observed a better degree of protection in children receiving vaccine which contained antigen type 3. I do not think that their conclusions are justified; other countries with vaccines which do not contain the type 3 factor have not made changes in order to include serotypes of prevalent type 3 antigen strains; nor have they considered that such changes were of any importance as far as vaccine efficacy is concerned, provided the vaccines were produced and standardized according to WHO requirements.

The incorporation of mineral adjuvants in British vaccines is based on a very small study by Butler, Voyce, Burland and Hilton[48].

Since the PHLS study of the mid 1960s[44] there has been no controlled study in the UK to measure the protection afforded by the current 1970 British vaccines by comparing the attack rates in family or of school contacts of vaccinated and non-vaccinated children. The evidence available on their efficacy rests on data from the PHLS Epidemiological Research Laboratory reported by Noah[49] and in a study by Miller and Fletcher[50]. In the former study covering the years 1972–74, the occurrence of notified whooping cough in children who were considered to be 'fully immunized' (i.e. had received at least three doses of vaccine at suitable intervals) was compared with 'not fully immunized children'. It was reported that in children born after 1969 there was a significant difference in the notification of whooping cough in 'fully immunized children' in all age groups but the data do not lend themselves to a precise measure of vaccine effectiveness because of lack of limits of confidence and because they include all sorts of biases. Of considerable interest, however, was the observation that in children born in 1968 and 1969 the differences in the attack rates in the 'fully immunized' were sometimes higher than in the 'not fully immunized' children. Noah's data indicate that current vaccines have some protective effect and that earlier ones were relative ineffective.

The study of Miller and Fletcher[50] related to the severity of illness in over 8000 cases of whooping cough notified in England and Wales, from October to March 1975, of whom 7317 were treated at home and 806 admitted to hospital. In this study the cases are classified as 'severe', 'moderate' and 'mild' on the 'judgement' of the writers from their perusal of hospital case summaries of patients admitted to hospital, and from a record card completed retrospectively by the doctor who notified the cases which were treated at home. Obviously, as previously noted, this type of study is full of biases such as observer bias, on the reason for admission to the hospital, on the accuracy of the diagnosis, on the 'judgement' of the writers, on their assessment of the severity of those admitted to hospital and of those treated at home, etc. Although this survey was not designed to assess the protection afforded by vaccine, Miller and Fletcher conclude that at all ages previous vaccination reduced the severity of the disease.

Of 459 cases in 'fully vaccinated' children only ten were admitted to hospital compared with ninety-four of the 575 unvaccinated group. Of the 'fully vaccinated' group treated at home only four had so-called 'severe' whooping cough compared with twenty-eight unvaccinated children. The other differences are shown in Table 3. Whilst the differences in admission rates could be merely a reflection of social class differences correlated with vaccination state, it is suggested[10] that such bias can be overcome by combining the two categories 'admitted to hospital' and 'severe illness treated at home' which *suggests* that vaccination had modified the severity of the disease in the individual. I do not think that the individual protection which pertussis vaccine may confer has ever been in serious dispute. The real problem relates to the community effect of routine immunization.

Table 3 Severity of illness in 1–2-year-olds according to vaccination state[9]

	No. of cases	*No. (%) admitted to hospital*	*No. (%) treated at home**		
			Severe	*Moderate*	*Mild*
Fully vaccinated	459	10 (2)	4 (0.9)	111 (24)	334 (73)
Unvaccinated	575	94 (16)	28 (5)	214 (37)	239 (42)

* Excluding those in whom the degree of severity was not known.

Like the study of Noah[49] the study of Miller and Fletcher[50] gives no precise measure of vaccine efficacy, so at the present time there are no accurate data on the efficacy of British whooping cough vaccine, nor of the frequency of any adverse effects. *However, all the available evidence indicates that current vaccines are better than those which were available when the controversy started, and secondly that untoward reactions of a serious nature are less than they were in the early 1960s.*

WHO ARE AT RISK?

Over the years (as shown in Table 4) notifications of whooping cough in England and Wales has been highest in those aged 1–4 years, and lowest in

Table 4 Notification per 1000 population (England and Wales)

Years	*Under 1 year*	*1–4 years*	*5–9 years*
1944–45	12.1	17.7	8.4
1946–49	14.6	22.4	11.0
1950–53	19.3	28.2	15.0
1954–57	12.1	16.5	9.7
1958–61	5.0	6.1	4.4
1962–65	3.1	3.5	2.1
1966–69	2.3	3.0	1.6
1970–73	1.6	1.3	0.9

the 5–9 year age-group. This was also applicable to the notifications for Scotland until 1957 when, as in England, there was a marked reduction of notification in all ages; but in Scotland the notifications in the under 1-year-olds exceeded that in the other age-groups. When deaths are considered it is found that the case fatality (deaths per 1000 notifications) is very much higher in the under 1-year-olds. The distribution of all deaths from whooping cough in infants and children in recent years is presented in Table 6. It may be seen that between 1970 and 1974 about 50% of the deaths from whooping cough occurred in infants under 3 months of age, and 75% of them were in infants under 6 months.

Table 5 Deaths per 1000 notifications (England and Wales)

Year	*Under 1 year*	*1–4 years*	*5–9 years*
1944–45	63.7	6.99	1.05
1946–49	42.6	4.07	0.40
1950–53	15.9	1.24	0.12
1954–57	8.8	0.55	0.09
1958–61	5.3	0.46	0.07
1962–65	9.2	0.60	0.04
1966–69	8.7	0.13	—
1970–73	8.2	0.24	0.14

Table 6 Number of deaths from whooping cough, 1970–74 (England and Wales) categorized according to age in months

Under 3 months	*3–5 months*	*6–11 months*	*12 months and over*	*All*
26	14	6	7	53

So those at greatest risk of death and of severity[50] are those in whom the disease is least likely to be influenced by immunization following the schedule recommended in the UK[51]. Because of this, some have suggested that immunization should be started much earlier. Unfortunately there are no adequate studies which show that whooping cough vaccine is effective when given to small infants, although it has been shown that they produce agglutinins following inoculation[48] but at a lower level than older children.

Secondly there is no information that current British Dip/Tet/Pert vaccines are as reactive in the first few months of life as they are in older infants (see p. 44). It is important that studies should be carried out on the efficacy and reactogenicity of current vaccines in young infants.

Melchior[52] has indicated that giving pertussis vaccines to infants at an early age does not seem to have produced any change in the age of onset of infantile spasms in Denmark. In the USA, a primary series of three injections, 1 month apart, is recommended by the American Public Health Association[5] beginning at 1–2 months of age. But the report of the Committee of Infectious Diseases of the American Academy of Pediatricians[54] notes that inoculation within the first few weeks of life is not usually recommended; but no reasons are given for this statement.

Meanwhile, in the UK, until further information is available it would seem sensible to continue to pursue the policy of immunizing older infants in those communities at risk, and thereby attempting to protect the small infants in the family environment from infection.

THE QUESTIONS

The question which was posed when the controversy started was 'Before accepting . . . severe and serious complications as a necessary evil of whooping cough vaccine, it would be interesting to know what benefits communities are deriving from their present programmes'[33]. Are we convinced 'that the community benefit of whooping cough vaccination outweighs the damage which it may be doing?'[27].

VIEW OF THE JOINT COMMITTEE

In reviewing all the available evidence, the Joint Committee on Vaccination and Immunisation of the Central Health Services Council and Scottish Health Services Planning Council[10] supported the continued use of whooping cough vaccine as a routine measure. It has pointed out that, on the available evidence, whooping cough is still a serious disease; and that immunization will not only reduce the attack rate, but also the severity of the disease. The committee was unable to make any wholly reliable estimate of the incidence of neurological complications after vaccination, but considered that the risk with current vaccines is slight.

The Joint Committee has voiced some concern on the future incidence of whooping cough in the UK, since the acceptance of whooping cough vaccine is much lower in 1977 than it was in 1974. It has been predicted[10] that the next wave of pertussis may be at least as serious as, and possibly more serious than, that in 1974–75 (see Figure 4). As has already been noted (p. 30) variations in notifications may be due to factors other than the incidence of the disease. When the course of pertussis and deaths from pertussis are followed over the years (see Figures) it is difficult to believe that all the forces, apart from immunization, which have been reducing the incidence and mortality from pertussis for more than 100 years, should be less efficacious in the next few years than they have been in the past. The history of pertussis until 1957 (see Figures) was not influenced by vaccine.

PERSONAL VIEW (DE OMNIBUS DUBITANDUM)

There is no doubt that effective vaccines can be produced which will give some individual protection against whooping cough. It is usually claimed that the approximate halving of the notifications in 1958–61 in England and Wales was due to the use of a vaccine which had an efficacy similar to that used in the MRC trials[1–4]. If much of the vaccine used in the early and mid 1960s was only about 20% effective, why did this downward trend continue? What conclusions would have been drawn as far as the effectiveness of the vaccine is concerned if it had been introduced in 1951 (Figure 3).

Reference has already been made to the fact that it was obvious that, at the beginning of this century, the same influences which had led to the decline of mortality from measles were leading to a decline of mortality from whooping cough. While the reasons are probably complex, anything which tends to postpone an attack of measles or whooping cough will tend to make the disease less mortal and much of the reduction in the incidence of measles from 1915 to 1935 was due 'to the reduction in the size of families, particularly poor families. This favourable influence operated in two ways. The older children who go to school pick up infectious diseases there, and bring them back to their younger brothers and sisters. When there are many younger brothers and sisters in the population, measles will tend to occur at an early age and will tend to be more dangerous'[55]. The situation is similar with whooping cough, but more so as far as the age of mortality is concerned. In 1931, mortality from whooping cough in babies 1 year old in social class V was about twenty times that of children of the same age in social class I[55]. This still seems to be the case and, for example, all the seven deaths from whooping cough in 1970 were in social class V. The important factor may not have been the social class *per se*, but the larger family size in social class V. (In spite of certain recent statements to the contrary, social class V still has an average family size above the national average and the most recent available data[56] indicate that in the 1974 General Household Survey it was discovered that class V had an average family size of about 15% above the national average.) The age of attack will be postponed in smaller families, and this will tend to make the disease less mortal.

Whilst it is difficult to identify social classes, it would seem that the greatest opportunity for protection should be offered where the risk of mortality (and presumably serious illness) is greatest. Not only is mortality greatest among the underprivileged but acceptance of immunization is lower in poorer sections of the community, and presumably also the need for admission of such children to hospital is greater when whooping cough occurs. The importance of these social factors was spelt out 20 years ago by the Chief Medical Officer who wrote in his annual report: 'A striking change has taken place in the whooping cough position in the past two years . . . We can point to better housing, good nutrition, ready access to medical nursing care and more efficacious therapy as factors'[57]. While in general I agree with the proposals of the Joint Committee[10], I feel that no unnecessary risk should be taken with any vaccine. We do not yet have a precise measure of the *reactions* associated with current vaccines (but they certainly seem to be much less than the media has implied, for it has unjustly related past complications with present vaccines). We do not have a precise measure of the *protection* offered by current vaccines, but they seem to be effective. Meanwhile I believe that every effort should be made to encourage the use of whooping cough vaccine in the underprivileged, living in overcrowded conditions with perhaps less available medical care than that of other members of the community. In this respect it is of interest that the Federal Health Office in Germany has the Standing Committee for Vaccination Problems of the Federal Health Office in Germany has recently proposed[58] that pertussis immunization should be removed from the programme of free (transl. 'free of charge') vaccinations, and that pertussis vaccination is indicated for infants in institutions, for those living under deprived social conditions (i.e. in large families, with poor or crowded living conditions) and for those considered to be at special risk (e.g. with diseases of the respiratory or cardio-vascular system).

In the UK selective immunization is practiced for BCG and for rubella and if it were practised more actively with pertussis vaccines[58] we might see more effect on the further reduction in the morbidity and mortality from whooping cough.

References

1. Medical Research Council (1951). The prevention of whooping cough by vaccination. An MRC investigation. *Br. Med. J.*, **2**, 1463
2. Medical Research Council. (1956a). Vaccination against whooping cough. Relation between protection in children and results of laboratory tests. *Br. Med. J.*, **2**, 454
3. Medical Research Council. (1956b). Poliomyelitis and prophylactic inoculation against diphtheria, whooping cough and smallpox. Report of the MRC committee on inoculation procedures and neurological lesions. *Lancet*, **ii**, 1223
4. Medical Research Council. (1959). Vaccination against whooping cough. The final report to the whooping cough immunisation committee of the MRC. *Br. Med. J.*, **1**, 994
5. Benenson, A. S. (1975). *Control of Communicable Diseases in Man*. 12th edn., p. 365. An Official Report of the American Public Health Association
6. Preston, N. W. (1977). Maternal antibody against pertussis. *Br. Med. J.*, **1**, 706
7. Islur, J., Anglin, S. C. and Middleton, P. J. (1975). The whooping cough syndrome: a continuing pediatric problem. *Clin. Pediatr. (Phila)*, **14(2)**, 171

8. British Society for the Study of Infection. (1977). Whooping cough – a retrospective study of hospital admissions. *J. R. Coll. Gen. Practit.*, **27**, 93
9. Miller, C. L. and Fletcher, W. B. (1976). Severity of notified whooping cough. *Br. Med. J.*, **1**, 117
10. Report (1977). *Whooping cough vaccination – Review of the Evidence on Whooping cough Vaccination by the Joint Committee on Vaccination and Immunisation, DHSS* HMSO
11. Leading article (1956). Measles. *Lancet*, **ii**, 1089
12. Nicol, C. G. M. (1956). Monthly Bulletin of the Ministry of Health Laboratory, vol. 15, p. 126
13. *General Practitioner*, 2nd September, 1977, p. 1
14. Kendrick, P. and Eldering, G. (1939). *Am. J. Hyg.*, **B29**, 133
15. McFarlan, A. M., Topley, E. and Fisher, M. (1945). Trial of whooping cough vaccine in city and residential nursing groups. *Br. Med. J.*, **2**, 205
16. Hopper, J. M. H. (1961). Illness after whooping cough vaccination. *Med. Off.* **106**, 241
17. Dane, D. S., Dick, G. W. A., Simpson, D. I. H., Briggs, E. M., McAlister, J., Nelson, R. and Field, C. M. B. (1962). New quadruple vaccine. *Lancet*, **i**, 939
18. Haire, M., Dane, D. S. and Dick, G. W. A. (1967). Reactions to combined vaccines containing killed bordetella pertussis. *Med. Off.* **117**, 55
19. Hannik, C. A. (1974). *WHO Conference on Whooping Cough, Utrecht.* WHO/BAC/75.1
20. College of General Practitioners (1960). A survey of the epilepsies in general practice. A report by the research committee of the College of General Practitioners. *Br. Med. J.*, **2**, 416
21. Van den Berg, B. J. and Yernshalmy. J. (1967). Studies on convulsive disorders in young children. *Paediatr. Res.*, **3**, 298
22. Harker, P. (1977). Primary immunisation and febrile convulsions in Oxford 1972–75. *Br. Med. J.*, **2**, 490
23. Berg, J. M. (1958). Neurological complications of pertussis immunization. *Br. Med. J.*, **2**, 24
24. Strøm, J. (1960). Is universal vaccination against pertussis always justified? *Br. Med. J.*, **2**, 1184
25. Strøm, J. (1967). Further experience of reactions, especially of a cerebral nature, in conjunction with triple vaccination: a study based on vaccination in Sweden 1959–1965. *Br. Med. J.*, **4**, 320
26. Malgrem, B., Vahlquist, B. and Zetterström, R. (1960). Correspondence Complications of immunisation. *Br. Med. J.*, **2**, 1801
27. Dick, G. W. A. (1974). Reactions to routine immunisation in childhood. *Proc. R. Soc. Med.*, **67**, 371
28. Ehrengut, W. (1974). Uber Konvulsive Reaktionen nach Pertussis-Schutzimpfung. *Dtsch. Med. Wochenschr.*, **99**, 374
29. Kulenkampff, M., Schwartzman, J. S. and Wilson, J. (1974). Neurological complications of pertussis inoculation. *Arch. Dis. Child.*, **49**, 46
30. Stewart, G. T. (1975). *Br. Med. J.*, **i**, 283
31. Stewart, G. T. (1977). Vaccination against whooping cough. *Lancet*, **i**, 234
32. Roden, A. T. (1974). Convulsived disorders in young children. *Proc. R. Soc. Med.*, **67**, 38
33. Dick, D. W. A. (1970). Proc. Conference on Application of Vaccines against Viral, Rickettsial and Bacterial Diseases of Man, Dec. 1970 PAHO Scientific Publication No. 226, 420, (1971)
34. Pollock, T. M. (1977). The efficacy of whooping cough vaccines (unpublished)
35. Stephenson, J. B. P. (1977). Vaccination against whooping cough. *Lancet*, **i**, 357
36. Ounsted, C. (1977). Vaccination against whooping cough. *Lancet*, **i**, 419
37. Dick, D. W. A. (1966). Edited Lecture, Toronto, Jan. 1964. *Can. J. Publ. Hlth*, **57**, 435
38. Pollock, T. M. (1976). (Personal communication)
39. Bousfield, G. (1952). A future for combined diphtheria and whooping cough prophylaxis? *Med. Off.*, **87**, 265
40. *Annual Report for 1976 of the Medicines Commission and the Committee on Safety in Medicine.* HMSO, 428
41. Wilson, G. S. (1967). *Hazards of Immunisation* (London: Athlone Press)

42. WHO (1964). Expert Committee on Biological Standardisation – 16th Report (*WHO Technical Report Series No. 274*) (Geneva: WHO)
43. Perkins, F. T. (1969). Correspondence, vaccination against whooping cough. *Br. Med. J.*, **4**, 429
44 Public Health Laboratory Service (1969). Efficacy of whooping-cough vaccines used in the United Kingdom before 1968. A preliminary report to the Director of the Public Health Laboratory Service by the PHLS Whooping-Cough Committee and Working Party
45 Preston, N. W. (1963). Type specific immunity against whooping cough. *Br. Med. J.*, **2**, 724
46. Preston, N. W. (1965). Effectiveness of pertussis vaccines. *Br. Med. J.*, **2**, 11
47. Preston, N. W. and Stanbridge, T. N. (1972). Efficacy of pertussis vaccines: a brighter horizon. *Br. Med. J.*, **3**, 448
48. Butler, N. R., Voyce, M. A., Burland, W. L. and Hilton, M. L. (1969). Advantages of aluminium hydroxide adsorbed combined diphtheria, tetanus, and pertussis vaccines for immunisation of infants. *Br. Med. J.*, **1**, 663
49. Noah, N. D. (1976). Attack rates of notified whooping cough in immunised and unimmunised children, *Br. Med. J.*, **1**, 128
50. Miller, C. L. and Fletcher, W. B. (1976). Severity of notified whooping cough. *Br. Med. J.*, **i**, 117
51. DHSS (1972). *Immunisation against Infectious Disease* DHSS, Scottish H H? and Welsh Office, July 1972, HMSO
52. Melchior, J. C. (1977). Infantile spasms and early immunisation against whooping cough. *Arch. Dis. Child.*, **52**, 134
53. Report (1974). *Report of the Committee on Infectious Diseases* 17th edn. (Evanston: American Academy of Sciences)
54. Gale, A. H. (1959). *Epidemic Diseases*, p. 98 (Harmondsworth: Penguin)
55. Fact Sheet (1977). Family Planning Information Service. 29th March 1977
56. CMO (1959). On the state of the public health. *The Annual Report of the CMO for the year 1959.* HMSO

5
Measles vaccines

ERLING NORRBY

The successful propagation of measles virus in tissue culture by Enders and Peebles in 1954 provided conditions for the development of measles vaccines. Almost 10 years later two different kinds of measles vaccines were licensed in the United States. These were a live attenuated measles virus vaccine (Edmonston B strain) and a formalin-inactivated aluminium-precipitated vaccine. The Edmonston B vaccine frequently caused clinical reactions, and in order to reduce these complications the live vaccine was given either after a primary vaccination with killed vaccine or after administration of γ-globulin. Considerable modifications were later introduced in the outlining of vaccine policies in different countries.

INACTIVATED MEASLES VACCINES

Vaccine products

Besides the formalin-inactivated crude measles vaccine produced by Chas. Pfizer & Co. (Terre Haute, Indiana) a semi-purified formalin-inactivated vaccine was developed at Connaught Medical Research Laboratories, Toronto. As an alternative to formalin-inactivation, vaccines were also prepared by splitting of virus material by treatment with Tween 80 and ether. An unpurified preparation was introduced into the market in West Germany by Behringwerke AG, either as an isolated product or combined with inactivated polio and DTP vaccines. Semi-purified haemagglutinin obtained from Tween–ether treated virus was also used in limited field trials in Sweden[10].

DURATION OF IMMUNITY

Three to four years after the introduction of inactivated measles vaccines it was found that the immunity obtained was not satisfactory. Both subclinical and clinical reinfections occurred after exposure to wild virus. Further, immunopathological complications were encountered in some cases after exposure to wild virus, and also after vaccination with live attenuated virus. The poor immunity produced by inactivated vaccines was unexpected, since it was known from long experience that passive immunization with γ-globulin provided a good protection against disease. Measured by conventional techniques (haemagglutination inhibition – HI – and neutralization tests) it was found that 50–100 times higher titres of antibodies induced by vaccination with killed vaccines as compared to antibodies provided by administration of γ-globulin were needed to provide a corresponding protection.

Recently the failure of the inactivated vaccines has been explained. It was demonstrated that both types of inactivation procedures used destroyed the immunogenicity of one component (the haemolysin, fusion factor) in the virus envelope[9–11]. Therefore only partial immunity was induced, which carried the disadvantage of establishing conditions for the development of immunopathological reactions.

Experiences made with hitherto-used inactivated vaccines have two implications. The first one is that by use of some alternative inactivation procedures it might be possible to develop an efficient inactivated measles vaccine. However, in view of the satisfactory results obtained with live measles vaccines it seems unlikely that any new type of inactivated measles vaccine will ever be produced. The second implication is that in attempts to develop inactivated or subunit vaccines from other enveloped viruses (e.g. herpes viruses, retro viruses, hepatitis B virus) it should be certified that the eventual vaccine product contains all the essential surface antigens needed to provide complete immunity. If this is not the case, then vaccination may put an immunized individual in a disadvantageous position compared with an unvaccinated individual.

As a consequence of the bad experiences with inactivated measles vaccines, all products of this kind were removed from the market. The Tween–ether vaccine produced by Behringwerke AG was used in West Germany until August 1976. It was used mostly as a combined vaccine and only for immunization prior to administration of live vaccine. No untoward clinical reactions have been encountered in children receiving both vaccines and the titres of, e.g., HI antibodies were higher than after immunization with the live vaccine only[13]. However, it was recently found that in spite of the potent HI antibody response, most vaccinees did not produce antibodies to the second major envelope component, the hemolysin[11]. Thus the combined procedure of vaccination cannot be recommended for use.

LIVE MEASLES VACCINES

Vaccine products

Live measles vaccines have been used extensively in different parts of the world, particularly in the United States and the Soviet Union. Several different vaccine products marketed by private companies or produced by governmental laboratories have been used (Table 1). Since the original Edmonston B strain was too reactive, further attenuated strains were developed. The first one to be introduced on the market was the Schwarz strain which is the one hitherto most extensively used. This strain was licensed for use in the USA in 1965 and is marketed by Dow Chemical Company (Indianapolis).

Table 1 Live measles vaccines used in different countries

Country	*Vaccine virus strain (production)*	*Government-sponsored programme*	*Remarks*
Canada	Moraten (MSD; import)	+	High frequency of vaccination
Holland	Moraten (MSD; import)	+ (from Jan. 1976)	Until 1975 only limited use of vaccine
Japan	CAM 70 (Biken Institute Osaka) Schwarz (Takeda Chem. Ind.)	−	About 50% of children vaccinated during 1971–75
Sweden	Schwarz (State production)	+	10–15% of children vaccinated
United Kingdom	Schwarz (Glaxo Lab.)	+	About 60% of children vaccinated
USA	Schwarz (Dow Chemicals) Moraten (MSD)	+	60–70% of children vaccinated (currently mostly combined live vaccines)
USSR	Leningrad-16 (State) production)	+	About 31 million doses distributed in 1967–72

It is produced on licence in several other countries. Another strain of further attenuated virus, named Moraten, was licensed and developed by the Merck, Sharp & Dohme Research Laboratories and licensed for the US market in 1968. In other countries further attenuated strains have also been derived from the original Edmonston B strain. In England the Beckenham strain 31 (later withdrawn) was developed at the Wellcome Research Laboratories and in the State Laboratories in Yugoslavia and USSR the Belgrad and Leningrad 16 strains were developed.

Conversion rates

Properly applied, the live measles vaccines give a high frequency of conversion in immunized individuals. Frequency figures between 90 and 95% are regularly reported[5]. However, improper storage of vaccine, a situation which may readily arise in tropical climates, may cause problems. Certain vaccine failures encountered in the USA have been explained by the use of live vaccines which contain insufficient remaining quantities of infectious virus. In some developing countries highly discouraging figures on conversion rates have been reported. Recently, technological developments have been introduced which have improved the temperature stability of vaccine products.

DURATION OF IMMUNITY

Immunity as measured by persistence of antibodies is highly satisfactory. Antibody titres are lower than after regular measles, but appear to persist; in most individuals devoid of detectable antibodies a state of sensitization remains. In several field trials protection against diseases upon exposure to wild virus in vaccinated individuals has been documented to be 90% or more. A certain number of cases have been reported where individuals contracted measles after prior immunization with live vaccine. In most cases these infections occur in individuals in whom vaccination has failed. This may be due either to the use of an improperly stored vaccine or to a restricted replication of vaccine virus because of the presence of maternal antibodies, simultaneously administered γ-globulin or prior immunization with inactivated vaccine.

Reinfections occur after vaccination but generally are subclinical. The number of clearly documented cases of clinically overt measles in individuals with a previous serologically defined take of vaccination are relatively few[7]. Some odd cases of aberrant measles in children previously receiving only live vaccine were described[3]. This kind of case need further analysis.

Revaccination

The possibility of revaccinating with live vaccine has been discussed and also tried in a few field studies[1]. It appears that the live vaccine can give a booster immunization provided the level of circulating antibodies is low. The general situation in vaccinated communities does not indicate a need for any large-scale revaccination.

Acute and late side-reactions

The acute side-reactions in connection with vaccination by use of further attenuated virus strains do not pose any problems. Vaccination only occasionally and transiently affects the general activities of children. Children with defective cell-bound immunity should not, however, be given live measles vaccine, since they may contract a fatal disease. These children might be given inactivated vaccine. A special interest has been devoted to complications in the central nervous system in connection with vaccination. The frequency of postvaccination encephalitis is very low and not distinguishable from the background frequency of encephalitis expected to occur even in the absence of vaccination[6]. Concerning the uncommon late sequelae of measles named 'sub-acute sclerosing panencephalitis', current data indicate that this complication shows a 5-fold reduction or more in vaccinated individuals[8].

Combined live vaccines

Live measles vaccine has been successfully combined with other live vaccines, e.g. rubella, mumps and smallpox vaccines. In the USA a triple live measles, rubella and mumps vaccine marketed by Merck, Sharp & Dohme is most commonly used[14]. Recently a corresponding product from the Dow Chemical Company was tested in field trials. Measles vaccine has also been combined with smallpox vaccine. The simultaneous replication of more than one live vaccine virus has not reduced the immunizing capacity of individual live vaccines. In certain European countries rubella immunization is performed at early adolescence instead of during childhood. In these countries combined live vaccines including rubella will not have any applicability, but the combination of measles and mumps vaccines may become increasingly interesting.

Measles epidemiology in vaccinated communities

The epidemiological consequences of introducing live measles vaccine have been extensively discussed. Since vaccine virus does not spread from vaccinees to other individuals, the possibilities for circulation of wild virus determines the absence, or endemic or epidemic occurrence of measles. Experience shows that the highly contagious measles virus can circulate in a community in which as much as 90% of the population is immune to the disease. Thus, eradication of measles is not as readily reached as was originally thought. Measles virus has continued to circulate within almost all vaccinated communities in the USA and in the USSR, but the massive immunization in both these countries has had a marked impact on morbidity and mortality secondary to measles. The importance of maintaining a high frequency of vaccination was exemplified by the resurgence of the disease in 1969 after removal of direct federal funds for measles vaccination in the USA in 1968. After re-institution of funds decreasing trends in measles were again seen in 1972.

Circulation of virus may stop in a community with more than 90% of individuals with immunity to measles as exemplified by the situation in Alaska[4] and in East Germany[12]. Under these conditions it is essential to maintain a high frequency of vaccination. Otherwise the fraction of non-immune individuals may run a risk of contracting measles at an increased age.

Benefit–cost analysis

In the USA and USSR a summary has been made of health and resource savings due to vaccination against measles during the periods 1963–72 and 1967–72, respectively. During these periods the numbers of vaccine doses distributed were 58.5 and 30.7 million. The net economical benefits for the year-period were calculated at $1.3 billion for the USA[15] and $244 million for the USSR[2].

Vaccination in industrialized countries and in developing countries

The indications for use of measles vaccines are distinctly different in these two different milieus. In industrialized countries the motivation is to prevent a distressing, but very seldom fatal, disease and its sequelae, in particular, postinfectious encephalitis. This indication has carried varying impact in different countries. In Sweden only about 15% of all children are vaccinated today, in spite of the fact that general vaccination of children is recommended and the cost of vaccination is carried by the State. Questions that have hampered the enthusiasm for vaccination among pediatricians are: (a) is the disease worth preventing? (b) is the immunity after vaccination durable?; and (c) is the vaccine infection harmless also with reference to late sequelae? As a contrast to Sweden it can be mentioned that the level of vaccination in Norway approaches 70%. Similar figures are also found in most countries with a governmentally sponsored vaccination programme (Table 1).

In developing countries the impacts of measles infections are much heavier than in industrialized countries. The disease is one of the major causes of death in children between the age of 2 and 10 years. A combination of undernourishment and/or simultaneous occurrence of other, e.g. parasitic, diseases with measles seems to be highly dangerous. The World Health Organization has underlined the importance of applying measles vaccine in developing countries in a proclamation for expanded programmes of immunization.

There are three major problems in using the vaccine in developing countries. One special problem concerns the fact that in these countries vaccination has to be carried out early to give optimal protection. In industrialized countries vaccination is not performed before the age of 14 months due to the risk of interference by maternal antibodies. However in certain developing countries it is recommended that vaccine be given before the age of 8 months. Another problem, which was already mentioned, is the risk of loss of infectivity of the vaccine product under the prevailing conditions of immunization. A final problem is the cost of introducing the vaccine. Although the costs for vaccine may be kept low, the expenses for a yearly distribution of vaccine may be a considerable burden to a developing country with restricted economical resources. To this should be added the fact that appropriate medical personnel to carry out vaccinations are frequently not available.

CONCLUSIONS

Remarkable medical progress has been made by application of live measles vaccines in different parts of the world. However, a lot of work still remains in seeing that vaccine is made available also to those parts of the world in which they are most urgently needed. Further technological development, as well as financial assistence, may help in reaching a proper use of a highly efficient vaccine product.

References

1. Bass, J. W., Halstead, S. B., Fischer, G. W., Podgore, J. K., Deal, W. R., Schydlower, M., Wiebe, R. A. and Ching, P. M. (1976). Booster vaccination with further live attenuated measles vaccine. *J. Am. Med. Assoc.*, **235,** 31
2. Burgasow, P. N., Andzaparidze, O. G. and Popov, V. (1973). The status of measles after five years of mass vaccination in the USSR. *Bull. Wld Hlth Org.*, **49,** 571
3. Cherry, J. D., Feigin, R. D., Lober, Jr., L. A. and Shackelford, P. G. (1972). Atypical measles in children previously immunized with attenuated measles virus vaccines. *Pediat.*, **50,** 712
4. Eisenberg, M., Crowe, J. D. and Anchorage, M. P. A. (1976). Measles and rubella eradication in Alaska. *J. Am. Med. Assoc.*, **235,** 179
5. Krugman, S. (1971). Present status of measles and rubella immunization in the United States: A medical progress report. *J. Pediat.*, **78,** 1
6. Landrigan, P. J. and Witte, J. J. (1973). Neurologic disorders following live measles-virus vaccination *J. Am. Med. Assoc.*, **223,** 1459
7. Linneman, C. Jr (1973). Measles vaccine: Immunity, reinfection and revaccination. *Amer. J. Epidem.*, **97,** 365
8. Modlin, J. F., Jabbour, J. T., Witte, J. J. and Halsey, N. A. (1977). Epidemiologic studies of measles, measles vaccine, and subacute sclerosing panencephalitis. *Pediat.*, **59,** 505
9. Norrby, E. (1975). Occurrence of antibodies against envelope components after immunization with formalin inactivated and live measles vaccine. *J. Biol. Stand.*, **3,** 375
10. Norrby, E. and Lagercrantz, R. (1976). Measles vaccination, VIII. The occurrence of antibodies against virus envelope components after immunization with inactivated vaccine. Effects of revaccination with live measles vaccine. *Acta Paediat. Scand.* **65,** 171
11. Norrby, E., Enders-Ruckle, G. and ter Meulen, V. (1975). Differences in the appearance of antibodies to structural components of measles virus after immunization with inactivated and live virus. *J. Infect. Dis.*, **132,** 262
12. Starke, G. and Rudinecz, S. (1975). Der Gegenwartige Stand des Masern-Eradikations-programms in der Deutschen Demokratischen Republik. *J. Hyg. Epidemiol. Microbiol. Immunol.*, **19,** 265
13. Stehr, K., Enders, G., Suschke, H. J. and Spiess, H. (1970). Klinische und immunologische Reaktionen nach Masernschutzimpfung mit Spaltimpfstoff und Lebendvaccine. *Monatschr. Kinderheilk.*, **118,** 383
14. Weibel, E., Buynak, B., Stokes, J. Jr., and Hilleman, M. R. (1972). Measurement of immunity following live mumps (5 years), measles (3 years) and rubella ($2\frac{1}{2}$ years) virus vaccines. *Pediat.*, **49,** 334
15. Witte, J. J. and Axnick, N. W. (1975). The benefits from 10 years of measles immunization in the United States. *Publ. Health Reports*, **90,** 205

6
Vaccines against influenza

C. HANNOUN

Influenza vaccines have been in use since the early 1940s. However, their controversial status is attested by a relatively low level of use. Although it has been improved during the last few years, the image of this type of vaccine has been poor for a number of reasons.

Firstly, flu is not always considered as a very dangerous agent, and it is not, as long as young healthy adults are concerned. Its virulence is so variable, however, that in some instances it can become a dreadful killer, such as in 1918–1919 when the 'Spanish flu' claimed 20 million victims. Even when not so dangerous, the disease is serious for all weaker individuals such as older people, patients with chronic diseases or organic deficiencies; especially when the heart, lungs or kidneys are involved. Such patients are described as 'high risk' not because they have a high risk of getting the disease, but because, if they get it, they have a much higher risk of its developing into a severe illness or death.

Secondly, the degree of effectiveness of the vaccine has frequently been questioned. In various experiments, it has been shown to vary from zero to more than 90% effective. This is surprising if compared with the results of other virus vaccines. The reason for this is mainly the existence of several types of influenza viruses (A, B, and C), to the many other viruses producing similar, although usually less severe, diseases, and to an intrinsic variability of the virus A (the most dangerous), which allows it to escape the effects of specific immunity.

Another problem is vaccine potency. To be efficient a vaccine should contain an adequate amount of a particular antigen. There are limits to the amount which can be inoculated without adverse reactions, and this makes it more difficult to prepare polyvalent vaccines. Each addition of a new component obliges one to reduce the amount of the others, so that the total dose does not exceed the tolerable limit. In addition, children are more susceptible to toxic reactions than adults, and they should receive smaller doses. Consequently, it is more difficult to provide efficient protection for them.

Finally, another problem is production. Influenza vaccines are made from chick embryos and the yield, especially with new strains, is generally such that one egg is not always enough to make one dose. Manufacturing millions of doses of vaccine means inoculating and harvesting millions of embryonated eggs, representing a high-cost operation. Influenza vaccine is, therefore, an expensive vaccine, a fact which constitutes another limit to its use on a larger scale.

In spite of these drawbacks and limitations, the use of influenza vaccines has increased markedly in the last few years, especially since 1969. At this time the Hong Kong epidemic was studied in detail and offered several explanations to some poorly understood aspects of influenza virus variation and evolution. Nevertheless, it seems that, for a few years at least, vaccine will still be the only useful measure against flu.

TYPES OF INFLUENZA VACCINES

Inactivated vaccines

Virus grown in embryonated eggs is inactivated by formalin or β-propiolactone, and more or less purified to prepare a suspension which is then titrated and diluted for injection.

Purified vaccines

Several techniques have been designed to improve the purity of the final product. They include adsorption–elution cycles on particulate substrates such as formalinized chicken red cells or mineral precipitates, high-speed pelleting in ultracentrifuge or, better, zonal centrifugation in sucrose gradients. Vaccines prepared by a combination of several of these techniques reach a high state of purity and hardly contain any foreign material except virus. They cause fewer side-reactions and can be used at higher dosages.

Split vaccines

An additional step can be used – splitting the viral particles by a lipid solvent or a detergent. The product thus obtained still contains all constituents of the virus but is less reactogenic. Such vaccines, however, are less immunogenic, especially under conditions of primary immunization. Their use in children, which would seem to be advisable because of their high sensitivity, is, therefore, disappointing since the level of immunity reached is not always satisfactory.

Adjuvated vaccines

Various types of adjuvants have been tried and used with influenza antigens such as mineral precipitates or vegetable oil emulsions. This type of material gave irregular results and has not yet passed into general use.

Live attenuated vaccines

Russian investigators have tried to attenuate influenza strains for use as live vaccine. It is difficult to find and stabilize the proper degree of attenuation. If not enough, the reactions are unacceptable. They can, in fact, reproduce the disease itself. If too much, no side-reactions occur, but no immunity either. After a period of empirical attenuation, other groups have started to study more carefully the genetics of influenza virus. There is a reasonable hope that the use of temperature-sensitive, cold-adapted, or inhibitor-resistant selected variants can eventually be used as locally administered live vaccines.

Many of the points mentioned above would deserve more detailed development. We will emphasize some of the main aspects that are important for an overall appreciation of the problem of influenza control by vaccination: definition of high-risk groups; vaccination policies; costs of the disease and of the vaccination; manufacturing time required for production.

DEFINITION OF HIGH-RISK GROUPS

Such a definition cannot be universal because evaluation of risk may vary according to circumstance and place. Some consider vital risk to be the most important, others the economical risk, and still others the social risk. Two main categories have to be differentiated:

A. Medical risk

In this sense, risk can be described as a net increase of the probability of a very severe evolution of the disease with complications and eventually death. All people above a certain age should be put into this group since relative mortality by influenza increases exponentially with age after 45. The risk is serious and much above the average mortality rate after 65, the limit uniformly accepted for high risk. This is especially true in people living in institutions. Another category with high medical risk contains people of all ages with chronic or debilitating diseases such as:

cardiovascular diseases: chronic rheumatic heart diseases, degenerative heart disease, hypertensive heart disease, congenital malformations or other diseases of the circulatory system;

bronchopulmonary diseases: asthma, chronic bronchitis, tuberculosis and other diseases of the respiratory system;
renal diseases: nephritis and nephrosis, infections and other diseases of the kidney, patients under haemodialysis, or those having had kidney transplants.
metabolic diseases: diabetes mellitus, Addison's disease.

Pregnant women also come into this category.

B. Socio-economic risk

This group includes all persons who are exceptionally exposed to contagion and who are essential to the social or economic life in a country. They do not necessarily personally risk severe disease, but their absence is detrimental to the community. They are in a situation where they can efficiently spread the disease and thus accelerate and amplify the diffusion of the epidemic. Medical and paramedical personnel are particularly exposed to infections since they have to take care of, and have direct contact with, patients. In addition, their unavailability, even temporarily, is a great inconvenience during an epidemic when hospitals are overcrowded. All public service professions in which people have contact with the public also have a high risk of contamination. These include the following services: transportation; police; post office; communications. Because of their confinement other communities are exposed to explosive outbreaks such as the armed forces and schools. In schools, the risk is even greater. Children not only contract flu easily from their infected schoolmates, but they will also, even with a mild disease, bring the infection home and contaminate their family, including older persons who have a high medical risk.

Table 1 General and high-risk populations, 1968–69, by age

Age-group	*Population (000)*	*High-risk population (percentage of total population)*	*High-risk population (percentage of total high-risk population)*
All ages	196 391	22.8	100.0
Under 17	66 970	7.4	11.0
17–44	70 504	17.3	27.2
45–64	40 423	22.8	20.6
65+	18 494	100.0	41.2

A quantitative evaluation of the number of people in medical high-risk groups in the USA is given in Table 6.

VACCINATION POLICIES

Public health agencies have a choice between several policies for influenza control.

1. Vaccination is provided to the previously defined high-risk groups to reduce excess mortality and the most dangerous forms of disease.
2. Vaccination is provided to the active working population. This will save economical losses in labour and efficiency.
3. Vaccination is provided to some key groups who play a major role in the dissemination of the agent, such as children of school age. This should stop or reduce epidemics.

Each of these policies is being used in some countries with irregular results (Table 2). A long-term evaluation of the results has not yet been obtained.

Table 2 Use of influenza vaccine in the USA

	Total population		*Population aged 65 and over*	
Year	*Number of persons immunized (000)*	*Percentage of total immunized*	*Number of persons immunized (000)*	*Percentage of total immunized*
1968–69	21 045	10.7	3506	19.0
1972–73	15 254	7.7	3209	15.8
1973–74	17 318	8.3	3628	17.4

Source: US Immunization Survey, 1969, 1973, 1974

There is, however, a fourth attitude towards influenza vaccination which consists of giving vague informal recommendations without trying to enforce them and without promoting any official programme of immunization. The decision is then left in the hands of private distribution circuits. An analysis of the reasons for not using the vaccine has demonstrated a very complex attitude.

People believe they are not personally sensitive to influenza.
They are not really concerned over the severity of the disease.
They lack confidence in the vaccines.
They are afraid of pain or side-reactions associated with vaccines.
They are unaware that there is a public programme in that field.
They have to pay for vaccine and they cannot afford, or they do not like it.

COST OF THE DISEASE, COST OF THE VACCINATION

A simple cost–benefit analysis of the effect of vaccination on a selected target population, the cohort of people aged 65 or more (about 10% of the total population), is shown in Tables 3 and 4 in conditions which could be observed in France. Different hypotheses are considered for the attack rate, from a mild epidemic to an average one (real attack rates might be as high as 40% in severe epidemics). The efficacy of the vaccine has been chosen at 80% (during recent epidemics in vaccinated institutions, rates of protection in comparison to control unvaccinated groups were more than 90%).

Table 3 Cost of influenza, France, 1973

Type of disease	*Cost in French francs**	*Treatment + labour losses*
Uncomplicated	976	(96 + 880)
Complicated	1859	(99 + 1760)
With hospital care	5510	(2870 + 2640)

* 1 FF, 1973 = 0.22 US dollar

Table 4 Effect of influenza vaccination

Attack rate (%)	*No. of cases for each 5 million older people*	*No of deaths*	*Minimal cost in French francs**	*With an 80% effective vaccine*		
				Cases prevented	*Deaths prevented*	*Cost saved in French francs**
5	¼ million	1250	250 million	200 000	1000	200 million
10	½ million	2500	500 million	400 000	2000	400 million
20	1 million	5000	1000 million	800 000	4000	800 million

* 1 FF, 1973 = 0.22 US dollar

The cost of the vaccine has been taken at the retail price (it would probably be cheaper in large vaccination programmes). Deaths have not been taken into consideration, since it is not possible to evaluate that type of intangible loss. Prevented deaths are an additional benefit. However, even with the lowest attack rate and with minimal evaluations, the balance is still quite positive.

MANUFACTURING

If one tries to evaluate how much time it would take to manufacture vaccine after isolation of a new strain of influenza, many assumptions have to be made about the time necessary for several important technical steps (adaptation, identification, clinical trials) or political steps (decision on choice of strain, licensing). Such an evaluation is shown in Table 5. A figure of 40 weeks is given between the original case and vaccine administration. This situation occurred in 1968 and, in fact, the actual time duration was much shorter since 1 million doses of vaccine had been manufactured within 20

Table 5 Estimate of the time necessary from the isolation of the strain to the vaccine

Operation	*No. of Weeks*	*Cumulative time (weeks)*
Isolation	1	1
Identification, decision, recombination, distribution	13	14
Production pilot experiments	3	17
Laboratory, clinical trials	6	23
Licence application	(2)	25
Production	6	31
Clinical trials, controls	7	38
Distribution to wholesale dealers and retail	2	40

Vaccination after 40 weeks, or about 9 months.

weeks (Table 6). The epidemic had already started at least 1 month before that time (November 25, 1968). Cases involving military personnel and outbreaks in civilian populations began in California during the third week of October and reached the East Coast in November. The peak of the epidemic in the USA, however, was observed between December 15 and January 4, 1969. At that time, 4 million people could have received the new vaccine.

This survey shows that influenza vaccines are clearly worthwhile from both the social and the economic standpoints.

Table 6 A real situation: Hong Kong epidemic, 1968

Isolation	4 days (instead of 1 week)
Identification, recombination, distribution of strain	8 weeks (instead of 13 weeks)
From seed strain to first release	10 weeks (instead of 26 weeks)
To production of first million doses	2 weeks
TOTAL	20 weeks (instead of 40 weeks)

5 million doses 22 weeks
20 million doses 29 weeks
Source: Murray

Bibliography

US Public Hlth. Surv., Center for Disease Control. US Immunization Survey 1969–1974
Murrary, R. (1969). Bull. WHO, **41**, 495
Selby, P. (ed.). (1976). Influenza: Virus Vaccines and Strategy. (London: Academic Press)

7
The New York Swine Influenza Immunization Program

P. J. IMPERATO

On March 24, 1976, President Ford announced a $135 million programme to immunize every man, woman and child against the swine flu in the USA. From the outset, the programme was surrounded by controversy and plagued by a series of problems, ranging from delays in vaccine production to malpractice liability insurance difficulties. It is beyond the focus of this paper to discuss these aspects of the programme. This programme was the largest mass vaccination programme ever undertaken in the USA, and can be effectively defended or criticized, depending on one's interpretation of the evidence and the implications of the evidence[1–11].

The United States Congress approved the President's programme and voted the necessary funds for vaccine production and delivery. Federal legislation provided for the vaccine and monies (0.14 cents) to be given to the local health departments to administer the programme. The actual average cost for administering a dose of vaccine in the USA is about 0.50 cents, so that local health departments had to absorb costs of 0.36 cents per dose. There was much criticism of the federal programme on this account by local health departments[4].

ORGANIZING A MASS VACCINATION PROGRAMME FOR NEW YORK CITY

The federal government set up broad guidelines for the programme, but left the organization, planning and administration up to the individual local State Health Departments[12]. The broad guidelines included a requirement for a coordinating committee, participation by the private medical sector, utilization of volunteers, engagement in public health education and public awareness programmes, training of personnel in cardiopulmonary resuscitation and the use of automatic jet injectors, the assessment of vaccine utilization, the obtaining of a signed informed consent on all immunized, and surveillance for the disease and for reactions to the vaccine.

The programme for New York City was discussed intensively within the executive level of the Department of Health in early April, and the following recommendations were made to the Mayor:

1. Establish a New York City Swine Influenza Immunization Task Force to include representatives from medicine, industry and commerce, etc.
2. Establish a special Swine Influenza Immunization Unit within the Department of Health to operationally administer the programme.

On April 4, 1976, the Mayor publicly announced the formation of the task force and asked the First Deputy Health Commissioner to be the Chairman, with 25 members.

The task force decided on a policy of immediate and detailed planning, organizing of a programme for the entire population, and approved of the following general guidelines:

1. Participation by private medicine

The private sector will be involved in the planning of the programme and part of the available vaccine will be administered by private physicians.

2. Participation of other health care providers

Vaccines will be made available for administration by hospitals, university health services, industrial medical units, etc. with the capability of administering the vaccines.

3. Utilization of volunteers and other community resources

Volunteers will be recruited to inform and motivate the communities, to stimulate and control the flow of persons into and within clinic sites and to assist in the compiling and tabulation of data relating to vaccine usage, vaccine reactions, etc. Whenever and wherever appropriate, volunteers will administer vaccines.

4. Coordination of the influenza programme with ongoing immunization activities

In great part, influenza immunizations will be carried out in District Health Centers and in schools where routine immunizations are provided. The staff of the existing vaccine-preventable diseases programme will be at the centre of the influenza programme.

5. Professional education

A continuous flow of information will keep the medical and allied professions abreast of the influenza programme via letters to be sent to all physicians in New York City over the signature of the First Deputy Commissioner.

6. Public awareness activities

It is anticipated that the news media will be active participants in the influenza programme. Radio, television and the daily newspapers will be presented with information for their use as the programme develops.

7. Training staff and volunteers

Personnel will be trained in the conduct of mass immunization clinics, the use of necessary forms, the operation and repair of jet injectors and in the practice of cardiopulmonary resuscitation (CPR).

8. Vaccine storage, supply and delivery

The Department of Health Bureau of Laboratories will serve as the repository for vaccines. It will supply vaccines to high-volume users such as industrial medical units, and will deliver vaccines to District Health Centers where clinics will be situated.

9. Programme for high-risk groups

In mid-October, a programme for immunization of high-risk groups will be implemented (e.g. persons in long-term care facilities and senior citizen centres). Mass clinics will be operated in District Health Centers for ambulatory high-risk patients, and persons aged 65 and over, and vaccines will be provided to private physicians and hospitals.

10. Programme for remaining susceptibles

When monovalent vaccine is available in October, vaccine will be provided for the remaining population. The vaccine will be offered in District Health Centers and in schools by jet injector teams. Vaccine will be provided to hospitals, universities, industrial medical units and private physicians.

11. Assessment of vaccine utilization

Age-specific vaccine use will be tallied and reported to the Center for Disease Control weekly by telephone and monthly in written form.

12. Surveillance of disease and vaccine reactions

Existing influenza surveillance mechanisms in New York City, including serological sampling, are believed to be quite good and will be continued.

Vaccine-associated reactions will be monitored, and appropriate response to such complaints will be made.

13. Informed consent

Appropriate information about the risks and benefits of vaccination will be provided to all persons (or parents or guardians) before they receive the vaccine.

PROGRESS OF PROGRAMME PLANNING AND ORGANIZATION

The national programme was initially scheduled to begin in July. In mid-June however, the four pharmaceutical firms producing the vaccine, announced that they were losing their liability insurance and so ceased producing it. Congress finally passed legislation indemnifying all the vaccine producers and programme participants from malpractice suits. The irresolution of this issue for 2 months and the production of 6 million doses of vaccine by one manufacturer from a wrong virus strain delayed the programme's beginning until October 15, 1976.

On June 21, 1976 the US Public Health Service announced the results of vaccine field trials. Recommendations were made for vaccine use in the high-risk population and in the remainder of the population above 18 years of age. Essentially these recommendations are as follows:

1. Bivalent vaccine containing killed A/Victoria/75 and A/New Jersey/Swine/76 is to be given to all individuals above 65 years of age and to all individuals of any age suffering from any of the following chronic debilitating medical conditions: diabetes mellitus, chronic bronchopulmonary disease, congenital, rheumatic, coronary or hypertensive heart disease, chronic renal disease and other chronic metabolic diseases.
2. The monovalent vaccine containing A/New Jersey/Swine/76 is to be given to all individuals 18 years and above who are not high risk.

NEW YORK CITY PROGRAMME DETAILS

The programme was designed to be as flexible as possible in the event that it was decided to immunize the school-age population, and included the following essential elements:

1. University graduates were hired and trained in the use of the automatic jet injectors and in cardiopulmonary resuscitation.
2. Sanitary inspectors and public health nursing assistants were given training on the automatic jet injectors and in cardiopulmonary resuscitation.
3. Hundreds of volunteers per day were recruited through the New York Chapter of the American Red Cross.
4. Forty-five Swine Influenza Immunization Clinics were established throughout the city, staffed by Department of Health personnel using automatic jet injectors.
5. Fifteen mobile teams, using automatic jet injectors, were established.
6. The mobile teams were then sent into areas of the city where there are large numbers of commuting workers, and into geographic areas from one of the fixed sites.
7. Vaccine was made available to private physicians in quantities of 100 doses of both types at a time and a cumulative total of 600 doses.
8. Vaccine was made available to large group medical practices in quantities of 1000 per request and a cumulative total of 5000. Requests above these quantities had to receive special approval.
9. Hospitals and industrial firms requesting vaccine received one-eighth per week of the total doses needed.
10. The department's sixty teams consisted of six persons, two vaccinators, a clinic supervisor, and three clerical and support personnel.
11. Malpractice coverage was provided to all 'participants'. Private physicians could charge an administration fee if they so wished but in doing so lost the federal malpractice coverage.
12. All participants had to obtain a signed informed consent which has to be retained for 3 years.
13. All vaccine recipients received an information sheet, informing them of the advantages and risks of vaccination, and possible side-reactions.
14. All participants had to send in a tally by age of all immunizations given and this was forwarded to the Center for Disease Control.
15. Because the vaccine was free of charge at Department of Health-operated facilities, Medicaid and Medicare providers could not bill for it.
16. All forms were printed in Chinese, Japanese, Italian, Yiddish, French, Spanish and Greek.
17. An extensive public health education programme was undertaken using radio, television and local newspapers.

SURVEILLANCE FOR THE DISEASE AND VACCINE REACTIONS

New York City has routinely conducted an influenza surveillance programme as part of a national and international effort. The elements of this effort are as follows:

(a) Hospital surveillance

When influenza enters a community, one of the first changes noted is an appreciable rise in the number of patients seen in outpatient clinics and emergency rooms. This is monitored in nine hospitals in the city, on a weekly basis.

(b) School absenteeism

Although influenza affects all age-groups, during epidemic periods, age-specific prevalence rates are highest among primary- and secondary-school children at the onset of an epidemic. Thus this population serves as a very good index for influenza activity. Geographically selected schools were chosen to participate in the weekly influenza surveillance activity, providing weekly absenteeism data.

(c) Virus isolation

During the entire year, nasal and pharyngeal secretions, as well as other materials, are submitted by private physicians and institutions to the virology laboratory of the New York City Health Department. Influenza virus can be isolated in such materials during the early febrile stage of the disease, and once isolated further laboratory studies can be conducted to accurately identify type, subtype and strain.

(d) Serological surveillance

Throughout the year, thousands of blood specimens are submitted to the Department's laboratories for a variety of studies. Random samples of these sera are tested for the presence of haemagglutination-inhibition antibodies to influenza virus. At the present time most sera tested possess demonstrable antibody, reflecting a level of immunity in the city to current influenza virus strain.

(e) Pneumonia mortality

The number of pneumonia deaths characteristically rises 2 weeks after the onset of influenza outbreaks. The number of deaths per week reflects the influenza situation 2 weeks before. The natural curve of this mortality statistic for the city is one in which there is a gradual rise during the month of October reaching a peak during the third week of January. An increased rise over the expected number of pneumonia deaths at a given point of time usually reflects influenza illness two weeks before.

Physicians, hospitals and others administering the vaccine were given special cards for reporting serious reactions, and a special Reaction Surveillance Unit was set up.

COST OF THE PROGRAMME

The federal government provided New York City with an allocation of 10 million doses of vaccine if the entire population had to be immunized. However, only those 18 years and older were immunized. In New York City this population projected by ageing from the 1970 census is about 6 million. New York City received about 4.0 million doses of vaccine, only enough to reach less than 70% of this population. The cost of the vaccine was 52 cents per dose amounting to $2 million. Eighty jet injectors were provided at a cost of eighty thousand dollars, supplies at some hundred and fifty thousand dollars and personnel costs at nine hundred thousand dollars. The total of federal funds was just under three and a half million dollars for immunizing the population over 18 years. If the entire population were immunized, additional vaccine costs would have brought the total cost up to about $6 million.

Because the amounts in the federal grant were originally calculated on the basis of 10 million vaccinations, the administering of only 6 million immunizations meant that the federal monies per does for administration were increased to about 23 cents per dose.

The direct costs to the Department of Health were $1 million, most of it consisting of personnel costs. Personnel were reassigned from other programmes to carry out this programme. Ongoing programmes had to be curtailed or suspended in order to do so.

DISCUSSION

A mass immunization programme such as the Swine Influenza Immunization Program conducted in a complex urban setting like New York City is not difficult to plan, organize and rapidly deliver, provided the appropriate strategies and tactics are employed. The New York City programme was centrally operated, in contrast to most health programmes today which are decentralized. Planning went smoothly from the outset because there was representation from all segments of the health care delivery system.

The presence on the department's steering committee of three individuals who had worked in West Africa directing mass immunization campaigns against smallpox, measles, cholera, and yellow fever was a great asset[13–15]. The American Red Cross which recruited thousands of volunteers and which maintained a Swine Flu Hotline telephone service for the general public contributed enormously to the success of the programme. The presence of twenty individuals in the department's immunization programme knowledgeable in the use and repair of automatic jet injectors capable of delivering 1000 immunizations per hour was an important asset.

Had the malpractice issue not been resolved by federal legislation, it is unlikely that the programme could have gone ahead.

However, the greatest problems confronting the programme were those which shaped public attitudes and resulted in people refusing to be immunized. The programme was plagued with problems from its inception in March 1976. Table 1 lists the chronology of major events affecting the

Table 1 Events affecting the swine influenza immunization programme prior to its commencement

Date	*Event*
January 1976	Outbreak of swine flu reported at Fort Dix in New Jersey. One recruit dies.
March 1976	Officials at Center for Disease Control announce that USA faces possible swine flu epidemic in the fall. Virus is likened to the influenza virus of 1918.
March 24, 1976	President Ford announces a \$135 million programme to immunize the entire population against swine flu. He acts on advice of officials of the Center for Disease Control.
April–May 1976	Four pharmaceutical companies begin production of swine flu vaccines. Tests of these vaccines begun on 5000 people. One company produces vaccine from an unacceptable strain of virus.
June 15, 1976	Vaccine manufacturers announce that they are losing liability insurance for swine flu vaccines. Government officials request that Congress pass Regulation to indemnify vaccine manufacturers. Request is denied by the House Sub-committee on Health.
June 21, 1976	US Public Health Service officials announce results of field studies of swine flu vaccines. Vaccine is declared safe for those above 24 years of age but not yet satisfactory for those below this age because of side-effects. Further studies planned.
July 9, 1976	President Ford announces that the programme will go ahead in spite of mounting opposition and doubts among experts and scientists.
July 13, 1976	Ford administration agrees to bear cost of defending law suits and requests the Congress to pass legislation indemnifying the vaccine producers.
August 1976	The Congress does not act on the President's request for liability legislation. The swine flu programme is at a standstill.
August 1976	The Congress passes legislation indemnifying the vaccine producers and those administering swine flu inoculations from malpractice.

programme prior to its operational phase which began in October 1976. To begin with there were always doubts both in scientific and lay circles about the swine flu virus, its epidemic potentials and the need for a mass immunization programme. The major impetus for the programme came out of the Center for Disease Control in Atlanta, Georgia, and from its then director, Dr David Sencer. On the basis of evidence presented in early 1976, the centre's proposal for a mass nationwide immunization programme was strongly endorsed by a number of non-governmental scientists, including Dr Albert Sabin and Dr Jonas Salk.

But as time went on, and no swine flu materialized during the winter season in the southern hemisphere, many began to doubt the need for a mass immunization programme. In November 1976, Dr Albert Sabin, who had been re-thinking his position since the announcement of the field trials in June, stated publicly that there was little possibility of a swine flu epidemic[16].

(a) Early problems

The loss of liability insurance on the part of the four vaccine manufacturers in June 1976 raised questions in the minds of ordinary citizens about the safety of the vaccines. The production of vaccine from a laboratory strain of swine influenza virus too weak to provide adequate protection magnified public concerns about the vaccines.

On June 21, 1976, a conference was held at the Clinical Center of the National Institute of Health at which the results of the vaccine field trials were presented. These trials involved the testing of four types of vaccine: bivalent whole virus, bivalent split virus, monovalent whole virus and monovalent split virus. The studies showed that antibody responses were very poor in those below 25 years of age and that reaction rates were unacceptably high in young people, especially children.

At this point the federal government could have shifted away from its commitment to a mass immunization programme for the entire population and have gone ahead with one for the high-risk group only. Many public health officials at this point favoured this approach. However, the Center for Disease Control resisted this kind of change. Thus as the summer drew to an end, with the liability issue as yet unresolved, there were still no immunization guidelines published for those below 25 years of age. Aside from the difficulties in programme planning and organization which this posed for local public health officials, it made the general public believe that the swine flu vaccines were so new and untried that experts didn't know as yet how and if they could use them in the younger age-groups. And if they weren't safe for young people, how safe could they be for older people?

The Congress finally passed legislation in August providing government malpractice coverage to the vaccine manufacturers and to those administering the vaccines. This was the first time in which the US Government assumed the role of insurer for medical malpractice purposes on such an enormous scale.

(b) The October crisis

The New York City programme began on October 12, 1976. The ceremonial opening of the programme was held at 9 a.m. that morning at one of the Department's sixty immunization stations. In other areas of the USA the programme had begun several days before. The turnout at all of the Department's sixty stations was excellent that morning. However, during the opening ceremonies, at which most of the New York City radio and television stations and newspapers were represented, news arrived over the Associated Press and United Press International wires that three persons had allegedly died in Pittsburgh, Pennsylvania, following swine influenza immunizations.

Because New York City is the media capital of the United States, where all of the major radio and television stations are headquartered, the local swine influenza programme received intense scrutiny. By midday, several state health departments had suspended their immunization programmes. But the decision of the New York City Department of Health was to continue. After an emergency meeting at midday, the staff of the Department recommended continuation of the programme, even though the lot of bivalent vaccine being used was the same as that alleged to have caused the deaths in Pennsylvania. The Department's staff could not see any causal relationship between the three cardiac deaths in Pennsylvania and the swine influenza vaccine based on their scientific and professional knowledge.

The Department's executive staff was keenly cognizant that a suspension of the programme in New York City would receive more intense media and press coverage than any other area of the country and was aware of what the national impact of this would be.

During this time, the Department's executive staff attempted to reach the Center for Disease Control in Atlanta, Georgia, in order to obtain more information and solicit advice. Numerous telephone calls went unanswered and we were not able to speak with anyone at the Center. Our colleagues across the country encountered the same problem. This led to local decisions which varied, depending on the degree of expertise in local health departments. Nine states suspended the programme, some states only suspended use of the vaccine lot in question and some continued.

Rubin, who has recently summarized press coverage of the swine flu programme, said the following of the October crisis: 'Many reporters complained about the CDC's level of cooperation during the October crisis. They realized that phones were ringing off the hook, but when calls did get through, reporters said they were treated in a haughty manner[17].' Had the CDC acted promptly and with decisiveness, a unified position across the country would have resulted. No comments were made by the Center on the issue until late in the day. By this time the epidemic of hysteria which began to develop at midday had mushroomed. By the time the CDC came out with a statement, the press and media had drawn their own conclusions in the vacuum created by the CDC, and headlines in New York City newspapers the following day included: 'The Scene at The Death Clinic' and 'Death Toll Mounting'.

After midday on October 12, 1976, the early morning turnout dwindled to a small number of people. After a week, media and press interest in the alleged deaths dwindled, when no correlation was demonstrated indicting the vaccine, and when other lots of vaccine were used. The concensus was that the other deaths, especially among the elderly with chronic cardiac disease, were not causally related to the vaccine, although many among the general public had their doubts.

(c) Other events in October 1976

On October 23rd, 1976, recommendations were made for immunizing the 3–18-year-old age-group. The recommendation for two inoculations, 4 weeks apart, was impractical. In addition, the advisory bodies making this decision at the national level decided that split virus monovalent vaccine was to be used in healthy youngsters of 3–18 years and whole virus monovalent in those aged 18–24 years. Whole virus bivalent was being used in those over 65 and high-risk individuals 25–65, but split virus bivalent was recommended for high-risk individuals aged 3–18 years.

In effect, then, the programme was administering four vaccines to different age-groups, two of whom required a booster after 4 weeks. Logistically it was virtually impossible to implement this complex protocol in a mass immunization programme.

This surfaced a long-standing problem in the USA. The federal agencies, such as the Center for Disease Control and the National Institutes of Health in this instance formulate national policy and programme procedures, but are not responsible for implementing them. This responsibility falls on the shoulders of cities and states, who must adhere to the national guidelines in order to qualify for the federal government monies which pay for such programmes. The majority of those at the national level, particularly in the Center for Disease Control, had no personal operational experience directing any type of public health programme, and their recommendations were not practical. State and city health departments then began to formulate different plans.

In November 1976, the New York City Health Department convened an Ad Hoc Expert Advisory Committee to advise the Task Force on swine influenza immunizations for children aged 3–18 years. In view of the poor antibody responses, the significant level of side-reactions, and the fact that the flu season was already well underway with no swine flu in sight, this committee recommended that healthy children in this age-group should not be immunized, unless an epidemic occurred. This then became the policy of the New York City Department of Health, a policy which was opposite to that recommended by the Center for Disease Control.

(d) Swine flu cases and their effects on the programme

On November 23, 1976, a non-fatal case of swine flu was reported in Missouri; this led to a dramatic rise in the daily number of immunizations given in New

Table 2 Events affecting the outcome of the swine influenza immunization programme after its commencement

Date	*Event*
October 12, 1976	New York City programme begins. Three persons alleged to have died in Pittsburgh from swine influenza inoculations. Nine states suspend the programme. The New York City Department of Health chooses to continue the programme.
October 13, 1976	Sharp fall in attendance at New York City clinics. Intense media and press coverage of deaths in Pittsburgh.
October 14, 1976	Programme resumed in some states after epidemiologic investigations, and tests of vaccine lots exonerate vaccine as cause of deaths. President Ford and his family receive inoculations.
October 15, 1976	In spite of assurances about vaccine safety from Center for Disease Control, few turn out for inoculations.
October 18, 1976	Press carries stories that swine influenza vaccines lack neuraminidase enzyme necessary for antibody production.
October 20, 1976	Press continues to carry stories tallying up, 'deaths due to swine flu vaccine'.
October 23, 1976	Federal officials recommend two doses 4 weeks apart for high-risk children aged 3–18 years. No recommendations given for healthy children in this age-group.
October 25, 1976	The *New York Post* and *Time* magazine report that mobster Carlo Gambino had died after a swine flu shot.
November 17, 1976	Ad Hoc Expert Advisory Committee on Immunizations for Healthy Children convened by New York City Health Department. Committee recommends against immunization of healthy children.
November 19, 1976	New York City Health Department survey reveals that 83.9% of interviewees had not received, and did not intend to receive, swine flu shots.
November 23, 1976	Non-fatal case of swine flu reported in Missouri. One-day rise in attendance at New York City clinics. Swine flu appears as a mild disease. Some 20 million inoculations given to date in the USA.
November 27, 1976	Press reports possible death of a man in New Jersey due to a swine flu shot.
December 8, 1976	Swine flu virus isolated in Wisconsin pig farmer. Disease confirmed as being mild. Assertions of opponents of programme that swine flu virus is present constantly, and periodically transmitted to man from pigs, are strengthened.
December 14, 1976	Guillain-Barré paralysis reported linked to swine flu inoculations.
December 16, 1976	National swine flu programme suspended because of concern that shots were linked to ninety-four cases of Guillain-Barré syndrome in fourteen states.
January 15, 1977	Advisory Committee on Immunization Practices of US Public Health Service recommends resumption of swine flu programme. The New York City Department of Health opts not to fully resume programme but to make vaccine available to hospitals and private physicians. Five clinics opened in each of five city boroughs. Attendance at each runs about four persons per day.

York City. When it became apparent that the disease was mild and did not spread, attendance fell once again. On December 8, 1976, swine flu virus was isolated from a Wisconsin pig farmer. This had no effect on the numbers immunized. By this time it was commonly accepted by the public that: (1) swine flu was mild; (2) it was always around in different places; (3) it spread occasionally from pigs to man. The threat of swine flu was increasingly seen as being very remote. The events affecting the outcome of the programme are summarized in Table 2.

(e) Survey of public's response to swine flu immunizations

By mid-November, less than 5% of the target population in New York City had been immunized. The widespread availability of the vaccine and the convenient location of the Department's sixty clinics, indicated that the vast majority did not wish to be immunized. In order to ascertain more precise data on public attitudes towards the programme, a 1-week interview survey was conducted. The results are summarized in Table 3.

On November 27, 1977, the Center for Disease Control, concerned by the poor turnout, especially in the larger cities, cited that those directing the programmes in large cities were failing minority populations. Such a statement erroneously presumed that the minority population desired immunization. But another intent of this statement was to shift responsibility for the programme's failing fortunes from those who had conceptualized it to those who had the burden of implementing it.

The New York City Department of Health responded to this CDC accusation by citing the results of its survey and by pointing out that of all the populations in the city, the poor had the best access to the Department's swine flu clinics.

Another survey, undertaken by *The New York News*, gave results similar to those obtained in the Department of Health survey.

(f) The Guillain–Barré syndrome and the suspension of the programme

On December 14, 1976, the Center for Disease Control reported that a number of cases of Guillain–Barré paralysis had occurred in individuals after receiving swine influenza immunizations. On December 16, 1976, the programme was suspended throughout the United States. Guillain–Barré can occur following immunizations and some cases were to be expected following swine influenza immunizations. At the time that the programme was suspended 40 million (17%) of the national target population had been immunized.

In a number of cases the diagnosis had been inaccurate and between October 1, 1976, and January 1, 1977, of the total of twenty-two persons who died in the USA from the Guillain–Barré syndrome, only half had received swine flu vaccine.

Table 3 Attitudes towards swine influenza immunizations, New York City, November 1976

	Reason for not being immunized								
	Not necessary		*Afraid to be immunized*		*Physician advised against it*		*No reason*		
Area of City	*No.*	*Percentage*	*No.*	*Percentage*	*No.*	*Percentage*	*No.*	*Percentage*	*Total No.*
Commuter	35	61.3	11	19.3	10	17.5	1	1.9	57
Inner-city	85	48.2	67	38.1	20	11.3	4	2.4	176
Total	120	51.5	78	33.5	30	12.8	5	2.2	233

Table 4 Swine influenza immunizations, New York City, 1976–77

	*Private organizations**			*Health department*			*Private physicians*			*Totals*		
	Mono-valent	*Bi-valent*	*Total*	*Mono-valent*	*Bi-valent*	*Total*	*Mono-valent*	*Bi-valent*	*Total*	*Mono-valent*	*Bi-valent*	*Total*
Doses administered	160 529	48 562	209 091	155,212	118,745	273,597	41 267	114 829	156 046	357 008	282 136	639 144
Doses distributed	672 180	268 670	940 850	437 000	600 050	1 037 050	71 170	148 060	219 230	1 180 350	1 016 780	2 197 130

* Includes nursing homes, industrial organizations, commercial organizations, hospitals and unions.

(g) The programme resumes

On January 15, 1977, the US Public Health Service Expert Advisory Committee on Immunization Practices recommended a partial resumption of the programme for the high-risk population. In New York City, the Department of Health once again made the vaccine available to private physicians, clinics and hospitals and opened an immunization clinic in each of the city's five boroughs. Fewer than half a dozen people showed up per day at each of the five clinics.

(h) Overall results of the programme in New York City

Table 4 presents the results of the swine influenza immunization programme in New York City. A total of 639 144 doses were actually administered. Among these there were 2366 untoward reactions constituting a ratio of 3.7 per 1000. A total of 2 197 130 doses of vaccine were distributed to the three principal groups of providers, but only slightly more than a quarter of these were actually administered. These results are far below the targets established at the inception of the programme, but they reflect the public's perception of the need for immunization. The largest number of immunizations were given in the 22–44 and 45–64-year age-groups.

While the results of the programme were far below what had been originally intended, the programme itself afforded the New York City Department of Health the opportunity of planning, organizing and implementing the largest single immunization programme in its history. The New York City swine influenza immunization programme was the largest in the USA. It was possible to demonstrate that a mass immunization programme can be quickly planned, organized and implemented in a complex urban environment. It also demonstrated that in a highly developed city like New York where the population is both knowledgeable and sophisticated, a mass immunization programme will not be successful unless the public perceives that there is a need to be immunized.

Acknowledgements

I would like to extend my sincerest thanks to Dr Anita Stiles Curran, to Mr Peter Backman, to the staff of the New York City Swine Influenza Immunization Program, and to the numerous groups and individuals who volunteered their time and resources, for their invaluable efforts in the New York City Swine Influenza Immunization Program. I wish to thank Mrs Earlene Price for preparing the typescript.

References

1. Cooper, T. and Millar, J. D. (1976). Gearing up for swine flu. *Medical Opinion*, V, 44

2. Killer 'flu, how real a threat? *U.S. News And World Report*, May 24, 1976, p. 57
3. Imperato, P. J. (1976). *What To Do About the Flu* (New York: E. P. Dutton and Co.)
4. Imperato, P. J. Flu program's flaw, *New York Times*, April 29, 1976, p. 38
5. Imperato, P. J. (1976). All about swine flu, *Ladies Home Journal*, **XCIII**, 70
6. Imperato, P. J. (1976). The deeper issues of swine flu. *Medical Opinion*, **V**, 51
7. Boffey, P. M. (1976). Anatomy of a decision: how the nation declared war on swine flu. *Science*, **192**, 636
8. Boffey, P. M. (1976). Swine flu vaccination campaign: the scientific controversy mounts. *Science*, **193**, 559
9. *Influenza In The United States: Rationale for Mass Immunizations in 1976*, Atlanta, Georgia, CDC, USPHS, June 1, 1976, p. 14
10. Marwick, C. S. (1976). Swine flu immunization: 'go' at last. *Medical World News*, September 6, p. 60
11. Hearings Before A Subcommittee of The Committee on Appropriations, House of Representatives, Ninety-Fourth Congress, Second Session. Emergency Supplemental Appropriation Bill, 1976, Swine Influenza Immunization Program, Washington D.C., U.S. Government Printing Office, p. 43
12. Influenza Vaccine – Preliminary Statement, Recommendation of The Public Health Service Advisory Committee on Immunization Practices, *Morbidity And Mortality Weekly Report*, 25: 165–6, 171, 1976, Supplemental Statement, *Morbidity And Mortality Weekly Report*, 25: 225–7, 1976
13. Imperato, P. J., Fofana, B. and Sow, O. (1975). Strategie et tactique pour la vaccination des populations du delta l'interieur du Niger. *Afrique Medicale*, **14**(129), 307
14. Imperato, P. J. (1969). The use of markets as vaccination sites in the Mali Republic. *J. of Trop. Med. Hyg.*, **72**(1), 8
15. Imperato, P. J. (1973). Mass campaigns and their comparative operational costs for nomadic and sedentary populations in Mali. *Trop. Geog. Med.* **25**(4), 416
16. Sabin, A. B. (1976). Washington and the flu. *New York Times*, November 5, op. ed. page
17. Rubin, D. M. (1977) Remember swine flu? *Columbia Journalism Review*, July–August, p. 42

8
Rabies vaccines

J. CRICK

INTRODUCTION

Rabies is different from the majority of the diseases to be discussed at this meeting because it affects most warm-blooded animals including man. Vaccination is a powerful tool in combating the disease, and immunization of domestic animals and humans is widely practised. However, there are differences in the application of veterinary and human vaccines. Veterinary vaccines are generally used for pre-exposure immunization of farm and pet animals; post-exposure treatment of animals is rarely applied as it is regarded as potentially too dangerous for man should the vaccine fail. In humans, most of the vaccine is used in post-exposure therapy, pre-exposure immunization being reserved for the relatively small number of people who run some risk of infection because of their occupation.

Until the early 1960s, rabies vaccines were prepared solely in mammalian nervous tissue or in avian embryo tissue, but in the last 10–15 years tissue culture vaccines have been available for veterinary use and, at last, are being produced for man. I shall discuss briefly the older types of vaccines, since they are still widely used, and then in more detail the newer tissue culture vaccines. Finally, I shall consider some of the advances and changes there may be in the future.

VACCINES

Nervous tissue vaccines

More nervous tissue vaccines are used than any other type for they are the most potent antigens yet developed for human or veterinary use. There have been many modifications of Pasteur's original vaccine and two are still manufactured (Table 1). The most widely used is the Semple type of vaccine[1] prepared from the brains of infected animals such as sheep, goats or rabbits in which the virus is inactivated with phenol. Fermi vaccine[2], similarly prepared but containing residual live virus, is still being used in some countries. The use of such a vaccine is clearly undesirable and the WHO Expert Committee on Rabies (1973)[3] states that 'no vaccine that contains living virus should be employed in man' and suggests that its production be discontinued. Nevertheless, large amounts of this vaccine were manufactured and used for animals in Poland and the USSR in 1974[4].

Table 1 Nervous tissue vaccines available today

Date	*Originator*	*Type of vaccine*
1908	Fermi	Mature CNS: partly inactivated
1911	Semple	Mature CNS: inactivated
1955	Fuenzalida and Palacios	Immature CNS: inactivated
1965	Svet-Moldavskij *et al.*	Immature CNS: inactivated
1965	Gispen *et al.*	Immature CNS: inactivated

The use of mature brain vaccines in man is associated with a risk of postvaccinal reactions and paralytic accidents because nervous tissue from adult animals contains an encephalitogen[5]. Their use is usually restricted to postexposure immunization.

The brains of very young animals which are almost free from the encephalitogenic factor are used in a number of countries for the preparation of inactivated vaccines. Suckling mouse brain vaccine (SMBV) has become the most widely produced vaccine in South America[6] where it is used for postexposure therapy and for pre-exposure vaccination of persons at high risk. In addition many thousands of doses are used each year for animals. It is also manufactured in the USA for use in dogs and cats and in France where it is used for pre- and post-exposure vaccination of humans and for animals. Similar vaccines are prepared in the USSR and South Africa from suckling rat brains[7,8] and in the Netherlands from suckling rabbit brains[9,10].

These vaccines, like those prepared from adult brain, are good immunogens and are easily and cheaply produced. They appear safer than mature brain vaccines but cases of neurological diseases following their use have been described[11]. Although investigations failed to identify the cause of these accidents, encephalitogenic factor was considered the most likely[12].

Avian embryo vaccines

Three live vaccines (MLV) prepared by growing virus in chick embryos are available (Table 2). The two best known, the Flury LEP and HEP vaccines[13,14] are manufactured in a number of countries and are widely used as veterinary vaccines. The LEP (low egg passage) vaccine consists of virus at the 40–50th egg passage level. It appears safe for adult dogs, but retains some pathogenicity for young puppies, cats and cattle. It has been shown to compare favourably with the more recently developed tissue culture vaccines and SMBV, and a single dose of vaccine in dogs provided a duration of immunity for 3 years[15]. It has been widely used in massive vaccination campaigns, notably in the USA between 1953 and 1968[15] and in Malaya, Israel and Rhodesia[16].

Table 2 Avian embryo vaccines

Date	*Originator*	*Type of vaccine*
1948	Koprowski and Cox	Chick embryo: MLV – (Flury LEP and HEP)
1953	Komarov and Hornstein	Chick embryo: MLV – (Kelev)
1956	Peck, Powell and Culbertson	Duck embryo: inactivated – (DEV)

Flury HEP (high egg passage) vaccine, which consists of virus at about the 180th passage level, is safe for puppies, cats and cattle. Hubbard[17] found that cattle inoculated with it were resistant to challenge 22 months later. Other trials have given less convincing proof of its efficacy and its repeated use in South America has also resulted in a number of cases of anaphylaxis[18]. The HEP vaccine was also tried for pre-exposure vaccination of man, but with disappointing results (see Ref. 19 for further reading).

The third chick embryo vaccine is manufactured from the Kelev strain of virus[20] and was used with the LEP strain for a rabies eradication campaign in Israel in the 1950s. It is recommended for use in dogs and cattle[3]. All three vaccines are cheap and easy to prepare but have the usual disadvantage of live vaccines in needing protection against inactivation during shipment and use in the field.

A major advance in rabies vaccine production for man was achieved when a vaccine was prepared from virus grown in duck embryos and inactivated with BPL[21]. The results of a clinical trial suggested that antibody was produced more rapidly in persons receiving the new vaccine than in those receiving Semple vaccine.[22] This was considered especially important with regard to post-exposure therapy. The freedom of this vaccine from the risks associated with brain vaccines also commended it for pre-exposure immunization. However, its use is often accompanied by local reactions and some serious cases of anaphylaxis and neural involvement have been reported. Nevertheless, duck embryo vaccine (DEV) is generally regarded as safe and it is widely used[23]. Unfortunately considerable doubts have been expressed concerning its immunogenicity[24,25], especially when used in conjunction with antiserum in post-exposure treatment[26]. However, it was for some years the only vaccine generally available for man in Great Britain and is still the vaccine usually given in the USA.

Tissue culture vaccines

For veterinary use (Table 3)

Considerable effort has gone into the application of tissue culture methods for the production of rabies vaccines, and a range of MLV and killed vaccines for veterinary use are produced in this way. The first experimental tissue culture vaccine was prepared in hamster kidney cells by Fenje at the Con-

Table 3 Tissue culture vaccines for veterinary use

Date	*Originator*	*Type of vaccine*
1964	Abelseth	Pig kidney – MLV – ERA
1973	Selimov	Hamster kidney – MLV – Vnukovo-32
1967	Peterman *et al.*	Hamster kidney cell line – inactivated – Rabiffa
1970	Barth and Jaeger	Pig kidney – inactivated – Madivak

naught Laboratories[27] and this led directly to the development in the same laboratories of the ERA vaccine[28]. This MLV produced from infected pig kidney cells has been widely used and was the first licensed in the USA for use in all species of domestic animals (see Refs. 18 and 29 for further reading). The original SAD strain of virus used by Fenje in 1960[27] and grown in primary hamster kidney cells, is used in the USSR as a MLV (Vnukovo-32) for domestic animals[30]. LEP and HEP vaccines produced in tissue culture are also available commercially[29]. However, Abelseth has commented that of the MLVs produced in tissue culture, only the ERA strain has proven effective through extensive laboratory and field evaluation[18]. The ERA vaccine multiplies in the recipient host because it can confer immunity even when diluted 1000-fold[28]. This is an important advantage for field work where storage and handling conditions may be far from ideal. However, most countries where rabies is not endemic will not use the ERA or any other MLV. Fortunately a number of inactivated tissue culture vaccines are now available.

With the exception of 'Madivak' which is produced from pig kidney cells by Behringwerke in Marburg, Germany[31], the killed vaccines are produced from hamster kidney cell supernatants[32]. In Europe the best-known of these vaccines is 'Rabiffa' produced in the NIL line of hamster kidney fibroblasts at the Institut Mérieux in Lyon, France[33]. This vaccine is used in France for dogs, cats and cattle and in Britain for dogs and cats to be exported or being held in quarantine kennels after arriving from abroad.

A new vaccine for use in cattle, particularly in areas where rabies is carried by vampire bats, has been developed in Mexico[34]. The vaccine is prepared from a vampire bat virus isolate grown in BHK21 cells and inactivated, like 'Rabiffa', with BPL. Other recent developments with hamster kidney cell vaccines include the use of different inactivating agents; for example, acetylethyleneimine[35] and ethyleneimine[36]. Suspended cultures of BHK21 cells have also been used to produce vaccines on an experimental scale[37,38]. The inactivated tissue culture vaccines are good antigens although duration of immunity studies in dogs suggested that they were inferior to live virus vaccines and to SMBV[15]. However, they are safe for all species, store well and are acceptable for use in areas where rabies is not endemic (unless vaccination is restricted or completely prohibited, for example, in countries like Britain). They may also be conveniently blended with other veterinary vaccines; for example, foot-and-mouth disease vaccine for use in cattle, and distemper, canine hepatitis and leptospirosis vaccines for dogs. These polyvalent vaccines are manufactured in Europe and the USA.

For human use (Table 4)

The requirements for a cell substrate for use in humans are much more exacting than for veterinary vaccines, and most licensing authorities will consider only primary cultures of embryonic tissue from carefully selected stock or strains of diploid cells of human origin for this purpose. In addition most authorities follow the advice of the World Health Organization Expert Committee on Rabies (1973)[3] and require that these vaccines contain only inactivated virus.

Table 4 Tissue culture vaccines for human use

Date	*Originator*	*Type of vaccine*
1964	Wiktor *et al.*	HDCV – inactivated
1971	Fenje *et al.*	Primary hamster kidney – inactivated

The first tissue culture vaccine extensively tested in man was developed in the USSR and has been used for both pre- and post-exposure vaccination in that country and in Czechoslovakia and the German Democratic Republic. The vaccine is produced by inactivating Vnukovo-32[30]. A similar vaccine is produced in Canada where it is used for pre-exposure immunization[39], and fetal bovine kidney cells have been used in France to produce a vaccine which appears to be satisfactory for the same purpose[40].

The most promising development is human diploid cell vaccine (HDCV) produced from concentrated supernatant fluids from the Wistar Institute (WI-38) strain of human diploid fibroblasts and inactivated with BPL[41–44], or tri-(*n*-butyl) phosphate[45], a detergent which inactivates and disrupts the virus. These vaccines are being tested extensively in several different countries and the first indications of their success as human immunogens were given at the Second International Colloquium on Rabies held in Lyon in 1972[46,47].

A number of other reports confirming the efficacy of HDCVs as antigens have appeared subsequently (see Ref. 48 for further reading). Two of these[49,50] concern a clinical trial of the BPL inactivated vaccine which is being conducted in Britain. In their first paper the British group of workers showed that a very economical pre-exposure course of vaccination could be provided by two 0.1 ml intradermal doses given 4 weeks apart[49] (Figure 1). Their second study[50], was concerned with vaccination schedules for rapid immunization. They found that antibody was produced most rapidly when subjects were given four intradermal doses of vaccine at separate sites on the first day (day 0) of the test. Other people given the same number of vaccine doses, but on days 0, 1, 2, 3 or days 0, 3, 7 and 14, showed a delayed response (Figure 1).

So far, only mild effects have been recorded in most people receiving HDCV by intradermal or intramuscular routes. However, adverse side-reactions observed in seven out of fourteen people receiving intradermal booster doses of the vaccine 12 or 18 months after primary inoculation caused Cox and Schneider[51] to express some reservations about the use of the intradermal route for the first inoculations. These workers suggest that the primary vaccinations should continue to be given by the intramuscular route recommended by the manufacturer. Nevertheless, it now seems that reliable pre-exposure protection can be offered to those at risk and that safe, effective and

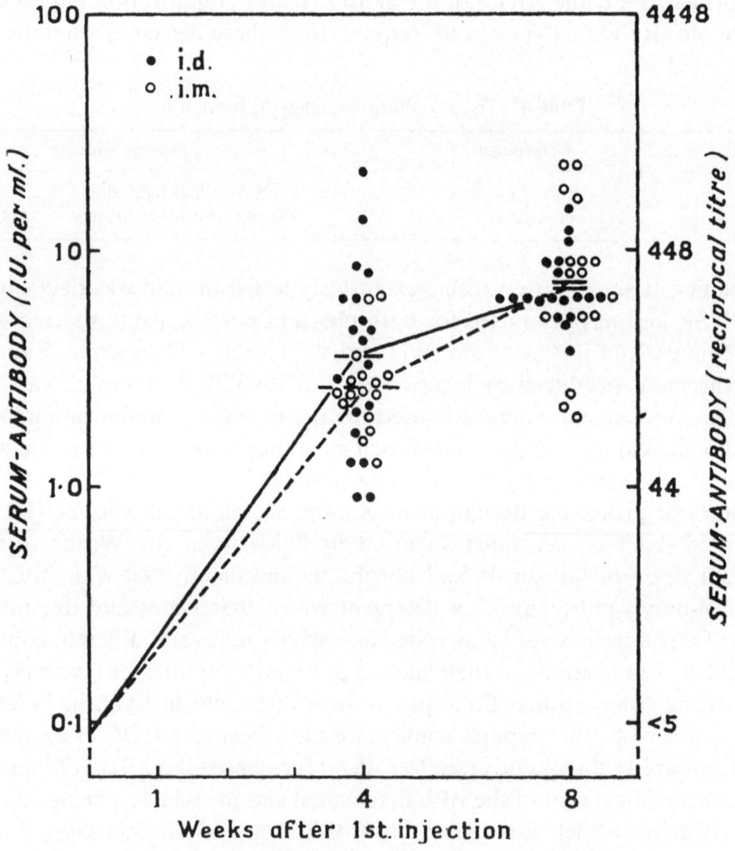

Figure 1 Rabies-neutralizing antibody in serum 0, 4 and 8 weeks after first injection of rabies vaccine

more acceptable post-exposure therapy is also possible. Already HDCV has been used, apparently successfully, for a number of post-exposure treatments in Germany, Iran and the USA (Kuwert and Hafkin, personal communications) and volunteers in Britain with high antibody levels following HDCV vaccination are donating serum so that stocks of human hyperimmune globulin are available to replace horse serum in post-exposure treatment.

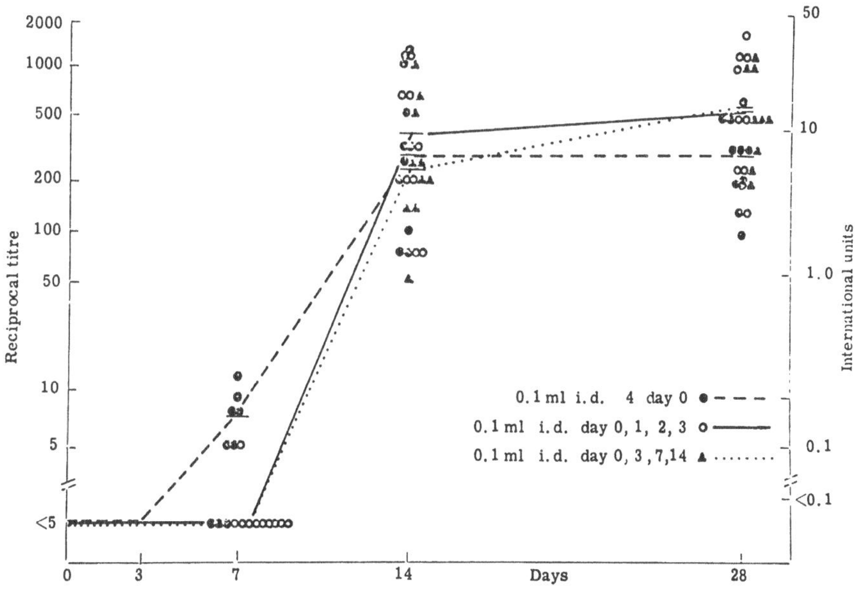

Figure 2 Antibody titres following three different rapid immunization schedules (based on ten subjects in each group)

The BPL inactivated vaccine is manufactured at the Institut Mérieux in Lyon and at the Behringwerke in Marburg, Germany. It is used in France for pre-exposure immunization and is licensed for similar use in Britain where it has replaced DEV for pre- and post-exposure vaccination (Gardner, personal communication). The subunit vaccine prepared by tri-(*n*-butyl) phosphate treatment of the virus is manufactured by the Wyeth Laboratories, Radnor, Pa. Recently there have been disquieting reports concerning future supplies of WI-38 cells and an alternative human diploid cell strain may be required[52,53]. Fortunately, the MRC-5 strain of cells, developed in London[54] is available, and at Pirbright has been found to produce rabies virus at least as efficiently as WI-38 cells. Recently trial batches of vaccine have been prepared in MRC5 cells both in Germany and the USA (Majer and Rosanoff, personal communications). However, all HDCVs are expensive to prepare, largely because the cells are relatively inefficient in their production of virus and concentration is necessary before use. Their cost may, therefore, preclude their use in the developing countries where rabies is a major problem and many thousands of doses of vaccine are required for post-exposure treatment each year.

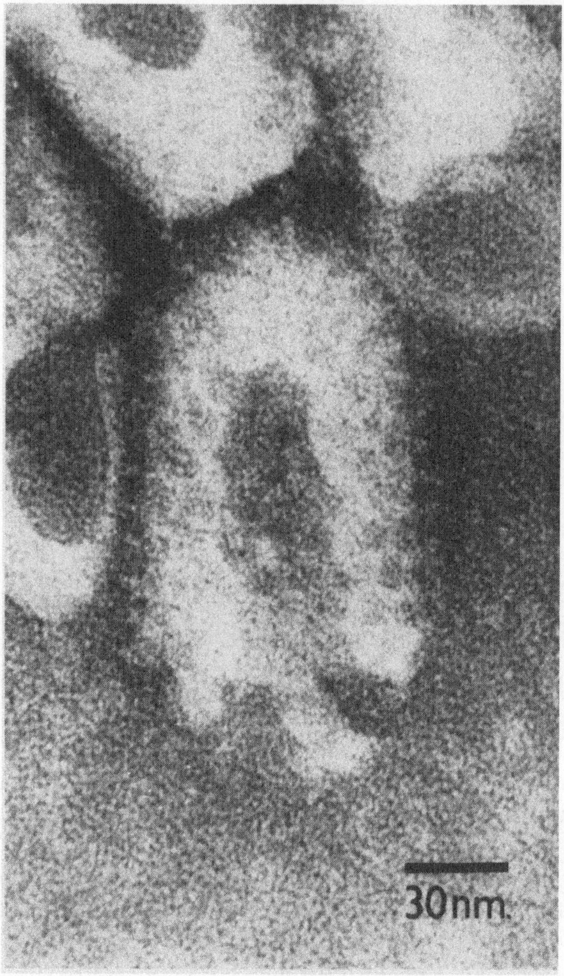

Figure 3 Electron micrograph of rabies virus

FUTURE CONSIDERATIONS

I should now like to mention four possible developments with regard to rabies vaccines and their application. These are subunit vaccines for man, more rational post-exposure therapy for man, polyvalent vaccines and the vaccination of wild animals.

Subunit vaccines

Before tissue culture vaccines for man had become a reality, Hummeler and Koprowski[55] described rabies vaccines as 'the worst biological products ever injected into the human body' and as I said earlier, even HDCVs occasionally produce undesirable side-effects[51].

At Pirbright, Dr F. Brown and I have frequently wondered whether a purified subunit vaccine prepared from virus grown in cells more productive but at present less acceptable than diploid cells, would be considered for human use. A vaccine of this type, free from extraneous host material and genetic information, would in fact consist of a chemically defined antigen and should be an ideal vaccine.

Experiments to elucidate the structure of rabies virus show that such a preparation could be made. Rabies virus is a member of the rhabdovirus group; that is, it has a characteristic bullet shape with spike projections covering the surface of the particle. These spikes consist of virus-specific glycoprotein, the antigen responsible for the production of neutralizing antibody. In several laboratories these spikes have been used to immunize experimental animals against rabies[56,57] and HDCV disrupted with tri-(*n*-butyl) phosphate has been shown to be a satisfactory antigen in man[46,58–60]. Since methods are available for the separation of the glycoprotein from the other constituents of the virus[57,61], it should be a relatively simple matter to prepare a purified subunit vaccine.

Unfortunately, there may be problems associated with the use of subunit vaccines for post-exposure treatment. In the first place it is unlikely that a purified protein, free from nucleic acid, would stimulate the production of interferon (see below). Second, and possibly more important, is an observation repeatedly made in our laboratory: we find that in both mice and guinea pigs given vaccine prepared from disrupted virus there is considerable delay in antibody production[62]. If the success or otherwise of treatment after exposure depends on rapid antibody production, such an effect could be disastrous for the patient.

More rational post-exposure therapy

Each year more than 1 000 000 people are vaccinated after known or presumed exposure to rabies[63]. Each person receives fourteen or more daily doses of vaccine, sometimes with antirabies serum or immunoglobulin included at the beginning of the treatment. Reservations have been expressed about this type of therapy (see Refs. 64 and 65 for further reading) but no alternative is yet available.

It is not known how the treatment works or how effective it is, since not everyone exposed to the virus and remaining untreated develops the disease. However, it has been assumed that the rapid production and/or administration of antibody is essential so that the infecting virus may be neutralized before it enters the central nervous system. Other responses may also be involved, including interferon production. Interferon will protect animals against rabies, but there is conflicting evidence as to whether all rabies vaccines stimulate its production[66] (and see Ref. 67 for further reading). In fact the experiments of Wiktor *et al.*[66] support the idea that the ability of a vaccine to stimulate interferon production could be crucial to its success in post-exposure therapy. However they do not share the view of Harmon and Janis[68] that a combination of interferon inducer and vaccine could be the preferred method of treatment in the future.

In our laboratory we have often questioned the standard practice of giving so many doses of vaccine so close together and indeed Rubin *et al.*[69] showed that in subjects receiving daily vaccination there was a prolonged IgM antibody response and delayed conversion to IgG antibody. They pointed out that since only IgG enters the tissues this is a serious disadvantage which could explain some of the treatment failures which have been reported. On the basis of their results they argued the need for more potent vaccines which would induce high levels of IgG antibody very rapidly after only one or two suitably spaced inoculations. In this connection, the experiments of Bahmanyar[47], Turner *et al.*[50] and Plotkin *et al.*[60] using only four or five inoculations of an HDVC are interesting, though no information on the IgM/IgG antibody ratios in their subjects is available.

Major changes in post-exposure therapy can only come when we have a better understanding of rabies pathogenesis. At the present time, despite the work of Baer and Cleary[70], and Murphy *et al.*[71] among others, our knowledge of this process is far from complete[69].

Polyvalent vaccines

Until recently rabies has been regarded as a serological entity unrelated to other members of the rhabdovirus group. Although isolates of rabies virus with different biological properties have been described, little antigenic variation has been found between them, and it is customary to use the same strains throughout the world for vaccine production[72].

However, Shope and Murphy and their colleagues (Refs. 73, 74, Shope, personal communication; Porterfield *et al.*, personal communication), have shown serological and morphological relatedness between rabies virus and six other viruses, four of which may be relevant to our discussion of rabies immunization (Table 5).

Schneider and Schoop[75] suggested that the Lagos bat, Nigerian horse and Mokola viruses are serotypes of rabies, in which case a broad efficacy of rabies vaccines should not be anticipated. Indeed, Tignor and Shope[76] found that mice vaccinated with rabies virus, for example, were only poorly protected against Mokola virus. This was an important observation, for while there is yet no known association of Lagos bat or the Nigerian horse virus with human disease, two strains of Mokola virus have been isolated from children, one of whom died[77].

Table 5 Rabies-related viruses from Africa

Virus	*Isolation*	
Lagos bat	Brain of fruit bat	Nigeria, 1956
Nigerian horse	Brain of horse with 'Staggers'	Nigeria, 1958
Mokola	Viscera of shrews	Nigeria, 1968
	Human CNS	Nigeria, 1968 and 1971
Duvenhage	Human brain	Transvaal, 1970

Shope and Tignor[78] have already suggested that a polyvalent or an appropriate combined vaccine regime might be suitable for areas such as West Africa in which more than one virus of the rabies group has been found, and the isolation of Duvenhage virus in the Transvaal[79] suggests that these considerations may apply equally to other parts of Africa. Further studies are required before we can decide how important the new viruses are to man and/or his domestic animals.

Wildlife vaccination

The attempted control of rabies in wildlife by the reduction in numbers of the appropriate vectors, has had only limited success and sylvatic rabies is on the increase, notably in North America and western Europe. Consequently the vaccination of wild animals, particularly foxes, is under active consideration[80,81]. The ERA MLV has been suggested as the most suitable vaccine for this purpose since it can be given by mouth (see Refs. 80 and 82 for further reading). Nevertheless, despite its good safety record in domestic animals, doubts have been raised as to whether it would be innocuous in all species likely to take the bait in which it was placed[80]. Until this question is resolved this use of vaccine cannot be contemplated except on an experimental basis.

CONCLUSIONS

In the last 10–15 years remarkable progress has been made in improving the quality of rabies vaccines. An outstanding achievement has been the production of high-quality tissue culture vaccines for veterinary use and also for the immunization of man. Sufficient information about the structure and controlled dissection of rabies virus is available for us to prepare subunit vaccines and new approaches to post-exposure therapy are being considered. However the discovery of hitherto unknown serotypes of rabies in Africa is disquieting and their relevance to the problems of disease has yet to be determined. Meanwhile the spread of sylvatic rabies is causing considerable concern in North America and western Europe, and in the foreseeable future we may be vaccinating foxes and other wild animals in order to protect ourselves and our domestic animals from the disease.

ACKNOWLEDGEMENTS

I would like to thank the World Health Organization, Geneva, for permission to quote data from the World Survey of Rabies No. XVI (1975), the WHO press release WHO/30 (1973) and an article by M. A. Selimov (WHO Publication VPH/RAB.RES/73.I). I am also grateful to Dr D. A. J. Tyrrell and the Editor of the *Lancet* for allowing me to reproduce Figures 1 and 2. Mr C. J. Smale kindly provided the electron micrograph in Figure 3.

References

1. Semple, D. (1911). *Scient. Mems. Offrs. med. sanit. Depts. India*, No. 44 (New Series, Calcutta)
2. Fermi, C. (1908). Über immunisierung gegen wut krankheit. *Z. Hyg. Infeckt. Krankh*, **58**, 233
3. World Health Organization Expert Committee on Rabies (1973). Sixth Report. WHO Technical Report Series No. 523. (Geneva: WHO)
4. World Health Organization (1975). World Survey of Rabies. XVI (for 1974) (Geneva: WHO)
5. Abdussalam, M. and Bögel, K. (1971). The problem of antirabies vaccination. In *International Conference on the Application of Vaccines against Viral, Rickettsial and Bacterial Diseases of Man.* Scientific Publication No. 226, pp. 54–59 (Washington DC: Pan American Health Organization, WHO)
6. Fuenzalída, E. and Palacios, R. (1955). Un método mejorado en la preparacion de la vacuna antirabica. *Bol. del. Inst. Bact. de Chile*, **8**, 3
7. Svet-Moldavskij, G. J. *et al.* (1965). An allergen-free antirabies vaccine. *Bull. WHO*, **32**, 47
8. Katz, W. (1976). Human rabies vaccines. *J. S. Afr. Vet. Assoc.*, **47**, 53
9. Gispen, R., Schmittmann, G. T. P. and Saathof, B. (1965). Rabies vaccine derived from suckling rabbit brain. *Arch. Ges. Virusforsch.*, **15**, 336
10. Gispen, R. and Saathof, B. (1965). Neutralizing and fluorescent antibody response in man after antirabies treatment with suckling rabbit brain vaccine. *Arch. Ges. Virusforsch.*, **15**, 377
11. Held, J. R. and Adaros, H. L. (1972). Neurological disease in man following administration of suckling mouse brain antirabies vaccine. *Bull. WHO*, **46**, 321
12. Trejos, A., Lewis, V., Fuenzalida, E. and Larghi, O. P. (1974). Laboratory investigations of neuroparalytic accidents associated with suckling mouse brain rabies vaccine. *Ann. Immunol.* (*Inst. Pasteur*), **125C**, 917
13. Koprowski, H. and Black, J. (1950). Studies on chick-embryo adapted rabies virus. II. Pathogenicity for dogs and use of egg-adapted strains for vaccination purposes. *J. Immunol.*, **64**, 185
14. Koprowski, H., Black, J. and Johnson, W. P. (1955). Rabies in cattle. IV. Vaccination of cattle with high egg-passage, chicken embryo-adapted rabies virus. *J. Am. Vet. Med. Assoc.*, **127**, 363

15. Sikes, R. K. (1971). Evaluation of canine rabies vaccines. In Y. Nagano and F. M. Davenport (eds.). *Rabies*, pp. 343–358 (Baltimore: University Park Press)
16. Bulletin of the World Health Organization (1954) **10** (Geneva: WHO)
17. Hubbard, H. B. (1969). Rabies immunity in vaccinated cattle. In *Proceedings of 73rd Annual Meeting of U.S. Animal Health Association*, pp. 307–322
18. Abelseth, M. K. (1975). Bovine vaccines – past and present. In G. M. Baer (ed.). *The Natural History of Rabies*, II, pp. 203–219 (New York, San Francisco and London: Academic Press)
19. Turner, G. S. (1969). Rabies vaccines. *Brit. Med. Bull.*, **25**, 136
20. Komarov, A. and Hornstein, K. (1953). Studies on the pathogenicity of an avianized street rabies virus. *Cornell Vet.*, **43**, 344
21. Peck, F. B. Jr., Powell, H. M. and Culbertson, G. C. (1956). Duck-embryo rabies vaccine. Study of fixed virus vaccine grown in embryonated duck eggs and killed with beta-propiolactone. *J. Am. Med. Assoc.*, **162**, 1373
22. Greenberg, M. and Childress, J. (1960). Vaccination against rabies with duck embryo and Semple vaccines. *J. Am. Med. Assoc.*, **173**, 77
23. Rubin, R. H., Hattwick, M. A. W., Jones, S., Gregg, M. B. and Schwartz, V. D. (1973). Adverse reactions to duck embryo rabies vaccine. *Ann. Int. Med.*, **78**, 643
24. Crick, J. and Brown, F. (1970). Efficacy of rabies vaccine prepared from virus grown in duck embryos. *Lancet*, **i**, 1106
25. Plotkin, S. A. and Clark, H. F. (1971). Prevention of rabies in man. *J. Infect. Dis.*, **123**, 227
26. Ellenbogen, C. and Slugg, P. (1973). Rabies neutralizing antibody: inadequate response to equine antiserum and duck-embryo vaccine. *J. Infect. Dis.*, **127**, 433
27. Fenje, P. (1960). A rabies vaccine from hamster kidney tissue cultures: preparation and evaluation in animals. *Can. J. Microbiol.*, **6**, 605
28. Abelseth, M. K. (1964). An attenuated rabies vaccine for domestic animals produced in tissue culture. *Can. Vet. J.*, **5**, 279
29. Sikes, R. K. (1975). Canine and feline vaccines – past and present. In G. M. Baer (ed.). *The Natural History of Rabies*, II, pp. 177–187 (New York, San Francisco and London: Academic Press)
30. Selimov, M. A. (1973). Live and inactivated tissue-culture rabies vaccine made from strain Vnukovo-32. VPH/RAB.RES/73.1 (Geneva: WHO)
31. Barth, R. and Jaeger, O. (1970). Vaccination trials with a new inactivated, tissue culture rabies vaccine. I. Vaccination of dogs and cats. *Deut. Tieraerztl. Wochenschr.*, **83**, 81
32. Ott, G. L. and Heyke, B. (1962). Preliminary trials of a new tissue culture rabies vaccine. *Vet. Med. and Small Anim. Clin.*, **57**, 158
33. Petermann, H. G., Lang, R., Branche, R. and Soulebot, J. P. (1967). Un nouveau vaccin antirabique préparé avec du virus fixe produit sur culture de cellules et inactivé. 18*ième Congrès Mondial Vétérinaire, Paris*, **1**, 227
34. Bijlenga, G., Hernandez, E. and Mar, C. R. (1971). *Resum. Octava. Reun. Ann. Inst. Nat. Invest. Pec. Mexico*, p. 33 and *19th World Vet. Congress, Mexico City, Mexico*
35. Crick, J. and Brown, F. (1971). An inactivated baby hamster kidney cell vaccine for use in dogs and cattle. *Res. Vet. Sci.*, **12**, 156
36. Larghi, O. P., Savy, V. L., Nebel, A. E. and Rodriguez, A. (1976). Ethyleneimine-inactivated rabies vaccine of tissue culture origin. *J. Clin. Microbiol.*, **3**, 26
37. Atanasiu, P., Ribeiro, M., and Tsiang, H. (1972). Vaccins antirabiques de culture cellulaire obtenus avec la souche Pasteur. Résultats de vaccination. *Ann. Inst. Pasteur, Paris*, **123**, 427
38. Chapman, W. G., Ramshaw, I. A. and Crick, J. (1973). Inactivated rabies vaccine produced from the Flury LEP strain of virus grown in BHK-21 suspension cells. *Appl. Microbiol.*, **26**, 858
39. Fenje, P (1971). The status of existing rabies vaccines. In *International Conference on the Application of Vaccines against Viral, Rickettsial and Bacterial Diseases of Man*. Scientific Publication No. 226, pp. 60–65 (Washington, DC: Pan American Health Organization, WHO)
40. Atanasiu, P., Tsiang, H., and Garnet, A. (1974). Nouveau vaccin antirabique humain de culture cellulaire primaire. *Ann. Microbiol. (Inst. Pasteur)*, **125B**, 419

41. Wiktor, T. J., Fernandes, M. V. and Koprowski, H. (1964). Cultivation of rabies virus in human diploid cell strain WI-38. *J. Immunol.*, **93**, 353
42. Wiktor, T. J. and Koprowski, H. (1965). Successful immunization of primates with rabies vaccine prepared in human diploid cell strain, WI-38. *Proc. Soc. Exp. Biol. Med.*, **118**, 1069
43. Wiktor, T. J., Sokol, F., Kuwert, E. and Koprowski, H. (1969). Immunogenicity of concentrated and purified rabies vaccines of tissue culture origin. *Proc. Soc. Exp. Biol. Med.*, **131**, 799
44. Wiktor, T. J. (1971). New vaccines and the future of rabies prophylaxis. In *International Conference on the Application of Vaccines against Viral, Rickettsial and Bacterial Diseases of Man*. Scientific Publication No. 226, pp. 66–75 (Washington, DC: Pan American Health Organization, WHO)
45. Tint, H., Dobkin, M. B. and Rubin, B. A. (1974). A new tissue culture (WI-38) rabies vaccine, inactivated and disaggregated with tri-(*n*)-butyl phosphate. In R. H. Regamey, W. Hennessen and F. T. Perkins (eds.). *International Symposium on Rabies*, II. *Symposia Series in Immunobiological Standardization*, **21**, pp. 132–143 (Basel: S. Karger)
46. Kaplan, M. (1974). Preliminary results on antibody profiles of humans receiving concentrated inactivated vaccine prepared in human diploid cells. In R. H. Regamey, W. Hennessen and F. T. Perkins (eds.). *International Symposium on Rabies*, II. *Symposia Series in Immunobiological Standardization*, **21**, pp. 226–230 (Basel: S. Karger)
47. Bahmanyar, M. (1974). Results of antibody profiles in man vaccinated with the HDCS vaccine with various schedules. In R. H. Regamey, W. Hennessen and F. T. Perkins (eds.). *International Symposium on Rabies*, II. *Symposia Series in Immunobiological Standardization*, **21**, pp. 231–238 (Basel: S. Karger)
48. Anon (1976). Pre-exposure prophylaxis of rabies. *Brit. Med. J.*, **2**, 197
49. Aoki, F. Y., Tyrrell, D. A. J., Hill, L. E. and Turner, G. S. (1975). Immunogenicity and acceptability of a human diploid cell culture rabies vaccine in volunteers. *Lancet*, **i**, 660
50. Turner, G. S., Aoki, F. Y., Nicholson, K. G., Tyrrell, D. A. J. and Hill, L. E. (1976). Human diploid cell strain rabies vaccine. Rapid prophylactic immunization of volunteers with small doses. *Lancet*, **i**, 1379
51. Cox, J. H. and Schneider, L. G. (1976). Prophylactic immunization of humans against rabies by intradermal inoculation of human diploid cell culture vaccine. *J. Clin. Microbiol.*, **3**, 96
52. Wade, N. (1976). Hayflick's tragedy: the rise and fall of a human cell line. *Science*, **192**, 125
53. Anon (1976). US scandal threatens vaccine supply. *New Scientist*, **70**, 126
54. Jacobs, J. P., Jones, C. M., Baille, J. P. (1970). Characteristics of a human diploid cell designated MRC-5. *Nature, London*, **227**, 168
55. Hummeler, K. and Koprowski, H. (1969). Investigating the rabies virus. *Nature, London*, **221**, 418
56. Crick, J. and Brown, F., (1970). Small immunizing subunits in rabies virus. In R. D. Barry and B. W. J. Mahy (eds.). *The Biology of the Large RNA Viruses*, pp. 133–140 (London and New York: Academic Press)
57. Atanasiu, P., Tsiang, H., Perrin, P., Favre, S. and Sisman, J. (1974). Extraction d'un antigène soluble (glycoprotéine) par le Triton X100 à partir d'un vaccin antirabique de culture tissulaire de premier explant. Résultats d'immunisation et pouvoir protecteur. *Ann. Microbiol. (Inst. Pasteur)*, **125B**, 539
58. Wiktor, T. J., Plotkin, S. A. and Grella, D. W. (1973). Human cell culture rabies vaccine: antibody response in man. *J. Am. Med. Assoc.*, **224**, 1170
59. Cabasso, V. J., Dobkin, M. B., Roby, R. E. and Hammar, A. H. (1974). Antibody response to a human diploid cell rabies vaccine. *Appl. Microbiol.*, **27**, 553
60. Plotkin, S. A., Wiktor, T. J., Koprowski, H., Rosanoff, E. I. and Tint, H. (1976). Immunization schedules for the new human diploid cell vaccine against rabies. *Am. J. Epidemiol.*, **103**, 75
61. Hayman, M. J. and Crumpton, M. J. (1972). Isolation of glycoprotein from pig lymphocyte plasma membrane using *Lens culinaris* phytohemagglutinin. *BBRC*, **47**, 923
62. Brown, F. and Crick, J. (1974). Antibody response to sub-units of rabies and vesicular stomatitis viruses. In R. H. Regamey, W. Hennessen and F. T. Perkins (eds.). *Inter-*

national Symposium on Rabies, II. *Symposia Series in Immunobiological Standardization*, **21**, pp. 119–122 (Basel: S. Karger)

63. World Health Organization (1973). Press Release WHO/30 (Geneva: WHO)
64. Hattwick, M. A. W. (1974). Human rabies. *Publ. Hlth Rev.* **III**, 229
65. Clark, H. F., Wiktor, T. J. and Koprowski, H. (1975). Human vaccination against rabies. In G. M. Baer (ed.) *The Natural History of Rabies*, **II**, pp. 341–365 (New York, San Francisco and London: Academic Press)
66. Wiktor, T. J., Koprowski, H., Mitchell, J. R. and Merigan, T. C. (1976). Role of interferon in prophylaxis of rabies after exposure. *J. Inf. Dis.*, **133**, Supplement, A260
67. Crick, J. and Brown, F. (1976) .Rabies virus and the problems of rabies vaccination in man. *Trans. R. Soc. Trop. Med. Hyg.*, **70**, 196
68. Harmon, M. W. and Janis, B. (1975). Therapy of murine rabies after exposure: efficacy of polyriboinosinic–polyribocytidylic acid alone and in combination with three rabies vaccines. *J. Infect. Dis.*, **132**, 241
69. Rubin, R. H., Dierks, R. E., Gough, P., Gregg, M. B., Gerlach, E. H. and Sikes, R. K. (1971). Immunoglobulin response to rabies vaccine in man. *Lancet*, **ii**, 625
70. Baer, G. M. and Cleary, W. F. (1972). A model in mice for the pathogenesis and treatment of rabies. *J. Infect. Dis.*, **125**, 520
71. Murphy, F. A., Bauer, S. P., Harrison, A. K. and Winn, W. C. Jr. (1973). Comparative pathogenesis of rabies and rabies-like viruses. Viral infection and transit from inoculation site to the central nervous system. *Lab. Invest.*, **28**, 361
72. Habel, K. (1966). Post-exposure vaccination and antiserum prophylaxis of rabies in man. In: *Proceedings of the National Rabies Symposium*. pp. 89–93 (Atlanta, Ga.: National Communicable Disease Center)
73. Shope, R. E., Murphy, F. A., Harrison, A. K., Causey, O. R., Kemp, G. E., Simpson, D. I. H. and Moore, D. L. (1970). Two African viruses serologically and morphologically related to rabies virus. *J. Virol.*, **6**, 690
74. Shope, R. E. (1975). Rabies virus antigenic relationships. In G. M. Baer (ed.) *The Natural History of Rabies*, I, pp. 141–152 (New York, San Francisco and London: Academic Press)
75. Schneider, L. G. and Schoop, U. (1972). Pathogenesis of rabies and rabies-like viruses. *Annls Inst. Pasteur, Paris*, **123**, 469
76. Tignor, G. H. and Shope, R. E. (1972). Vaccination and challenge of mice with viruses of the rabies subgroup. *J. Infect. Dis.*, **125**, 322
77. Kemp, G. E., Causey, O. R., Moore, D. L., Odelola, A., and Fabiyi, A. (1972). Mokola virus. Further studies on IbAn 27377, a new rabies-related etiologic agent of zoonosis in Nigeria. *Am. J. Trop. Med. Hyg.*, **21**, 356
78. Shope, R. E. and Tignor, G. H. (1971). Rabies and serologically-related viruses from Africa. In Y. Nagano and F. M. Davenport (eds.), *Rabies*, pp. 53–56 (Baltimore: University Park Press)
79. Meredith, C. D., Rossouw, A. P. and Van Praag Koch, H. (1971). An unusual case of human rabies thought to be of Chiropteran origin. *S. Afr. Med. J.*, **45**, 767
80. Baer, G. M. (1975). Wildlife vaccination. In G. M. Baer (ed.), *The Natural History of Rabies*, **II**, pp. 261–266 (New York, San Francisco and London: Academic Press)
81. Anon (1976). La vaccination antirabique des renards. *Rec. Méd. Vet.*, **152**, 57
82. Winkler, W. G. and Baer, G. M. (1976). Rabies immunization of red foxes (*Vulpes fulva*) with vaccine in sausage baits. *Am. J. Epidemiol.*, **103**, 408

9
Rubella vaccines

C. HUYGELEN

Rubella was reported initially by German authors in the eighteenth century; but not until 1938, was its viral nature established by Japanese workers and its transmissibility shown by the injection of throat washings. Before 1941, rubella was known as a mild disease of children and young adults, being characterized by lymphadenopathy and by an acute rash that lasts for about 3 days; it had been reported to be more severe in adult females, since about half of them experienced some form of arthralgia or arthritis. Rubella is considered to be less infectious than measles and the risk of infection is greatest following household contacts.

Table 1 Milestones in history of rubella 'prevention'

Eighteenth century	Description of disease (Rötheln)
1938	Proof of viral origin
1941	Recognition as cause of congenital malformations
1962	Isolation of virus (Weller & Neva; Parkman *et al.*)
1964	Large epidemic in the US
1968	International rubella conference (IABS) at London
1969	International rubella conference (NIH) at Bethesda
1969	First rubella vaccine licensed (Switzerland)

In 1941, McAlister Gregg, an ophthalmologist in Sydney, observed an unusual number of cases of congenital cataract coming from widely separated areas in Australia. In almost all cases, a history was obtained of the mother having had rubella in her pregnancy, most frequently in the first or second month. The epidemic in Australia occurred in wartime when many young women were employed in factories and offices. During the next two decades, several reports confirmed Gregg's observations, but apart from the 'rubella parties' organized in some countries for young girls, no further progress was made in the prevention of the disease, because the causal agent could not be propagated in the laboratory.

In the 1960s, several major events occurred. In 1962, rubella virus was isolated by two independent groups in the USA. Laboratory techniques thus became available for serological and virological studies just before a devastating rubella epidemic occurred in the US in 1964. This permitted detailed studies to be made on many malformed children. After the initial isolation of the virus, attempts to develop vaccines started immediately. Initially, most attempts were directed towards the development of killed vaccines, but they were all abandoned after some time because it soon became clear that these killed preparations were not sufficiently immunogenic. All efforts were then oriented towards live vaccines, and this resulted in 1969 in the licensing of two vaccines, first the Cendehill in Switzerland, and then the HPV-77 in the US (Table 1).

Rubella virus affects the division of the embryonic cells and results in severe lesions of the eye, the ear, the brain and the cardiovascular system. The risk of infection decreases with the age of the fetus. It is very high in the first 2 months of pregnancy and decreases rapidly thereafter. Congenital rubella patients require lifelong care.

The number of children damaged as a result of the 1964 epidemic in the US has been estimated at 20 000 to 30 000. In non-epidemic years, the incidence of congenital rubella infections lies in most countries around 1 per 1000 live births, whereas in epidemic years, this figure can be as high as 22 per 1000 live births. Recently, Schoenbaum *et al.*[1] calculated that without vaccination, lifetime expenditure for congenital rubella syndrome is more than $35 for every female in the population.

It has been claimed that the Japanese strains of rubella virus are only mildly teratogenic or non-teratogenic, as compared to strains of American or European origin. However, I have been unable to find any confirmation of these claims.

For the development of rubella vaccines in the 1960s, methods were used which had previously been shown to result in the attenuation of other human and animal viruses; i.e. serial passages of the virus in cell culture systems. Three different systems were used for the attenuation of rubella virus: primary rabbit kidney cells at RIT, Rixensart (Belgium); primary monkey kidney cells at NIH, Bethesda, Maryland, USA; and human diploid cells at the Wistar Institute, Philadelphia, USA. These serial passages led to the development of the Cendehill, HPV-77 and RA 27/3 strains respectively. These are the only strains that have undergone extensive evaluation before licensing and are now licensed in several countries.

As shown in Table 2, the Cendehill strain was obtained by making fifty-one passages in primary rabbit kidney cells[2]; it is produced at RIT, a subsidiary of SmithKline Corporation, located in Rixensart, Belgium. The vaccine is produced in primary rabbit kidney cell cultures and is sold under the tradename Cendevax or Ervevax.

Table 2 Rubella vaccines

Research Laboratory developing strain	*Substrate used*	*Name of strain*	*Manufacturer*	*Substrate for production*	*Trade name*
RIT (Huygelen and Peetermans)	Rabbit kidney (51 passages)	Cendehill	RIT (SmithKline)	Rabbit kidney	Cendevax (Ervevax)
NIH (Parkman and Meyer)	Monkey kidney (77 passages)	HPV-77	Merck, Sharpe & Dohme	Duck embryo HPV-77 DE 5	Meruvax
			Philips–Roxane	Dog kidney HPV-77 DK 12	Withdrawn from market
Wistar (Plotkin)	Human diploid (25 passages)	RA 27/3	Burroughs-Wellcome	Human diploid	Almevax
			Institut Merieux	Human diploid	Rudivax

The HPV-77 strain was attenuated by Parkman and Meyer through seventy-seven passages in primary green monkey kidney cells. Because of the frequent contamination of these cells with simian viruses, other substrates were subsequently used for the production of the strain. Merck, Sharpe & Dohme passed the strain five times through duck embryo cells (HPV-77 DE 5) and the resulting vaccine is sold under the trade name of Meruvax. Philips–Roxane made twelve passages of the strain in dog kidney cell cultures (HPV-77 DK 12); this strain was later withdrawn from the market because it induced a significantly higher degree of side-reactions, even in children.

The RA 27/3 strain was obtained by twenty-five passages in human diploid cells (WI-38 strain) by Plotkin. It is produced by Burroughs-Wellcome and by Institut Mérieux and sold as Almevax and Rudivax respectively. All three vaccines have been shown to meet the criteria of live attenuated rubella vaccines. These criteria are summarized in Table 3.

I would like to discuss very briefly the laboratory criteria first. A virus vaccine has to be produced in a 'clean' cell substrate. All three substrates mentioned, primary rabbit kidney cells, primary duck embryo cells and human diploid cells, have been accepted as a substrate for virus vaccine production after thorough testing in the absence of adventitious agents.

Rabbit kidneys and duck embryos are obtained from closed colonies under specific pathogen-free conditions. Human diploid cells are derived from healthy human fetal tissue and checked for the absence of contamination and of karyological abnormalities.

Table 3 Criteria for live rubella virus vaccines

LABORATORY CRITERIA
Production in an acceptable cell substrate
Stability during storage
Virological markers
CLINICAL CRITERIA
Absence of spread
Attenuation
Immunogenicity
Ideally: absence of teratogenicity

Rubella virus is very stable in the freeze-dried form and under normal conditions of storage, if a suitable stabilizer and freeze-drying cycle are used during the production process. Samples of many individual batches of Cendevax were kept at different temperatures and the virus content titrated at intervals. At +4 °C, no detectable loss of virus potency was observed after 5 years, the longest period tested. At room temperature, a gradual decrease was observed over several months. At incubator temperature (37 °C), a similar loss was observed over a period of a few weeks, but the virus titre was still above the required minimum after one month. Even after a whole year in the incubator, all vials still contained viable virus[3].

Markers of attenuation for live vaccine virus strains allow differentiation of these strains from wild viruses and can be extremely useful for two reasons:

(a) during the production process, they make it possible to have a reliable check on the absence of accidental contamination with rubella virus; and
(b) they allow identification of a vaccine virus isolated from humans and its differentiation from naturally occurring virus.

Several marker systems have been tested for rubella vaccine but only one has been found to be sufficiently reliable and reproducible to be used routinely and this is the rabbit marker[4]. Unfortunately, it is applicable only to the Cendehill strain and not to the other strains. In our laboratories, this marker system has given consistent results on every batch of vaccine produced over the last 8 years.

Non-communicability of the virus from vaccinees to contacts is a highly desirable property of any live vaccine; this applies particularly to rubella vaccines because of the potential risk of virus transmission from a vaccinated subject to a susceptible pregnant woman. The absence of spread was checked for the various vaccine strains by leaving vaccinated and non-vaccinated susceptible subjects in close contact for a period of several weeks and by checking their serological status at the end of the observation period. In our own studies in various groups, more than 1300 vaccinees were left in contact with an equal number of contacts and no transmission was observed[5].

The lack of spread can be explained by the synergistic effect of several factors: the percentage of virus excretors after vaccination is much lower than in natural infection; the excretion period of vaccine virus is much shorter than that of wild virus (1–2 days versus 10–14 days); the titre of the excreted virus is much lower (Table 4). Another important factor is the low infectivity of the Cendehill and the HPV-77 strains for the nasal mucosa. Even very high doses (up to 10 000 $TCID^{50}$ for the Cendehill strain) of these attenuated viruses do not infect when given intranasally. This lack of infectivity, together with the low excretion pattern, create a very wide margin of safety. In this respect, the RA 27/3 differs from the two other strains in that it infects readily by the nasal route.

Table 4 Factors in non-transmissibility of rubella vaccine virus

	Virulent virus	*Vaccine virus*
Titre of virus excreted	High	Low
Duration of excretion	Long	Short
Percentage of virus excretors	High	Low
Infectivity of virus for nasal mucosa	High	Low

Attenuation is another criterion to be met by live vaccines in general. It may be of less importance in rubella because of the mildness of the wild virus. Nevertheless, whenever possible, a vaccine should not cause illness or discomfort.

All three strains now in wide use have been shown to have an acceptable level of attenuation for children and young girls. Reactions do occur in some vaccinees, but are mild. One strain however, the HPV-77 DK 12, derived from HPV-77, caused significantly more symptoms in children. These symptoms consisted of arthritis and peripheral neuropathy in some cases; this strain is not available on the market any more.

Reactogenicity of rubella vaccines increases with the age of the vaccinees. Adult women seem to be particularly prone to develop joint symptoms after vaccination. A difference between the three virus strains has been noticed, the HPV-77 strain being the most reactogenic in adult women and causing joint problems in up to 30–50% of those more than 25 years old[6]. The Cendehill strain seems to be the best-tolerated strain in adult women, including those vaccinated during the post-partum[7] period.

Protection of the fetus is the ultimate objective of all rubella vaccinations, and this protection is provided by the presence of circulating antibodies in the blood of the mother; by this mechanism, viraemia and transplacental passage of the virus are prevented. All available evidence today suggests that if antibodies are present, there is no risk to the fetus even if a local reinfection of the nasopharynx occurs.

All three rubella vaccines have been shown to induce antibodies in a very high percentage of vaccinees. The seroconversion rates in almost all studies have varied between 90 and 100%, and mostly between 95 and 100%. These results have been confirmed in large numbers under many different conditions in persons of different age, sex and race. They have been so reproducible that one can safely say that in those exceptional cases where an investigator found a significantly lower seroconversion rate, there was either something wrong with the serological techniques used, or with the storage of the vaccine. Lack of sensitivity of the test system used is probably the most frequent cause of so-called vaccination failures in some studies. Recently, Fox *et al.*[8], reported results of a trial carried out in Washington State. They found about 10% non-responders in an adult population using the HI test. However, when the sera were retested, using a more sensitive method, all prevaccination sera of the non-responders were shown to contain antibodies.

No differences were found between the three vaccine strains with regard to the rate of seroconversion induced.

The antibody levels induced by vaccination are lower than those occurring after natural infection, they are about fourfold lower for the Cendehill and HPV-77 De 5 strains and about twofold for the RA 27/3 strain. This applies more particularly to the antibody levels measured 6–8 weeks post vaccination at a time when the maximum titre was not reached for part of the HPV-77 and Cendehill vaccinees. This finding is in line with the general observation that attenuated viruses induce lower antibody levels than natural infection. In rubella, where the objective is a long-lasting immunity, it is not so much the level of the antibodies as their persistence, which is important. Higher antibody titres have a greater tendency to drop to a lower level. In a large-scale study organized in Hawaii by the CDC, Herrmann *et al.*[9] found that the loss of antibody over a 4-year observation period was directly related to the antibody level achieved 12 weeks postvaccination. More than half of the children with vaccine induced titres of at least 1:160 experienced a fourfold or greater decline in antibody, while children with titres of 1:40 or less rarely lost antibody. These results suggest that antibody titres at low level may plateau in rubella vaccinees, after which little further decline in titre may take place.

In another large-scale trial organized in Scotland and involving 1072 girls enrolled in a 20-year programme, Zealley[10] found that although very few girls had lower antibody titres by the end of the first year of the study, this was observed more often in those given RA 27/3 vaccine than in groups with naturally acquired immunity or with immunity due to Cendehill vaccine. This suggested, according to the author, that the HAI antibody induced by RA 27/3 had reached its peak at the time of the first postvaccination blood tests 2 months after vaccination and that the titre in a few girls had subsequently begun to fall. Black *et al.*[11] reported a twofold decrease in antibody titre between 4 months and 2 years postvaccination in subjects vaccinated with RA 27/3. This was also confirmed in a recent study in Malmö, Sweden (Kullander *et al.*, unpublished) in which the authors found that the initial differences in the antibody levels induced by the three vaccines had disappeared 2 years postvaccination.

The actual persistence of antibody over longer periods of time has now been studied in several groups. In a group of young adult women in Switzerland vaccinated with Cendehill, Just[12] found persistence of antibody in all of 164 vaccinees whose serological status was checked $6\frac{1}{2}$ years postvaccination. The results were similar $7\frac{1}{2}$ years postvaccination (Just, personal communication). As mentioned earlier, Herrmann *et al.*[9] organized a long-term study including over 7000 children in Hawaii. The results after 4 years were published recently: the results after 5 years are now available and are essentially the same as after 4 years (J. Witte, personal communication). The vaccines included in the trial were HPV-77 DE 5, HPV-77 DK 12 and Cendehill (Table 5). All sera taken after 4 years were tested simultaneously with the prevaccination samples. To reduce the possibility that variations in antibody titre resulted from chance, all fourfold or greater rises or falls in titres were repeated. These are extremely important precautions, because all too often wrong conclusions have been reached in the past by investigators who neglected to test the sera simultaneously.

Table 5 Changes in antibody titres, Hawaii study (CDC)

Subjects	*HPV-77 DK 12* (%)	*HPV-77 DE 5* (%)	*Cendehill* (%)	*Total* (%)
Stable titre	62.3	56.1	68.7	62.1
⩾ fourfold rise	0.2	0.3	0.5	0.3
⩾ fourfold fall	37.5	44.6	30.8	37.6
Titre fall to <1:10	0.0	1.8	0.4	0.7
Vaccinees with persisting detectable antibodies	100.0	98.2	99.6	99.3

Source: Herrmann *et al.*

The immediate postvaccination sera of 5153 subjects showed seroconversion rates of 99.9% for HPV-77 DK 12, 97.5% for HPV-77 DE 5 and 99.8% for Cendehill. The GMT was 222, 118 and 95 respectively. After 4 years, the percentage of those showing a fourfold or greater titre fall was 37.5% for HPV-77 DK 12, 44.6% for HPV-77 DE 5 and 30.8% for Cendehill. Only 0.4% of those who initially seroconverted to the Cendehill strain had lost measurable antibody 4 years later; this figure was 1.8% in the HPV-77 DE

5 group. Overall measurable antibody persisted in 99.3% of all vaccinees. In total, 98.4% of the children had antibodies 4 years after vaccination. It should be mentioned that, during this period, there was no significant wild rubella activity in this area; this explains why only a negligible number of subjects showed antibody rises.

These results indicate that antibody induced by vaccination is long-lasting in spite of levels which are lower than those observed after natural infection. Although less information is available on the long-term persistence of antibodies after RA 27/3 vaccine, the data obtained so far are encouraging.

In other studies, during the long-term follow-up of several groups of vaccinees, a boost of antibodies was observed in some of the subjects. This was attributable to a local reinfection of the nasopharyngeal area with natural virus. Reinfection also occurred in naturally immune subjects, but to a lesser extent than in vaccinated individuals.

However, the important matter is that reinfection has no serious consequences since it has not been characterized either by clinical disease or viraemia. Since there is no viraemia, it is extremely unlikely that there could be spread of virus to the fetus. During reinfection also, very minimal or no virus can be detected in the throat and a reinfected person is much less likely to be a source of infection to susceptible contacts.

Intranasal vaccination has been suggested as a means of inducing local as well as systemic immunity to rubella, and trials have been done in this respect with the RA 27/3 strain, which is the only strain with a high enough infectivity for the nasal mucosa, which could be used intranasally. However, a high variability has been encountered in the seroconversion rates obtained. Very high titres had to be used to overcome the high number of vaccine failures. Although local antibodies could be observed[13] in RA 27/3 vaccinees, the titres were lower than those seen after natural disease. This is probably related to the lower replication rate of the attenuated virus. Since local IgA antibodies have a tendency to decrease much more rapidly than circulating antibodies, the stimulation of the local immune system by intranasal vaccination may present little advantage as far as long-term protection of the future pregnant woman is concerned. Unlike respiratory diseases, where local immunity is important, the prevention of congenital rubella is based on the presence of circulating antibodies.

Further follow-up is required to study the role of natural reinfection in the maintenance of natural and of vaccine-induced immunity. In almost all groups of vaccines followed so far, an antibody boost by natural reinfection has been observed in a variable percentage of individuals. Only time can tell whether a booster injection of vaccine will be necessary in those whose antibody levels decrease to a very low or undetectable level. Generally, rubella vaccines have been rather ineffective in boosting immunity in subjects with pre-existing naturally induced antibody[14]. In this connection, it is interesting to note that in girls who had not responded with a detectable antibody level in a Swedish study, a second dose induced an anamnestic-type response. This may indicate that a booster injection in the future may be helpful in those in whom it may be desirable, i.e. those whose level of immunity has dropped below the detectable level[15].

In the field, the various vaccines have been shown to be highly effective in preventing rubella in vaccinated subjects, as shown by the initial studies of Meyer *et al.*[16], using the HPV-77 strain and confirmed later by other studies such as that by Ladrigan *et al.*[17], who observed a 93.5% efficacy in adolescents vaccinated with Cendehill.

Ideally, rubella vaccines should be non-teratogenic or, to go one step further, should contain viruses which, when given inadvertently to a pregnant woman, would not replicate in the fetal tissues.

In cases of natural rubella during the first weeks of pregnancy, the virus can be isolated with very high frequency from the embryonic tissues. The isolation rate can be as high as 90% when cell cultures are made directly from these tissues. In comparison, the vaccine viruses are much less invasive for the fetal tissues, as shown in a few cases where susceptible women, in the beginning of pregnancy and scheduled for therapeutic abortion, were vaccinated and their products of conception examined for the presence of virus. However, virus could be found in the placenta and, in some cases, in the fetus.

Recently, Modlin *et al.*[18] published a report of all cases compiled by CDC and in which rubella vaccine was given inadvertently just before or after pregnancy. The study included 343 women. The pregnancies of 145 women were terminated and rubella virus was recovered from the products of conception of nine women, including six of the twenty-eight known to be sero-negative to rubella at the time of vaccination. Of these nine women, six had received HPV-77; one received Cendehill; and in three cases the vaccine given was unknown. None of the 172 infants carried to term had either clinical or serologic evidence of rubella infection, including thirty-eight infants of women known to be susceptible and twelve additional women estimated to be susceptible at the time of vaccination. The maximal calculated risk of rubella infection is therefore 5–10%, and the actual risk is probably much less. In contrast, the risk in natural infection is estimated at 10–66%. In Australia, Allan *et al.*[19] reported inadvertent vaccination with Cendehill in pregnant women; in thirty-six, the pregnancy was terminated; three aborted spontaneously; nineteen were delivered of normal infants.

We may conclude from these reports, and also from earlier studies in small numbers of pregnant women, that the Cendehill and the HPV-77 strains are undoubtedly much less teratogenic than wild rubella virus, and may even have lost their teratogenicity, but the recommendation that vaccination be avoided during pregnancy must be continued.

Very little is known of the teratogenic potential of the RA 27/3 strain, since this strain was not included in the large-scale CDC survey. In contrast to the other strains, the RA 27/3 strain is the only one which has been serially passed in human fetal cells, and it is difficult to speculate on the effect this may have had on its teratogenic properties.

Table 6 Immunization policy

Area	*Target groups*	*Objective*
North America	Young children of both sexes	Indirect protection of pregnant women
Europe	Girls at puberty Selective vaccination of adult women	Direct protection of those at risk

Two different approaches have been taken in the prevention of congenital rubella by vaccination. In North America, young children of both sexes are vaccinated whereas in Europe the target groups are young girls at the time of puberty and also adult women, but the latter on a selective basis. The US programme was revolutionary in the sense that, for the first time, the target population of an immunization programme was not the one at risk, i.e. susceptible women of childbearing age, but the age group from 1 to 12, including boys (Table 6).

The objective of the programme was to build up a herd immunity high enough to minimize the risk of infection to susceptible pregnant women. So far, 70 000 000 doses of vaccine have been distributed and there has been a substantial decline in the occurrence of rubella and congenital rubella (Figure 1). Furthermore, the pandemic that many epidemiologists predicted for the early 1970s has not materialized.

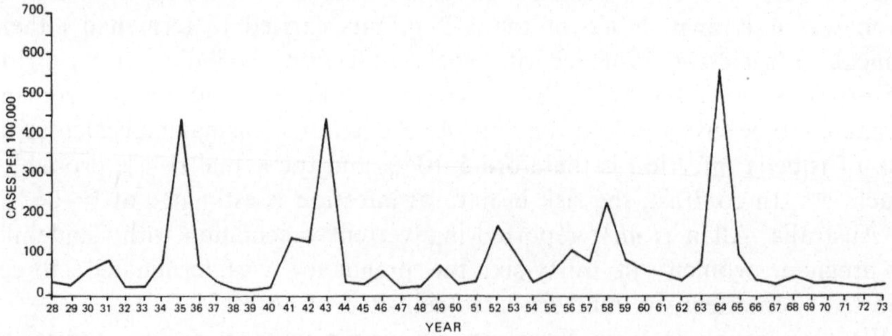

Figure 1 Rubella incidence in ten selected areas in the US, 1928–75 (From Witte, 1976)

A number of criticisms has been raised. Two recent studies[20,21] have cast doubt on the hypothesis that children are the major source of rubella infection for pregnant women; this doubt is based on the fact that a very high percentage of children with congenital rubella were born to primiparae. Also, according to some authors, attempts to demonstrate herd immunity for rubella have been unconvincing[22], and the opponents of the CDC policy claim that the reduction in congenital rubella can be accounted for by the infrequency of epidemics, declining birthrates and markedly increased availability of induced abortion.

Recently, Schoenbaum *et al.*[1] calculated benefits and costs of prevention of rubella, and came to the conclusion that for a more immediate return on investment, either single vaccination of females at 12 or vaccination at two ages would be better than the current practice of vaccinating children once at an early age. A major criticism, however, against the study by Schoenbaum *et al.* is that it disregards the very principle on which the whole vaccination campaign is based, i.e. that of herd immunity.

In most European countries, rubella vaccine policy has been to delay immunization until about 12 years of age. This allows natural infection to immunize about 75–80% of girls before this age. Girls are offered vaccine regardless of their immune status. This is because it would be prohibitively expensive to test them beforehand; moreover, testing poses considerable problems because the tests are not always completely reliable. The disadvantage of this approach is that it allows virulent wild virus to circulate among younger girls and the whole male population.

The group of individuals most in need of immunization against rubella are women of 20–25 who are non-immune, since this is the age-group to whom most children are born. The seronegatives in this group need vaccination but it has to be done under cover of adequate contraception. Vaccination of women in the post-partum period is recommended in several countries and is undoubtedly very useful for the protection of the next pregnancy. However, because of the high incidence of affected firstborn children, Marshall *et al.*[21] point towards the need for identification of susceptible women and their vaccination before their first pregnancy. This programme is seen as complementary to the vaccination of young girls, which takes about a decade to have a significant effect on the incidence of congenital rubella. Because of the risk of pregnancy, the vaccination of adult women has, of course, always to be done on a selective basis and preferably after examination of their serological status.

Whatever the programme used, there is a great need for rubella vaccine, not only for the age-groups growing up, but also for the adult women at risk. By far the largest number of doses of rubella vaccines have been used in the US where, in 1973, about 56% of the 1–4-year-old children and about 65% of those 5–9 years old had received the vaccine (Figure 2). Apart from the UK, Australia and New Zealand, vaccination programmes have been slow to start. In some countries, this is due to public apathy; in others, the public health authorities do not do enough to stimulate interest or to organize vaccination campaigns. The adverse publicity against vaccination organized by some groups probably has also had a negative impact. It is obvious that in the end, immunization of the whole prepubertal and susceptible post-pubertal female population, perhaps combined with childhood vaccination, is the only answer to the problem of congenital rubella, but much inertia and apathy has to be overcome to reach that objective.

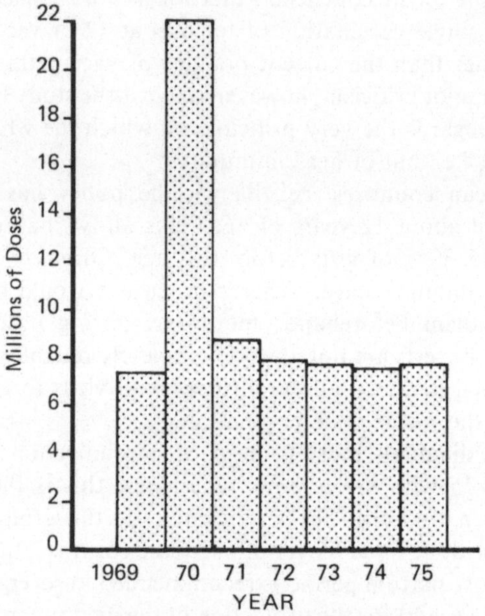

Figure 2 Net doses of rubella vaccine distributed in the US, 1969–75 (from Witte)

Finally, I would like to mention also that at least two rubella viruses, HPV-77 and Cendehill, can be given together with mumps and measles; the immunity induced is comparable to that induced by each vaccine given separately. Inclusion of rubella vaccine in combined vaccines is compatible only with a vaccination programme in early childhood.

References

1. Schoenbaum, S. C., Hyde, J. N. Jr., Bartoshesky, L. and Crampton K. (1976). Benefit–cost analysis of rubella vaccination policy. *N. Engl. J. Med.*, **294**(6), 306
2. Huygelen, C. and Peetermans, J. (1967). Attenuation of rubella virus by serial passage in primary rabbit kidney cell cultures. II. Experiments in animals. *Arch. Ges. Virusforsch*, **21**(3–4), 357
3. Peetermans, J., Colinet, G. and Huygelen, C. (1973). Stability of freeze-dried rubella virus vaccine (Cendehill® strain) at various temperatures. *J. Biol. Stand.*, **1**, 179
4. Zygraich, N., Peetermans, J. and Huygelen, C. (1971). In vivo properties of attenuated rubella virus Cendehill® strain. *Arch. Ges. Virusforsch.*, **33**, 225
5. Prinzie, A., Huygelen, C., Gold, J., Farquhar, J. and McKee, J. (1969). Experimental live attenuated rubella virus vaccine: clinical evaluation of Cendehill strain. *Am. J. Dis. Child.* **118**(2), 172

6. Weibel, R. E., Stokes, J., Buynak, E. B. and Hilleman, M. R. (1972). Influence of age on clinical response to HPV-77 duck rubella vaccine. *J. Am. Med. Assoc.*, **222**(7), 805
7. Grillner, L. Hedström, C. E., Bergström, H., Forssman, L., Rigner, A. and Lycke, E. (1973). Vaccination against rubella of newly delivered women. *Scand. J. Infect. Dis.*, **5**, 237
8. Fox, J. P., Rainey, H. S., Hall, C. E., Ray, C. G. and Patterson, M. J. (1976). Rubella vaccine in postpubertal women: experience in Western Washington State. *J. Am. Med. Assoc.*, **236**(7), 837
9. Herrmann, K. L., Halstead, S. B., Brandling-Bennet, A. D., Witte, J. J., Wiebenga, N. H. and Eddins, D. L. (1976). Rubella immunization: persistence of antibody four years after a large-scale field trial. *J. Am. Med. Assoc.*, **235**(20), 2201
10. Zealley, H. (1974). Rubella screening and immunization of school girls: a long-term evaluation. *Brit. J. Prev. Soc. Med.*, **28**, 54
11. Black, F. L., Lamm, S. H., Emmons, J. E. and Pinheiro, F. P. (1976). Reactions to rubella vaccine and persistence of antibody in virgin-soil population after vaccination and wild-virus-induced immunization. *J. Infect. Dis.*, **133**(4), 393
12. Just, M. (1974). Rötelnimpfung. *Ther. Umsch.*, **31**(8), 553
13. Cradock-Watson, J. E., McDonald, H., Ridehalgh, M. K., Bourne, M. S. and Vandervelde, E. M. (1974). Specific immunoglobulin response in serum and nasal secretions after the administration of attenuated rubella vaccine. *J. Hyg.*, **73**, 127
14. Freestone, D. S., Reynolds, G. M., McKinnon, J. A. and Prydie, J. (1975). Vaccination of schoolgirls against rubella: assessment of serological status and a comparative trial of Wistar, RA 27/3 and Cendehill strains live attenuated rubella vaccines in 13-year-old schoolgirls in Dudley. *Brit. J. Prev. Soc. Med.*, **29**, 258
15. Böttiger, M. and Heller, L. (1976). Experience from vaccination and revaccination of teenage girls with three different rubella vaccines. *J. Biol. Stand.*, **4**, 107
16. Meyer, H. M., Parkmann, P. D. and Panos, T. C. (1966). Attenuated rubella virus. II. Production of an experimental live virus vaccine and clinical trial. *N. Engl. J. Med.*, **275** (11), 575
17. Ladrigan, P. J., Stoffels, M. A., Anderson, E. and Witte, J. J. (1974). Epidemic rubella in adolescent boys: clinical features and results of vaccination. *J. Amer. Med. Assoc.*, **227**(11), 1283
18. Modlin, J. F., Herrmann, K., Brandling-Bennett, A. D., Eddins, D. L. and Hayden, G. F. (1976). Risk of congenital abnormality after inadvertent rubella vaccination of pregnant women. *N. Engl. J. Med.* **294**(8), 972
19. Allan, B. C., Hamilton, S. M., Wiemers, M. A., Winsor, R. H. and Gust, I. D. (1973). Pregnancy complicated by accidental rubella vaccination. *Aust. N.Z. J. Obstet. Gynaecol.*, **13**, 72
20. Schoenbaum, S. C., Biano, S. and Mack, T. (1975). Epidemiology of congenital rubella syndrome; the role of maternal parity *J. Amer. Med. Assoc.*, **233**(2), 151
21. Marshall, W. C., Peckham, C. S., Dudgeon, J. A., Sheppart, S., Smithells, R. W. and Weatherall, J. A. (1976). Parity of women contracting rubella in pregnancy: implication with respect to rubella vaccination. *Lancet*, **i**(7971), 1231

10
Vaccination against poliomyelitis

J. SALK AND D. SALK

INTRODUCTION

Effective immunization against poliomyelitis has been achieved with two different vaccines. An injectable killed, or inactivated, poliovirus vaccine was introduced in the mid-1950s, and an oral live, attenuated poliovirus vaccine was introduced in the late 1950s and early 1960s. In areas of the world where only the killed virus vaccine has been used, poliomyelitis has been brought fully under control; however, in areas where the live virus vaccine is in use, problems in the control of poliomyelitis continue to exist. Experience in recent years has revealed two particular difficulties related to the use of live, attenuated poliovirus vaccine:

1. The live virus vaccine is occasionally associated with paralytic disease, and in countries where paralytic poliomyelitis has been brought under control, it may be a more frequent cause of polio than the wild virus. The attenuated virus has been shown to revert to neurovirulence, and can reseed the natural virus reservoir, becoming established in a human population. This will be discussed in detail in the "Effect of Vaccination Programme" section.
2. In underdeveloped countries with warm climates, where poliomyelitis is still prevalent, antibody response to the live virus vaccine is uncertain because unexplained inhibitors in the intestinal tract interfere with vaccine virus implantation (Tables 1 and 2). In some countries four or more doses of the live virus vaccine have failed to protect against paralytic poliomyelitis[1,2]. There are the separate problems of loss of vaccine potency due to the need to maintain the live vaccine in the frozen state, and its uncertain booster effect, even in temperate climates such as England[86].

Table 1 Experience with live poliovirus vaccine, Mexico, 1975[62]

SEROCONVERSION IN 127 CHILDREN		
No. doses	*No. tested*	*Seroconversion (Titre ⩾ 1:8 to Type I)**
1 (T-I)†	53	23 (43.4%)
2 (T-I)	24	11 (45.8%)
3 T-I + 1 TOPV‡	50	25 (50.0%)
	127	59

VACCINATION STATUS IN PATIENTS WITH PARALYTIC POLIO		
No. doses‡	*No. cases*	*Percentage of total cases*
0	344	33.4
1	181	17.6
2	146	14.3
⩾3	221	21.5
Unknown	135	13.2
	1027	100.0

†Monovalent type I oral poliovirus vaccine.

‡Trivalent oral poliovirus vaccine.

*In other studies it has been found that approximately 20% of individuals have antibody titres between 1:4 and 1:8. Therefore, if a titre of 1:4 had been used to define seroconversion in this study, the figures for one, two and three doses would likely have been approximately 63%, 65%, and 70% respectively.

Table 2 Live virus vaccination status of non-Jewish patients with poliomyelitis in Israel, 1971–76[2]

No. doses	*No. cases*	*Percentage of total*
0	23	38.9
1	10	16.9
2	7	11.9
3	9	15.3
4	10	16.9
TOTAL	59	100.0

Additional data from Gaza and the West Bank of the Jordan river indicate that cases have occurred in children who had received three or four doses of oral vaccine, as well as in some who had not received the vaccine. When some of the vaccinated children who later developed polio were examined for neutralizing antibodies, they were found to have developed antibodies only to the type causing their disease. Thus, vaccination in these children had not induced antibodies against any of the three poliovirus types. Some children were given oral polio vaccine 6 months after the onset of paralysis and still failed to form antibody to the other types.

These problems can be avoided by the use of inactivated (killed) poliovirus administered parenterally[3–5]. The killed poliovirus vaccine will not cause paralytic poliomyelitis when properly prepared, induces immunity without passage through the gut (Tables 3 and 4), maintains potency with normal refrigeration, and reliably boosts antibody levels.

In addition, the killed poliovirus vaccine can be effectively combined with other vaccines to simplify schedules of routine immunization, and to avoid

Table 3 Percentage seroconversion rates in the tropics for live poliovirus vaccine compared with those for killed poliovirus vaccine[3]

Vaccine	*Trial*	*Percentage seroconversion rates to:*		
		Type I	*Type II*	*Type III*
Live	Mexico, 1960	55	83	37
	Nigeria, 1964	22	69	46
	Singapore, 1964	50	98	59
	Nigeria, 1966	48	92	50
Killed	Nigeria, 1966	93	89	93

Table 4 Comparison of antibody response of Nigerian babies to live and killed poliovirus vaccines[63]

	Percentage lacking antibody		
	Type I	*Type II*	*Type III*
Live poliovirus vaccine (at age 2, 3, 5 months)	52	8	48
Killed poliovirus vaccine (at age 2, 3, 5 months)	2	4	0
Post-booster (at age 15 months)	0	3	0

Table 5 Comparison of utilization of diphtheria–tetanus–pertussis (DTP) and oral live poliovirus vaccine (LPV) in the United States, 1974. The data are shown as percentages of the age groups that received three doses of DTP by injection and the percentages that received three doses of LPV by mouth [64]

	United States total		*Inner city areas*	
Age group (years)	*DTP*	*LPV*	*DTP*	*LPV*
<1	33%	21%	29%	22%
1–4	74	63	70	60
5–9	85	74	83	71
10–13	86	70*	83	68*

* Age group of 10–14 years.

the cost of separate immunization programmes. Combined diphtheria-tetanus–polio (DT–polio) and diphtheria–tetanus–pertussis–polio (DTP–polio) vaccines are used in Canada, Holland, Denmark, France, and other countries[6–8]. Vaccines given by injection are well accepted, as shown by the 1974 utilization rates of DTP vaccine and of live poliovirus vaccine in the United States: the utilization rate was higher for three or more doses of DTP given by injection than for three or more doses of live poliovirus vaccine given by mouth, even in the hard-to-reach inner-city population (Table 5).

IMMUNE RESPONSE TO KILLED POLIOVIRUS VACCINE

The potency of killed poliovirus vaccine can be adjusted to provide any desired immune response[9,10]:

1. The levels of antibody following both primary and booster doses of vaccine each depend on the quantity of antigen used for primary immunization (Tables 6 and 7);

Table 6 Percentage of subjects with type I poliovirus antibody titres at or above levels indicated, 2 weeks after a single intramuscular injection of killed poliovirus vaccine. Subjects were divided into groups which received different volumes of reference vaccine A. The pattern of response to poliovirus types II and III was similar[65]

*Antibody titre**	*Volume of reference vaccine A*					
	2 ml	*1 ml*	*1/2 ml*	*1/4 ml*	*1/8 ml*	*1/16 ml*
⩾4	100	100	96.2	93.4	87.2	77.2
⩾8	100	100	80.9	73.4	65.7	57.2
⩾16	94.2	88.3	61.7	50.1	37.6	40.1
⩾32	64.8	58.9	38.7	16.8	15.8	11.6
⩾64	32.5	17.8	8.0	10.2	6.5	0
⩾128	12.0	6.1	0	0	0	
⩾256	3.2	0				
⩾512	0					
Antibody mean†	36	26	12	10	9	7
Subjects (No.)‡	34	34	26	30	32	35

*Reciprocal of serum dilution capable of neutralizing 100 $TCID_{50}$ (tissue culture infective doses, 50 percent effective) type I virus.

†Geometric mean antibody titre.

‡Number from whom serum samples were available.

2. Immunologic memory, as demonstrated by the secondary-type antibody response to a booster dose, is induced even by quantities of antigen which are too small to induce persistently detectable levels of antibody (Table 8);
3. The rate and duration of faecal excretion of poliovirus can be reduced by

Table 7 Percentage of subjects with type I poliovirus antibody titres at or above levels indicated before (pre) and 2 weeks after (post) a third dose of killed poliovirus vaccine. Primary immunization administered 1 year earlier with two equal doses (2 weeks apart) of reference vaccine A. Subjects were divided into groups which received different volumes of reference vaccine A per dose. The third dose consisted of 1 ml of vaccine J for all groups[65–67]

Antibody titre*	*Percentages after a primary immunizing dose of:* 2 ml		1 ml		1/2 ml		1/4 ml		1/8 ml		1/16 ml		None	
	Pre	*Post*	Pre	*Post*	Pre	*Post*	Pre	*Post*	Pre	*Post*	Pre	*Post*	Pre	*Post*
⩾4	92.0		84.7		60.0		72.8		45.2		35.3		0	*78.8*
⩾8	84.0		61.7		40.0		45.6		29.1		14.8			*51.6*
⩾16	68.0		42.5		30.0	*100.0*	22.9		13.0	*100.0*	6.0	*100.0*		*33.5*
⩾32	24.0		11.8		15.0	*96.2*	9.3		3.4	*93.4*	3.1	*96.2*		*6.3*
⩾64	8.0		8.0		0	*92.4*	0	*100.0*	0	*80.1*	0	*80.9*		*3.3*
⩾128	0	*100.0*	0			*80.9*		*96.3*		*56.8*		*34.8*		*0*
⩾256		*95.9*		*100.0*		*73.3*		*70.4*		*33.5*		*15.6*		
⩾512		*91.8*		*95.3*		*69.5*		*40.8*		*16.9*		*4.1*		
⩾1024		*83.5*		*85.8*		*46.5*		*29.7*		*10.3*		*4.1*		
⩾2048		*75.2*		*52.5*		*19.6*		*14.9*		*7.0*		*0*		
⩾4096		*54.4*		*28.7*		*15.8*		*11.2*		*3.7*				
⩾8192		*25.3*		*14.5*		*12.0*		*7.5*		*0*				
⩾16000		*8.7*		*9.8*		*4.4*		*7.5*						
⩾32000		*4.6*		*5.1*		*0*		*3.8*						
⩾64000		*0*		*0*				*0*						
Antibody Mean†														
Pre	13		9		5		5		<4		<4		<4	
Post		*2534*		*1846*		*573*		*423*		*128*		*78*		*6*
Subjects	26	*24*	26	*21*	21	*26*	22	*27*	31	*30*	24	*26*	33	*33*

* Reciprocal of serum dilution capable of neutralizing 100 $TCID_{50}$ type I virus.

† Geometric mean antibody titre.

‡ Number from whom serum samples were available.

high levels of circulating antibody, and therefore faecal, as well as pharyngeal, transmission of poliovirus can be affected by killed poliovirus vaccine (this will be discussed more fully in the following section).

Practical and societal considerations will influence the choice of killed virus vaccine potency and the schedule of immunization preferred in different countries[10].

Table 8 Comparative estimation of type I immune status: detectable serum antibody *vs.* secondary-type responsiveness. (Data taken from Tables 6 and 7)

*No. subjects**	*Primary dose†*	*Percentage of group with detectable antibody (⩾1:4)*		*Percentage of group with secondary-type antibody response (⩾1:32)§*
		2 weeks after one dose	*1 year after two doses*	*2 weeks after booster dose‡*
33	None	—	—	6
24	2	100	92	100
21	1	100	85	100
26	1/2	96	60	96
27	1/4	93	73	100
30	1/8	87	45	93
26	1/16	77	35	96

*In the 2 weeks post-booster group.

†ml of reference vaccine A given in each of two doses 2 weeks apart.

‡1 ml of vaccine J.

§Antibody titre of 1:32 arbitrarily chosen as criterion for hyper-reactive secondary-type antibody response.

Table 9 Calculation of expected effectiveness rates for killed poliovirus vaccines of different hypothetical potencies, based on data and relationships shown in Figure 1. The potency of vaccine shown in Figure 1 is approximately 0.55. The potency of vaccine currently available[7,30,68,99] is greater than 0.8

*Vaccine potency**	*Effectiveness rate† after each dose*				*Doses required for desired effectiveness*	
	First	*Second*	*Third*	*Fourth*	⩾90%	⩾95%
1.0	100				1	1
0.9	90	99	99.9		1	2
0.8	80	96	99.2		2	2
0.7	70	91	97.4	99.2	2	3
0.6	60	84	93.6	97.6	3	4
0.5	50	75	87.5	93.8	4	‡
0.4	40	64	78.4	85.4	‡	‡
0.3	30	51	64.7	75.3	‡	‡

*Single-dose effectiveness rate divided by 100%.

†Expressed as cumulative percent of vaccinated individuals expected to be effectively immunized against paralysis.

‡Impractical.

There is a linear relationship between the number of doses of vaccine administered and the protection provided against paralysis in the United States in 1959 (Figure 1). Killed poliovirus vaccine used prior to 1959 was of low potency, and the vaccine which is now available produces a steeper dose-response curve than that shown in Figure 1. The effect of vaccines of different potencies is shown in Table 9, and it can be seen that a high-potency vaccine protects a greater proportion of individuals with fewer doses than a lower-potency vaccine.

The relationship shown in Figure 1 resembles a first-order chemical process such as the inactivation of virus particles, and suggests that vaccination protects against paralytic disease by 'inactivating susceptibility to paralysis'. Higher-potency vaccines produce steeper inactivation curves, resulting in a greater margin of safety in the inactivation of susceptibility throughout a

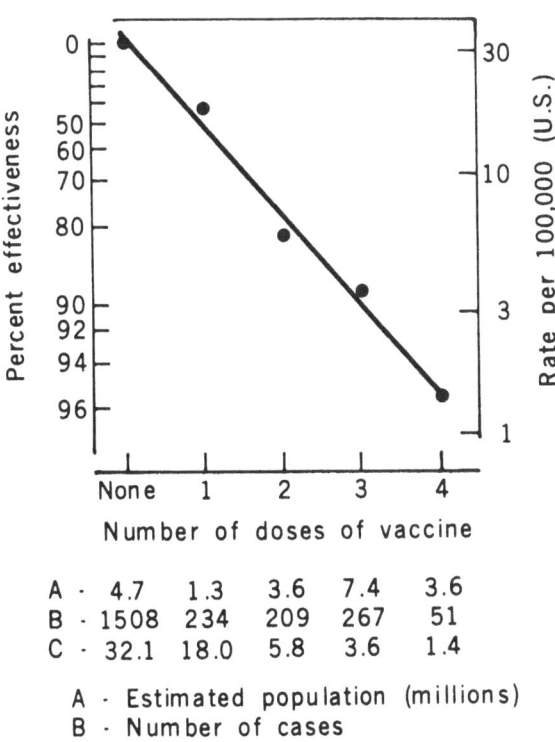

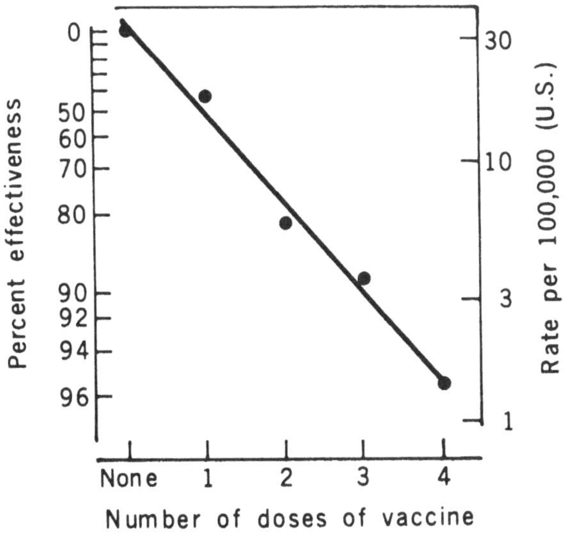

A ·	4.7	1.3	3.6	7.4	3.6
B ·	1508	234	209	267	51
C ·	32.1	18.0	5.8	3.6	1.4

A · Estimated population (millions)
B · Number of cases
C · Rate per 100,000

Figure 1 Relationship between killed poliovirus vaccination status and paralytic poliomyelitis attack rates in the 0–4-year-old age group in the United States in 1959. (The vaccine used in the United States between 1955 and 1959 was of low potency.) This inverse linear relationship on a semi-logarithmic plot suggests that with each succeeding dose the remaining susceptibles were reduced by the same proportion as by the first dose; or, in other words, it suggests first-order kinetics in the 'inactivation' of susceptibility to paralysis. (Adapted from Salk[13]; courtesy of *The Lancet*.)

population. The occurrence of paralytic polio in individuals with normal immune systems who have received several doses of vaccine (so-called 'vaccine failures') is a reflection of less than optimal vaccine potency, rather than a failure of the principles of vaccination.

Circulating antibody titres against poliovirus remain stable after an initial decline during the year following killed virus vaccination (Figure 2)[9,11,12].

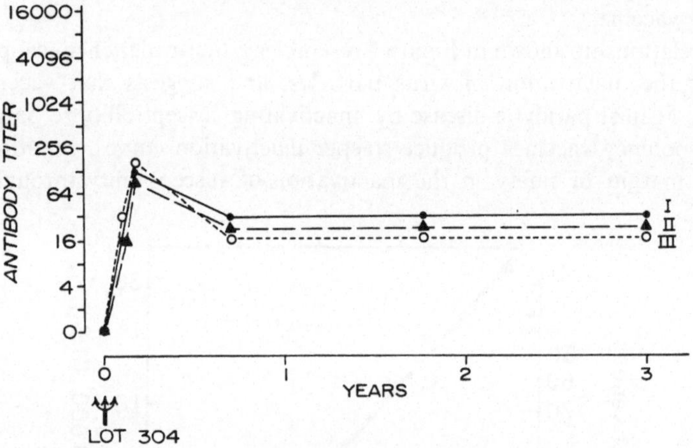

(a)

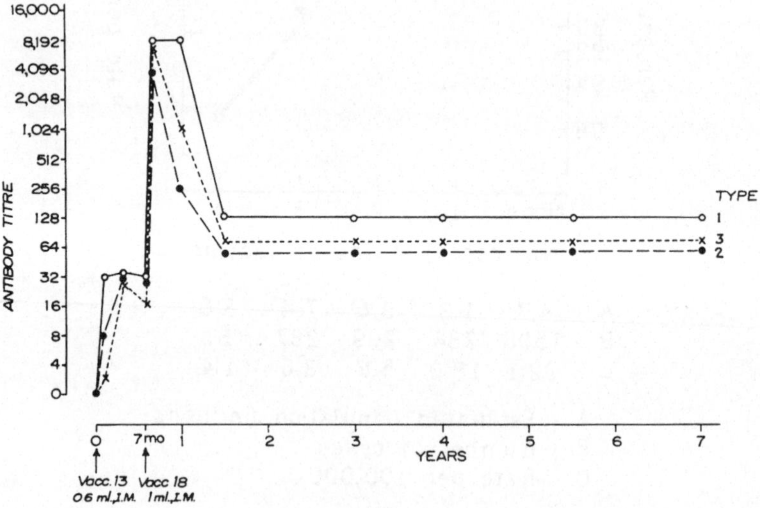

(b)

Figure 2 (a) Persistence of antibody 3 years after primary vaccination in a 7-year-old girl (from Salk[71]; courtesty of *Annals of Internal Medicine*); (b) Pattern of antibody response and persistence following a primary and booster immunization in a 10-year-old child followed for 7 years (from Salk[13]; courtesy of *The Lancet*). Response is typical of that seen in many children and is not an isolated finding

A plateau in level of antibody has been observed for at least 6 years following primary vaccination alone, as well as after a booster dose (Figures 3 and 4). Such persistence can be attributed to vaccination, and not to restimulation by infection, because infection in a vaccinated individual would result in a characteristic secondary-type antibody response against the infecting poliovirus type but not against the other two. Antibody persistence following killed poliovirus vaccine has been documented for as long as 12 years without booster doses; longer follow-up studies have not been done [13–16].

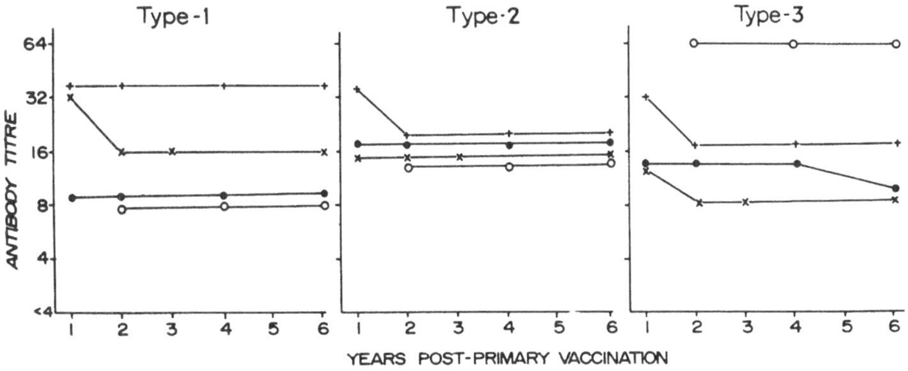

Figure 3 Antibody levels at 1–6 years after primary vaccination in triple-negative children. (Three doses 2 weeks apart; field trial vaccine, 1954). (From Salk[13]; courtesy of *The Lancet*.)

Immunologic memory persists even though circulating antibody may be undetectable (Figure 5); this has been observed as long as 7–8 years after the last dose of killed poliovirus vaccine[14]. Persistent immunologic memory alone, without detectable circulating antibody, appears to be effective in providing protection against paralysis. The rapid increase in circulating antibody titre, which is produced by a secondary-type immune response during the incubation period of poliomyelitis, will prevent transmission of poliovirus from its primary site of infection (the intestines) to its secondary site of infection (the central nervous system) (Figure 6)[17,18]. Although booster doses of vaccine reveal the presence of immunologic memory by eliciting a secondary-type antibody response, booster doses are not required in order to maintain immunologic memory[14].

The idea that persistent immunologic memory is sufficient for the prevention of paralysis is supported by serological and epidemiological data which demonstrate antigenic crossing between poliovirus types II and I, but not between types III and I[17,19]. Protection against paralysis from type I poliovirus is observed in individuals with detectable antibody against type II poliovirus only. Because of antigenic crossing, infection with type II wild poliovirus induces sufficient type I sensitization to result in a subsequent rapid secondary-type antibody response, even though there was no detectable type I antibody.

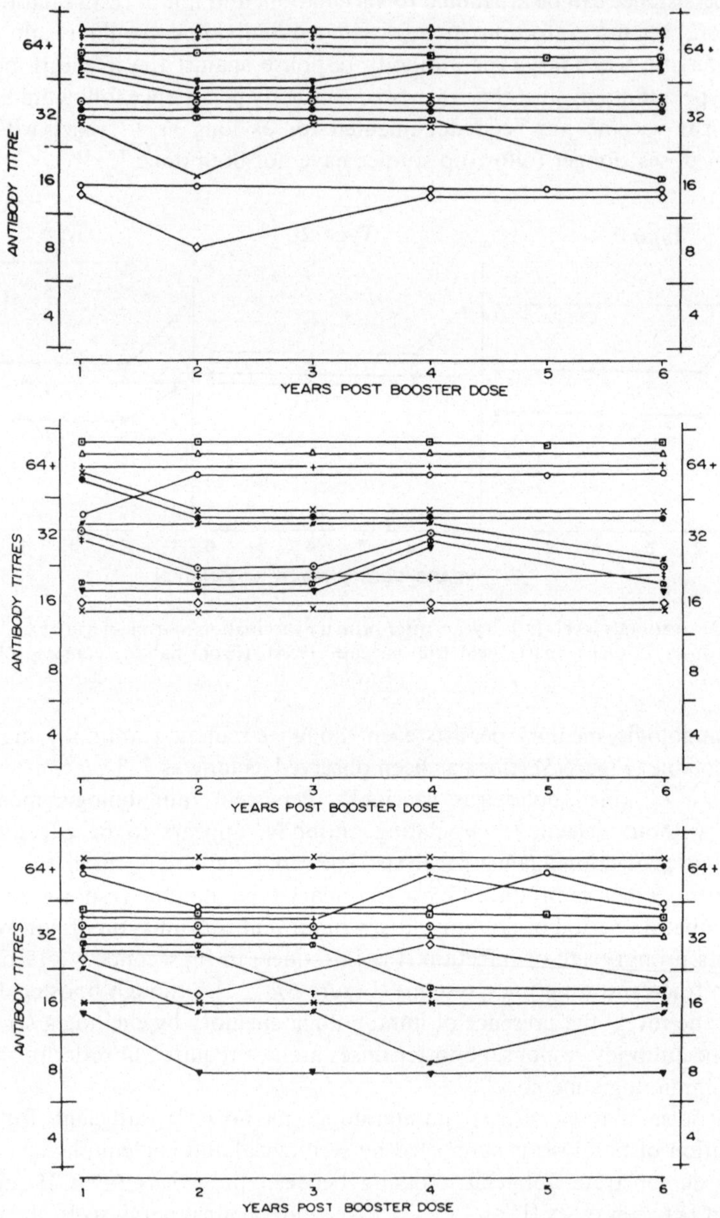

Figure 4 Types I, II, and III antibody levels at 1–6 years after booster in triple-negative children. The top, middle, and bottom portions of the figure refer to data for types I, II, and III, respectively. Two primary doses 2 weeks apart; a third dose (booster) 7 months to 1 year later. (From Salk[13]; courtesy of *The Lancet*.)

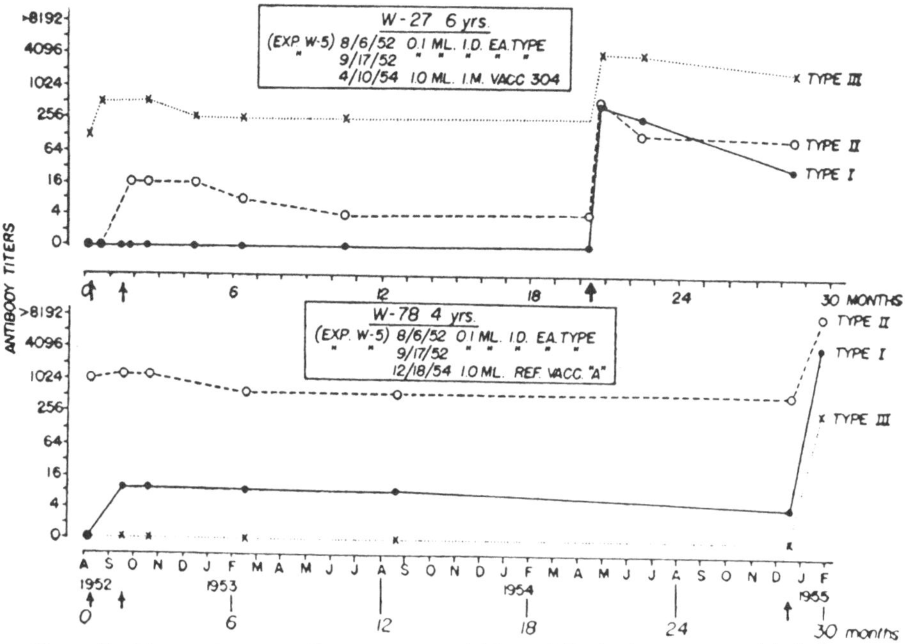

Figure 5 Observations over $2\frac{1}{2}$ years in two children of the first group inoculated. (From Salk[65]; courtesy of the *Journal of the American Medical Association.*)

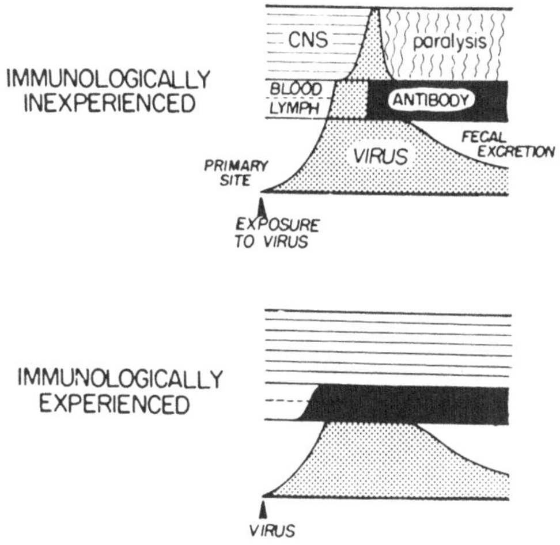

Figure 6 Schematic representation of the influence of previous immunological experience (infection or vaccination) on the prevention of paralysis from polio. In the immunologically experienced individual, the antibody response occurs sufficiently rapidly to block central nervous system invasion even without detectable antibody at the time of exposure. (From Salk[18]; courtesy of the *American Journal of Public Health.*)

COMMUNITY PROTECTION – HERD EFFECT

One of the principal reasons given in the past for favouring the use of a live poliovirus vaccine was its greater effect in reducing the quantity and duration of faecal virus excretion following a later feeding of attenuated virus. Because sufficiently high titres of circulating antibody were not induced by the low-potency killed vaccine initially used for testing, it appeared that the vaccine had little effect on the rate of faecal virus excretion[20]. Although subsequent studies demonstrated that killed poliovirus vaccine can reduce faecal excretion of virus[21–24], live poliovirus vaccine was still favoured because infection with attenuated live virus induces the formation of secretory immunoglobulin A (IgA) in the intestinal tract, whereas parenterally administered killed poliovirus vaccine does not (Figure 7). Although the serum immunoglobulin G (IgG) response to the killed virus vaccine is the same as the serum IgG response to the live virus vaccine, it was reasoned that the induction of IgA in the intestinal tract would more effectively reduce wild virus transmission; and that the use of the live virus vaccine could therefore lead to eradication of wild virus from the population, whereas the use of the killed virus vaccine could not[25].

This was a reflection of the belief that the principal mode of virus transmission was by the faecal–oral route. In countries with improved sanitation, however, pharyngeal transmission is probably more important; while in some of the underdeveloped countries where faecal–oral transmission may be significant, the antibody response to the live virus vaccine is irregular.

'Intestinal immunity' does not seem to be significant epidemiologically in view of the herd effect observed in areas where killed poliovirus vaccine alone has been widely used[3,15,16,22,26–28]. A sharp decline in the incidence of poliomyelitis in the United States followed the introduction of killed poliovirus vaccine in 1955 (Figure 8). By 1961 only about 54% of the total American population had received three or more doses of vaccine[29], and although the youngest age groups represented the majority of those vaccinated (Figure 9), the occurrence of a herd effect extended protection equally to non-vaccinated individuals of all ages (Figure 10). In each age group there was a 90–95% reduction of incidence of disease among the unvaccinated in 1961 when compared with the attack rates prior to the introduction of killed poliovirus vaccine. This indicates that there was a 90–95% reduction in the dissemination of wild poliovirus.

There is also evidence for the occurrence of a herd effect in European countries. Age-specific data from The Netherlands reveal a reduction in the incidence of polio in the unvaccinated population compared with the incidence prior to the start of killed virus vaccination programmes in late 1957 (Table 10). Children 1–9 years of age represented 74% of the poliomyelitis cases prior to 1957, and 67% of the cases between 1958 and 1965[30], and in this

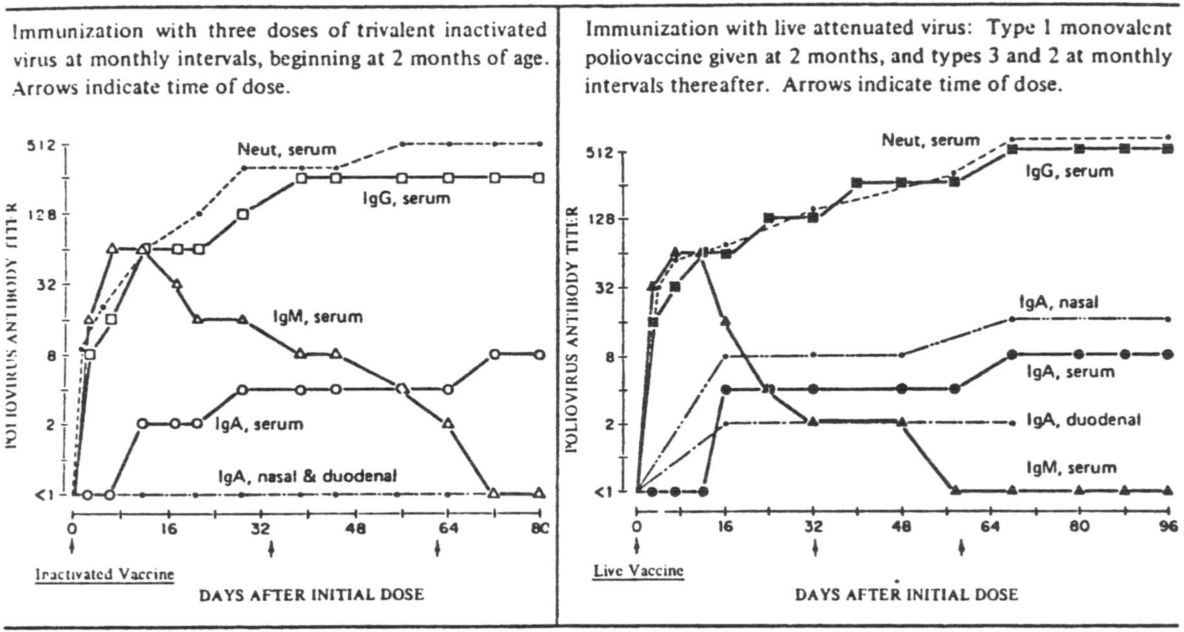

Figure 7 Comparison of responses to live oral and inactivated parenteral (Parke, Davis & Co. polio vaccine; 1967) poliovirus vaccines. Graphs show the detailed sequence of immunoglobulin G (IgG), immunoglobulin M (IgM), and immunoglobulin A (IgA) poliovirus antibody formation in serum and secretions after immunization. The serum neutralizing antibody response (Neut, serum) has been recorded for comparison. (From Ogra, *et al.*[72]; courtesy of Massachusetts Medical Society.)

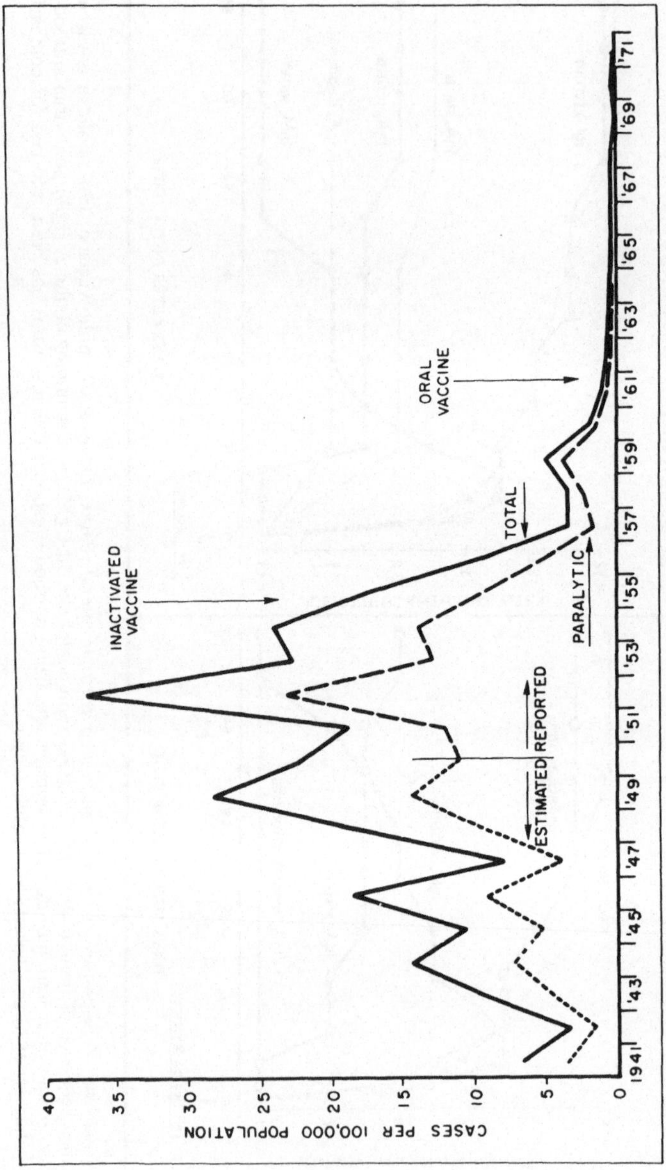

Figure 8 Polio incidence in the United States. Killed poliovirus vaccine (inactivated vaccine) introduced in 1955, and live poliovirus vaccine (oral vaccine) introduced in 1961–62. Broken line: paralytic polio only. Solid line: both paralytic and non-paralytic polio. (Courtesy of the Center for Disease Control (Atlanta)[73].)

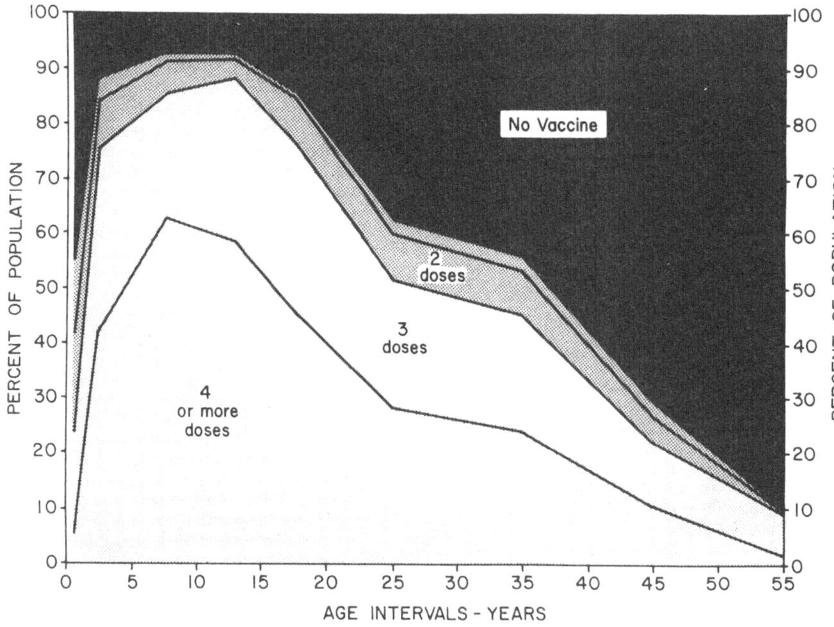

Figure 9 Estimated poliomyelitis vaccination status through September 1961. Of the American population below the age of 60, 53.6% had received three or more doses of killed poliovirus vaccine[29]. (From Salk[27]; courtesy of *Zentralblatt fur Bakteriologie*.)

Table 10 Evidence of a herd effect in The Netherlands after introduction of killed poliovirus vaccine in late 1957[30]. Percentage reduction in morbidity rates in 1958–65 compared with two pre-vaccine periods (1950–53 and 1954–57)

Age (years)	*Nonvaccinated: Percentage reduction compared with:*		*Three or more doses of vaccine: Percentage reduction compared with:*	
	1950–53	1954–57	1950–53	1954–57
<1	>89	>90	—	—
1–4	75	77	98.9	99.0
5–9	71	74	98.1	98.3
10–14	86	69	98.5	96.8
15–19	95	91	—	—
≥20	95	94	—	—

highly susceptible group, there was a reduction of approximately 75% in the incidence of disease among the unvaccinated.

Data from The Netherlands also show that the circulation of wild poliovirus was markedly decreased after the introduction of killed poliovirus

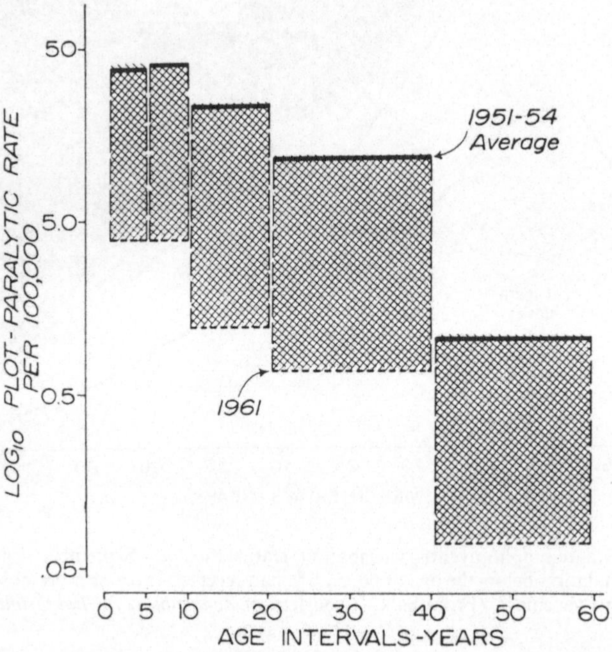

Figure 10 Herd effect induced by killed poliovirus vaccine in the United States. Age-specific paralytic poliomyelitis attack rates in the unvaccinated in 1961 compared with the average rates in 1951–54 before vaccine was available. (From Salk[55]; courtesy of the University of Toronto Press.)

vaccine (Figure 11). Unvaccinated children born since the start of significant vaccination programmes in 1960 (12 years of age or less in 1972) were not often exposed to wild virus and therefore did not develop anti-polio antibody.

After 1961–62 when the oral, live poliovirus vaccine was introduced into the United States, it was not possible to evaluate the potential of a killed poliovirus vaccine for eradicating wild virus from the population. However, experience in European countries where *only* a killed poliovirus vaccine has been used, has shown that it is possible to do so[15,16,31].

The pattern of polio decline in Finland and Sweden, for example, is shown in Figure 12. In these countries they have had essentially no domestic cases of polio since 1964 and 1966, respectively. In January 1977, one case of poliomyelitis with slight paresis occurred in an unvaccinated 2-year-old girl in Sweden. She belonged to a group believing in natural resistance to infection,

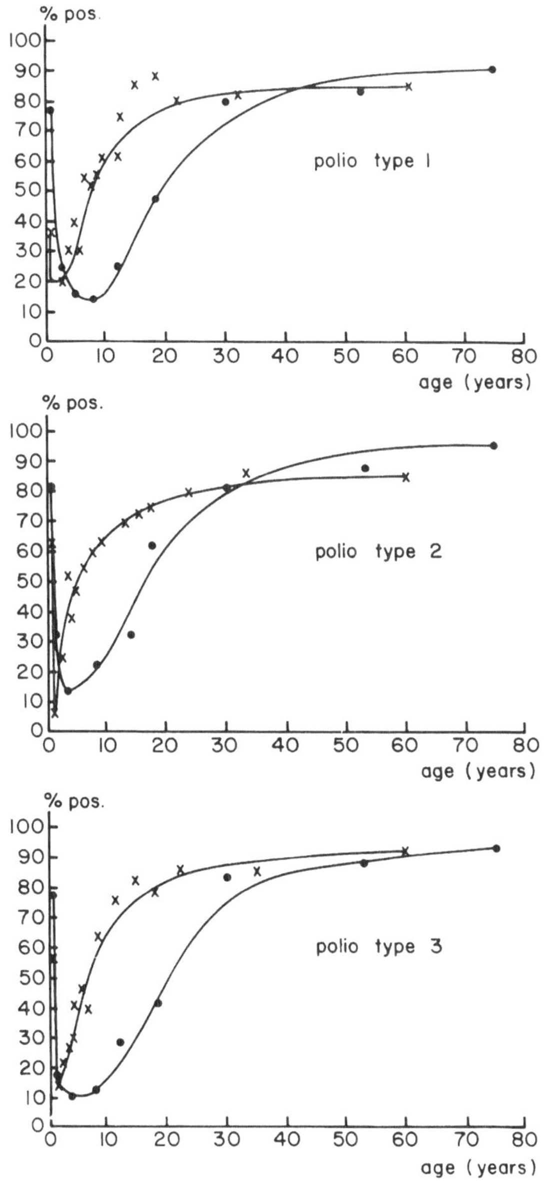

Figure 11 The effect of killed poliovirus vaccine on the circulation of wild poliovirus in The Netherlands. Spontaneous development of polio antibodies according to age – 1972 compared with 1960. × = 1960 (before significant vaccination programmes); ● = 1972 (unvaccinated population). (From Hoffman and Hekkens[74].)

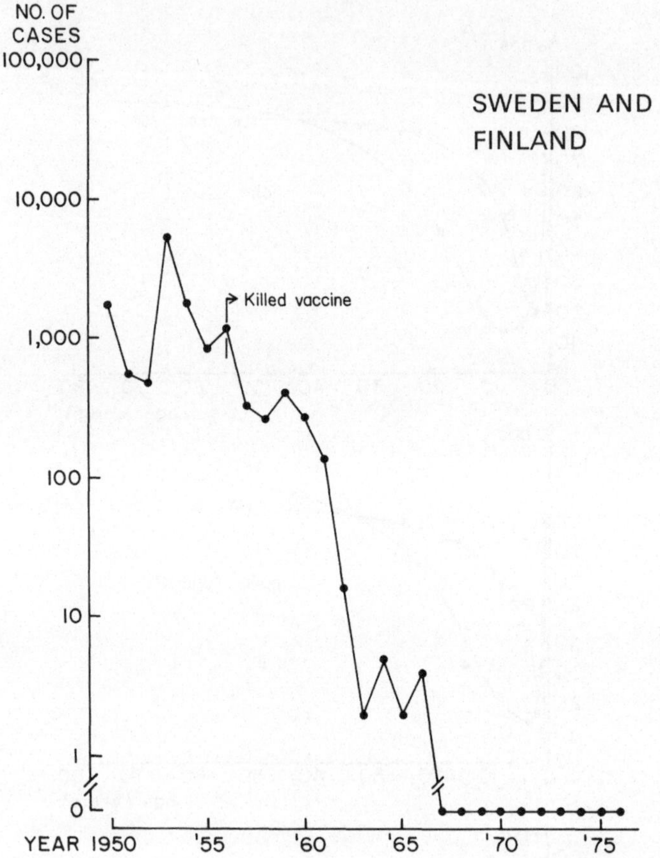

Figure 12 Total reported cases of poliomyelitis – Sweden[32] and Finland[75], 1950–1976. Data for 1950–1952 are for Sweden only

Table 11 Search for poliovirus in Finland, April 1972 to December 1974[33]

Source	*Number*	*Polio-virus*	*Other viruses (percentage)*
Patients Aseptic meningitis and meningo-encephalitis	308	0	52
Healthy children Preschool – 40 faecal samples per week	4878*	0	8–18
Helsinki sewage One sample per week	132	0	65

* Total number of samples from 4868 different children.

and many members of her community were not vaccinated. In addition, there was frequent contact with group members from elsewhere in Europe. Among 500 persons who were later investigated, 19 carriers were discovered[32]. Data soon to be published by Lapinleimu[33] from intensive poliomyelitis surveillance in Finland between April 1972 and December 1974 revealed no cases of poliomeylitis and no evidence of poliovirus (Table 11). Their experience indicates that they 'have not only eradicated poliomyelitis but have also eradicated the live virus'[31].

It is apparent that effective vaccination programmes using a killed poliovirus vaccine can reduce poliovirus dissemination to the point of eradication of domestic wild virus. A mechanism for this effect is suggested by studies demonstrating the absence of pharyngeal virus in individuals vaccinated with killed poliovirus vaccine and exposed to either wild-type or attenuated poliovirus. It is known that the period of highest communicability of naturally occurring paralytic poliomyelitis is more closely related to the presence of virus in the pharynx[34–38] than to the excretion of virus in the faeces (Figure 13), and these findings all suggest the importance of the oral–oral route of virus dissemination, especially when sanitation conditions are generally good.

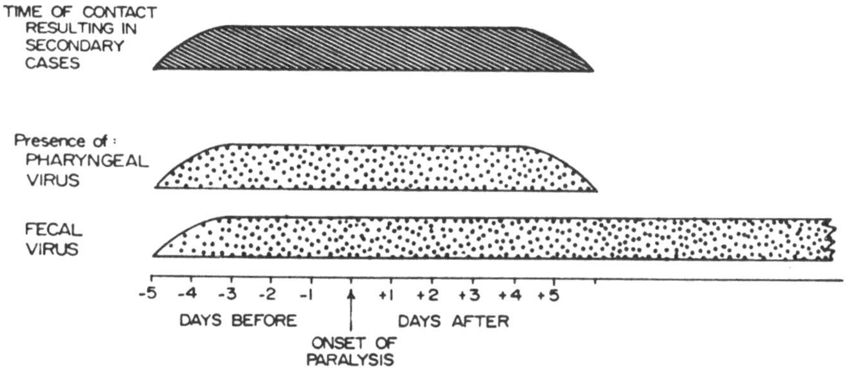

Figure 13 Approximate relationship of secondary cases of poliomyelitis to time of exposure to known paralytic cases. (From Salk[71]; courtesy of the *Annals of Internal Medicine*.)

Studies done in 1958[20], with individuals exposed to cases of paralytic polio, revealed a lower incidence of positive tests for virus in the pharynx of those who had been vaccinated with the killed poliovirus vaccine, compared with those who were unvaccinated. In other studies[39], tests for pharyngeal virus were uniformly negative after large amounts of attenuated strains were fed to children previously vaccinated with a killed poliovirus vaccine, although tests for pharyngeal virus were positive in 80% or more of unvaccinated controls.

The high incidence of pharyngeal virus in patients with wild or attenuated poliovirus infection is apparently due to secondary localization of virus from the blood, rather than to primary localization of ingested virus. Antibody in the blood blocks this secondary localization of 'viraemic' poliovirus in the throat, just as it blocks the secondary localization of poliovirus in the central nervous system (Figure 6). The idea that similar mechanisms are involved in community protection and protection against paralysis is supported by a comparison of Figures 1 and 10; three doses of the killed poliovirus vaccine then in use in the United States reduced community spread to the same degree that it reduced the rate of paralysis in individuals (approximately 90%).

In 1961, when the live virus vaccine was introduced into the United States, it was felt that the intestinal route of immunization was preferable, not only because of the induction of 'intestinal immunity', but also because the transmission of attenuated virus from vaccinated to non-vaccinated individuals would improve community protection by 'spreading immunity'. However, now that wild virus disease has been controlled in the United States, it has become apparent that the transmission of vaccine virus actually places the community at increased risk. The occurrence of vaccine virus-induced paralytic disease will be discussed more fully in the following section.

EFFECT OF VACCINATION PROGRAMME

The importance of the choice of vaccine and of vaccination programme in effectively eliminating paralytic poliomyelitis is shown by a comparison of the incidence of polio in Finland and Sweden (Figure 12) with the incidence in the United States and Great Britain (Figures 14 and 15).

The killed poliovirus vaccine was introduced in all these countries in the mid-1950s. In 1961 and 1962, the United States and Great Britain began using live poliovirus vaccine, while Finland and Sweden continued using the killed poliovirus vaccine exclusively. As already noted, there was a sharp decline in the incidence of paralytic poliomyelitis in the Scandinavian countries following the introduction of killed poliovirus vaccine, and they have had only a single case of paralytic polio in the last 11 years. In contrast, there was a slowing in the rate of decline in the United States and Great Britain beginning in the mid-1960s, and there has been a relatively constant number of cases since the beginning of this decade (Figure 16).

The slowing in rate of decline in the United States, England, and Wales after 1964–65 reflects both the presence of wild poliovirus activity in relatively unvaccinated subpopulations, and the occurrence of live virus vaccine-associated cases of paralytic poliomyelitis.

It is known that the live poliovirus vaccine can occasionally cause paralytic disease, but since the risk of acquiring polio from the attenuated virus is small, paralytic cases are less frequently observed in small populations and are less evident when wild poliovirus disease is prevalent. In the United States

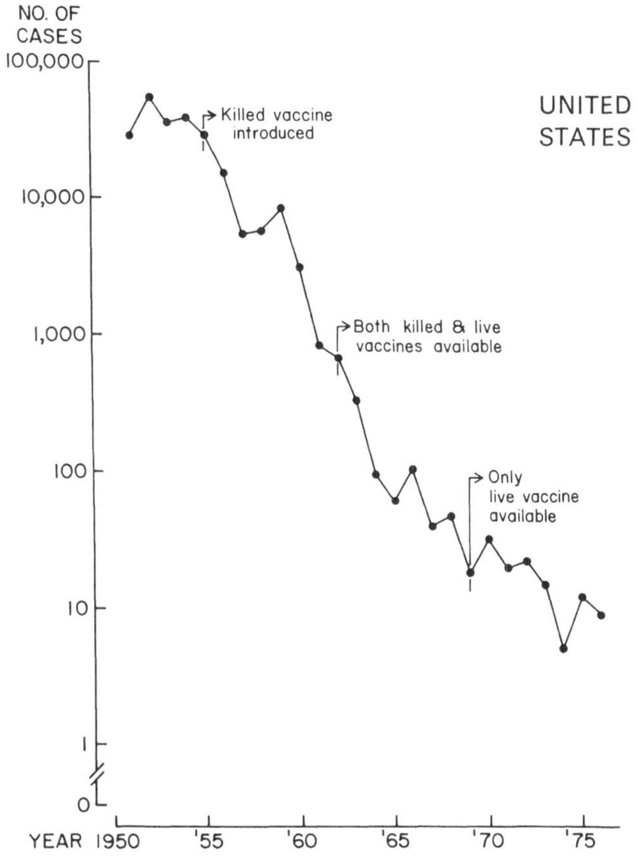

Figure 14. Poliomyelitis in the United States, 1951–76. These data reflect the total reported cases of poliomyelitis between 1951 and 1960[54,85], and the final revised count of paralytic poliomyelitis cases between 1961 and 1976[85]. On the scale in this figure, the numbers of total reported cases after 1961 (including non-paralytic and unspecified cases) do not differ significantly from the number of paralytic cases. The final revised paralytic case count is used since it represents the most accurate number for calculating the comparison discussed in Figure 17. Killed poliovirus vaccine was introduced in 1955, and live poliovirus vaccine in late 1961. After 1968, the killed poliovirus vaccine was not commercially available in the United States, except in the state of Michigan

since 1961, there have been more than 150 cases of paralytic poliomyelitis associated with the use of live poliovirus vaccine – an average of 10 or 11 per year. These cases have occurred at a relatively constant rate since the live virus vaccine was introduced in 1961–62, while the incidence of paralytic disease due to wild poliovirus has continued to decline (Figure 17). In 1976, all seven cases of domestically arising paralytic polio in the United States were vaccine-associated (Table 12).

The initial high incidence of live virus vaccine-associated polio in 1962–64

Table 12 Domestically arising paralytic poliomyelitis in the United States, 1976; all cases were live virus vaccine-associated[50,54]

	Age	*Sex*
Three immune-deficients		
Two recipients	9 months	Male
	7 months	Female
One contact	29 years	Female
Three household contacts	24 years	Female
	30 years	Male
	31 years	Female
One recipient	6 months	Female

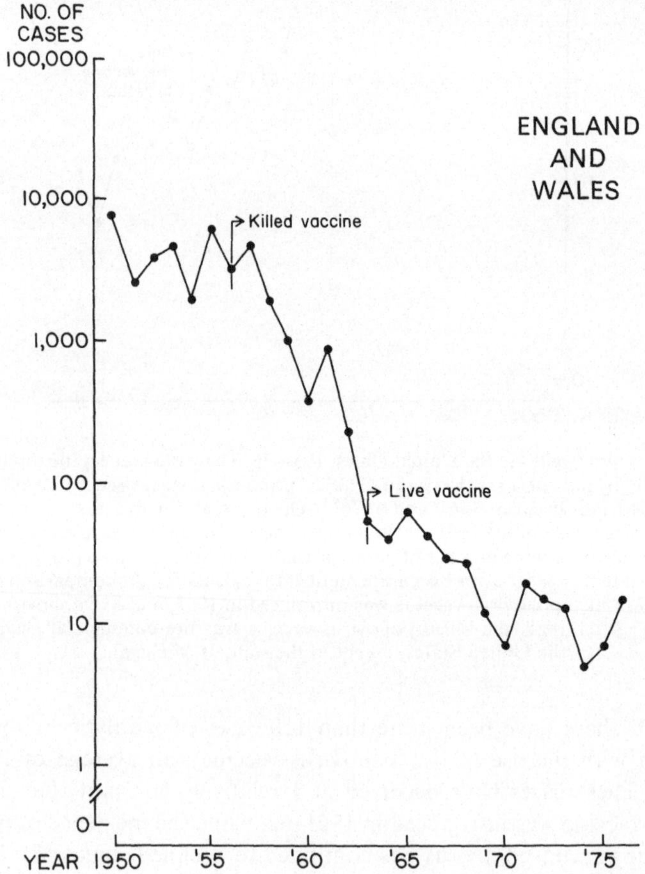

Figure 15 Total reported cases of poliomyelitis – England and Wales, 1950–76[76]. Killed poliovirus vaccine was introduced in 1956. The live poliovirus vaccine was introduced in 1963, and was essentially the only available vaccine in England and Wales after that time

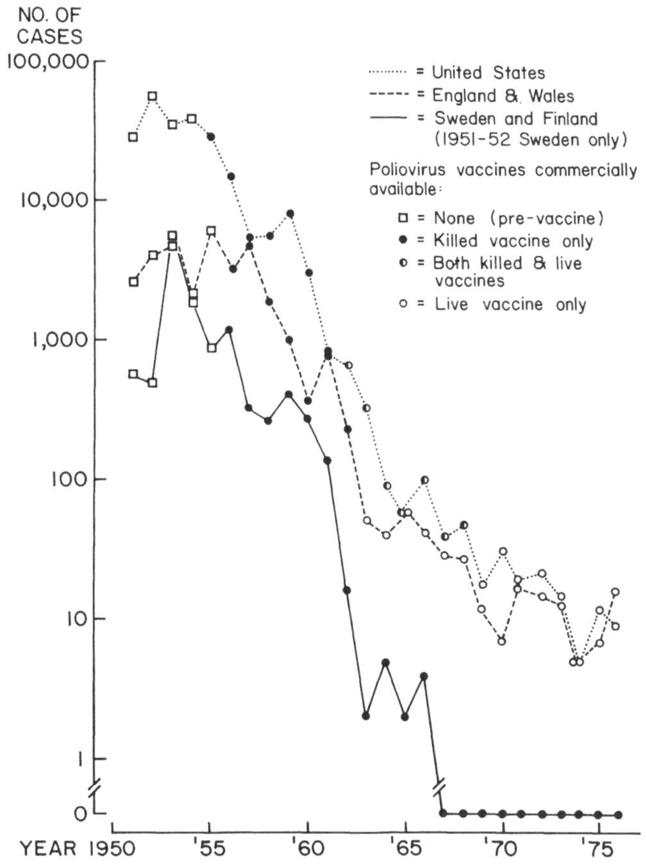

Figure 16 Poliomyelitis, 1951–76; composite of Figures 12, 14, and 15

reflects the mass immunization campaigns which included adults, many of whom were not previously vaccinated with the killed virus vaccine. After 1964 routine vaccination of adults was discontinued in the hope of avoiding vaccine-associated paralytic disease, but this change in policy had very little effect (Figure 17): disease continued to occur in adults exposed to vaccinated children, as well as in children who either received vaccine or were in contact with vaccinees. In addition, it became apparent in 1972 that vaccine-like virus was sometimes isolated from patients with paralytic polio who had had no known contact with the live virus vaccine[40]. These 'indirect community contact' cases had been observed frequently from 1965 to 1970, but had not previously been identified as vaccine-associated[41–45,78,79].

The identification of vaccine-associated paralytic polio is further complicated by the observation that the attenuated poliovirus can lose the antigenic characteristics which distinguish it from wild poliovirus, and 'wild-type' virus

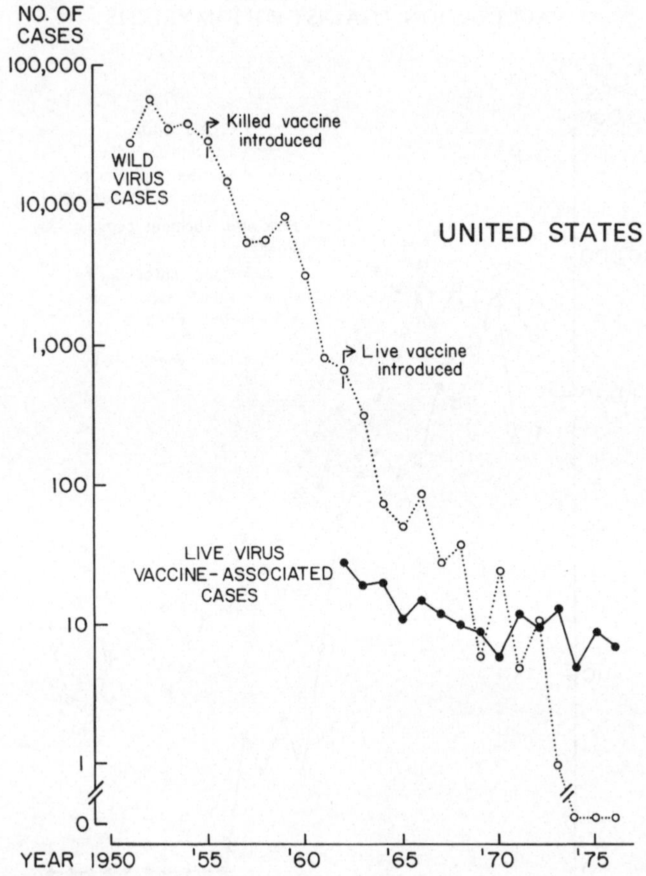

Figure 17 Poliomyelitis – United States, 1951–76. Wild virus cases: 1951–60, total reported cases; 1961–68, final revised paralytic case count; 1969–76, domestically arising paralytic cases. Live virus vaccine-associated cases: paralytic only. On the scale in this figure, the numbers of total reported cases after 1961 (including nonparalytic and unspecified cases) do not differ significantly from the number of paralytic cases. The final revised paralytic case count after 1961, and the domestically arising parayltic case count after 1969 are used since they represent the most accurate numbers for making a comparison with the number of live poliovirus vaccine-associated cases of paralytic poliomyelitis. In addition to cases defined as vaccine-associated by the Center for Disease Control (Atlanta), these data include previously unrecognized 'indirect community contact cases'. These cases are defined as those without a known history of contact with the live virus vaccine, which occur outside of areas where there is an epidemic outbreak of wild virus disease, and from which a virus has been isolated which can reasonably be considered to be vaccine-derived: type I poliovirus with vaccine-like or intermediate antigenic characteristics, or non-vaccine-like with negative temperature markers; type II, antigenically vaccine-like or intermediate; type III, antigenically vaccine-like with negative temperature markers[79]. Between 1965 and 1976 inclusive, there were 2, 6, 5, 4, 4, 4, 0, 2, 0, 1, 3, and 0 of these cases, respectively. One case in 1970 was in a patient with known exposure to the live virus vaccine, but was originally classified as 'not vaccine-associated' because the type I virus isolated was 'non-vaccine-like'; this case did not occur during an outbreak of wild virus disease, and probably represents loss of vaccine-like antigenic characteristics. Of the 1305 'wild virus cases' that occurred between 1962 and 1976, only 42 have studies reported on viral isolates which confirm the 'wild-type' antigenic characteristics of the virus[40–46,49,54,70,77–80]

has been isolated from known cases of vaccine-associated disease[47–51]. During multiplication in the intestinal tract, the attenuated poliovirus can apparently revert to the antigenic, temperature-sensitivity, and/or neurovirulence characteristics of the wild poliovirus. Thus, sporadic cases of paralytic poliomyelitis from which 'wild-type' virus is isolated, and for which there was no known exposure to either live virus vaccine or a source of wild poliovirus, may represent antigenic reversion of vaccine virus obtained by 'indirect community contact'.

In this regard, it is of interest to examine the last outbreak of polio in the United States, which occurred among unvaccinated students at a Christian Science boarding school in Connecticut in 1972. Eleven students (nine males and two females) developed poliomyelitis within 3–6 weeks of returning from vacation. Although virus characterized as wild-type was isolated from most of the paralysed individuals, a source of wild poliovirus was never identified, and vaccine-like virus was isolated from one male. This raises the question of whether the original source of virus in this outbreak might have been attenuated vaccine virus in the home community which one of the students visited during vacation. During multiplication and passage through the unprotected dormitory population at the school, the reverted neurovirulent virus could have lost the remaining genetic markers associated with 'vaccine-like virus'. It is known that the type I vaccine virus is particularly unstable: 97% of viral isolates from vaccine recipients are vaccine-like 1 week after feeding, but after 4 weeks only 11% are vaccine-like, 22% are intermediate, and 67% are non-vaccine-like[51].

The attenuated virus can become established in a human population. A recent study in Great Britain has reported isolation of vaccine-like strains of poliovirus from asymptomatic carriers and from patients with neurological disease more frequently than isolation of wild-type strains[52]. Cossart points out that 'about one-third of all of the strains studied came from persons without any definite contact with vaccine, so it is clear that, far from being eliminated, polioviruses are still circulating widely' (Ref. 52, p. 1623).

Because the live poliovirus vaccine produces infection in the human intestinal tract, use of this vaccine reseeds the natural virus reservoir. In an editorial commenting on Cossart's results, the *British Medical Journal* stated:

> This all suggests that at least some and perhaps most of the poliovirus strains causing disease in Britain today are vaccine strains that have reverted to some degree of virulence. The old, classic, virulent, wild strains may be on the way out, but they are being replaced by a new regiment apparently derived from vaccine strains (Ref. 53, p. 1617).

Although a population which is more fully vaccinated will contain fewer poorly immunized individuals who might be exposed to reverted vaccine virus, increasing the use of live poliovirus vaccine will not solve the problem of vaccine-associated polio. The spectrum of reported vaccine-associated cases indicates that there will be continued risk in the future (Table 12). As in the case of the 6-month-old girl in 1976, infants with normal immune status occasionally develop vaccine-associated paralytic disease[40-43,46,49,54], and as was true with vaccination against smallpox, immune-deficient individuals will always be at risk. Infants are routinely vaccinated before immune deficiency may be recognized, and known immune-deficient individuals, such as the 29-year-old woman in 1976, will be exposed to vaccine virus in the community.

The decline of polio incidence in the United States after 1961, and in Great Britain after 1962, cannot be attributed solely to the introduction of the oral, live poliovirus vaccine. By the time the live virus vaccine was introduced, use of the killed virus vaccine had resulted in a decline in incidence of disease of almost two orders of magnitude (approximately 90%) – poliomyelitis was already being brought under control.

Even after the introduction of the live virus vaccine, the proportion of individuals in the United States under the influence of the killed poliovirus vaccine was substantially greater (Figure 18); and moreover, the live virus vaccine was initially used largely by the segment of the population previously

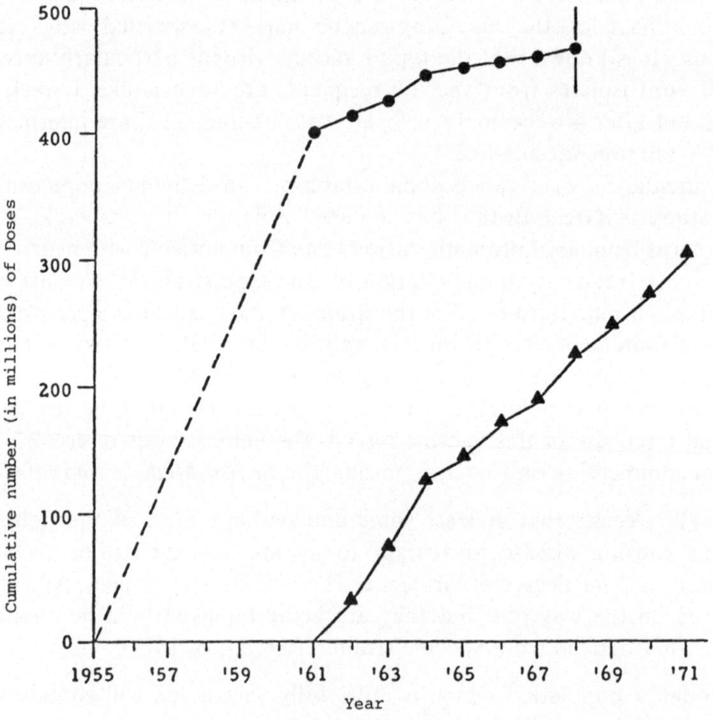

Figure 18 Cumulative number of doses of poliovirus vaccine distributed in the United States, 1955–71[73]. ● = killed virus vaccine; ▲ = live virus vaccine (Type 1 monovalent and trivalent)

immunized with the killed virus vaccine (Table 13). The majority of children who received three doses of live virus vaccine during the first 3 years of its use in the United States had previously received three or more doses of killed virus vaccine: 62% of the infants (ages 1–4 in 1964) and 82% of the young children (ages 5–9 in 1964 were 2–6 years old when the live virus vaccine was introduced).

Table 13 Killed poliovirus vaccination status (number of doses of KPV) of children who received 3 doses of live poliovirus vaccine (LPV) from 1961 through 1964[70]

Age in 1964 (years)	*No. (in thousands) and percentage of children who received three doses of LPV and who had previously received:* *Three or more doses of KPV*	*Less than three doses of KPV*	*Total children who received three doses of LPV*
1–4	4808 (62%)	2951 (38%)	7759 (100%)
5–9	9335 (82%)	1995 (18%)	11330 (100%)
1–9	14143 (74%)	4946 (26%)	19089 (100%)

Both in the United States and Great Britain, the effect of the live virus vaccine merely added to the effect of the killed virus vaccine: its introduction did not significantly *increase* the slope of the decline in the incidence of paralytic disease (Figures 8, 14 and 15) and, as already discussed, live virus vaccine-associated polio contributed to the relative *decrease* in slope after 1964–65 (Figure 16). There was no change in the decline of the incidence of disease caused by *wild* poliovirus after the live virus vaccine was introduced in the United States (Figure 17), and the decline in attack rate of wild virus disease is remarkably similar to the decline in Sweden and Finland where only the killed poliovirus vaccine was used (Figure 19).

As seen in Figure 19, there was a decrease in the rate of decline of wild poliovirus disease as the incidence became low: after 7 years of vaccination in the Scandinavian countries, and 9 years in the United States. This was predicted on theoretical grounds[27,55], and reflects both the relatively lesser role of the herd effect when more than 50% of a population is immunized, and the continued presence of pockets of wild poliovirus activity in relatively unvaccinated subpopulations.

The Scandinavian countries eradicated wild virus disease before the United States, and this was also predictable, based on their different geographical and population sizes[27]. Finland and Sweden are smaller than the United States, and they were therefore able to reach a critical level in the eradication of latent foci of infection more rapidly. They stressed vaccination of the highly susceptible age groups, and there were fewer poorly vaccinated groups in the Scandinavian countries. The single case of paralytic polio in Sweden in 1977 occurred in a child who was living in a group which was poorly vaccinated and which acted as a potential reservoir of wild virus. It is likely that this reservoir was seeded from outside, since the group was in frequent contact with members from elsewhere in Europe.

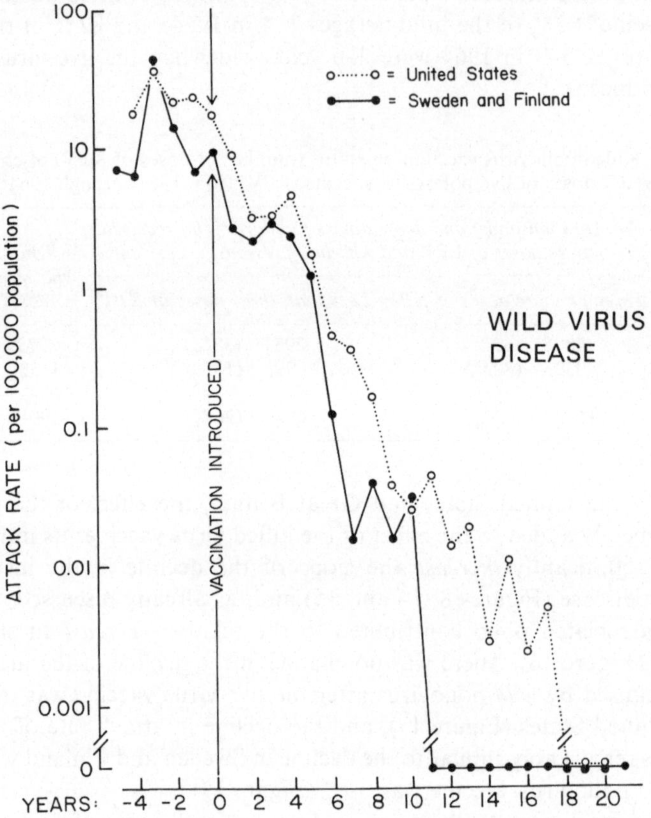

Figure 19 Attack rate (per 100 000 population) of wild poliovirus disease in Sweden and Finland compared with the United States. Rates calculated on the basis of data in Figures 12 and 17: United States population from the Bureau of Census mid-year estimates; for Sweden and Finland, rates calculated on the basis of a combined population of approximately 12.4 million

The increased risk for poorly vaccinated subpopulations in the United States is demonstrated by data collected during an outbreak of polio in Detroit, Michigan in 1958 which demonstrate that poliovirus activity was highest in the non-white community (Figure 20). The Chicago epidemic of 1956, the northern New Jersey epidemic of 1958, and several large and small outbreaks in the late 1950s all reflected a similar association with socio-economic and vaccination status[56–59,84]. Outbreaks of paralytic polio in Texas in 1970 and in a Christian Science boarding school in Connecticut in 1972 demonstrate that unvaccinated groups are at risk whether live or killed poliovirus vaccine is primarily in use.

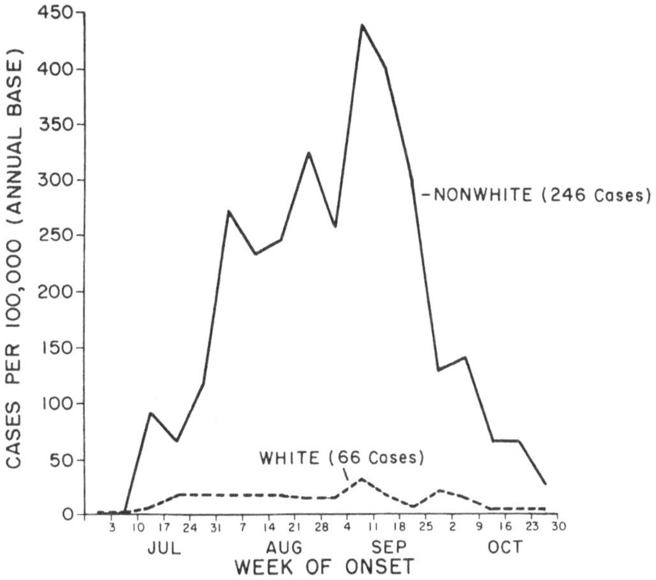

Figure 20 Paralytic poliomyelitis attack rates – Detroit, 1958. Population estimates: white = 1 480 000; non-white = 420 000; total = 1 900 000. (From Salk[81]; courtesy of the Royal Society of Health.)

The effect of choice of vaccine and vaccination programme has been demonstrated by the comparison of the decline in incidence of poliomyelitis in Finland and Sweden with the incidence in the United States and Great Britain. Two factors account for the differences observed:

1. Greater penetration of health care delivery in the smaller more homogeneous populations in the Scandinavian countries accounts for the more rapid elimation of wild virus disease observed there; and
2. Live virus vaccine-associated cases of paralytic poliomyelitis account for the relatively constant number of cases of paralytic poliomyelitis which continue to occur in the United States and in Great Britain.

INACTIVATION OF POLIOVIRUS

The inactivation of infectivity of poliovirus in formalin (37% formaldehyde) follows pseudo-first-order kinetics (Figure 21)[60,61]. The rate of inactivation of poliovirus is dependent on the concentration of formalin (Figure 21) and on the temperature, with deviation from first-order kinetics at lower temperature (Figure 22). Virus particles which are trapped in sediment may be protected from contact with formalin (Figure 23), but proper filtration removes these potentially infectious particles without significantly decreasing the amount of antigen present.

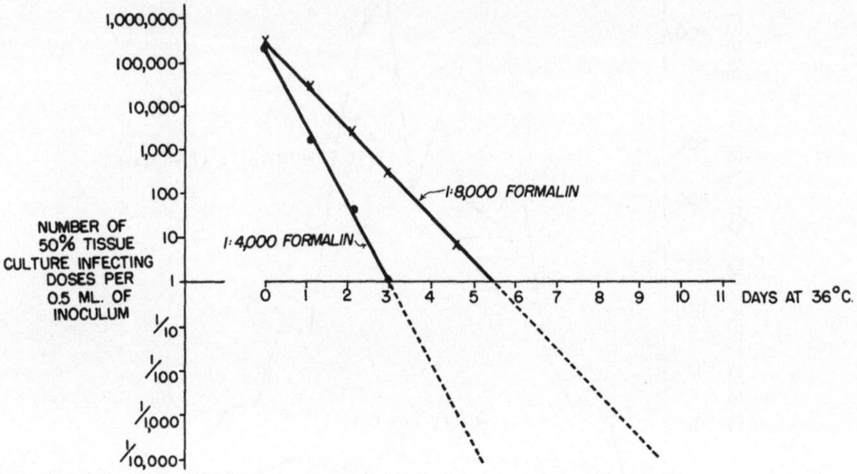

Figure 21 Rate of destruction of the infectivity of poliovirus in tissue culture fluid. Virus was treated with formalin at 36 °C and at pH 7.0. (From Salk and Gori[60]; courtesy of the New York Academy of Science.)

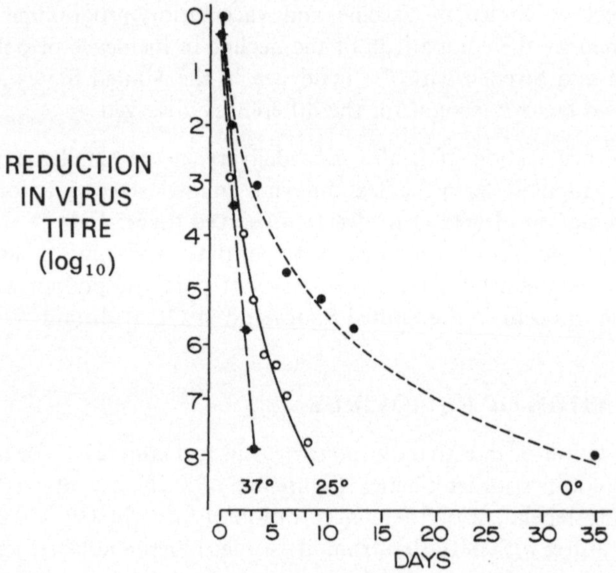

Figure 22 Effect of temperature on inactivation of poliovirus. (From Salk and Gori[60]; courtesy of the New York Academy of Science.)

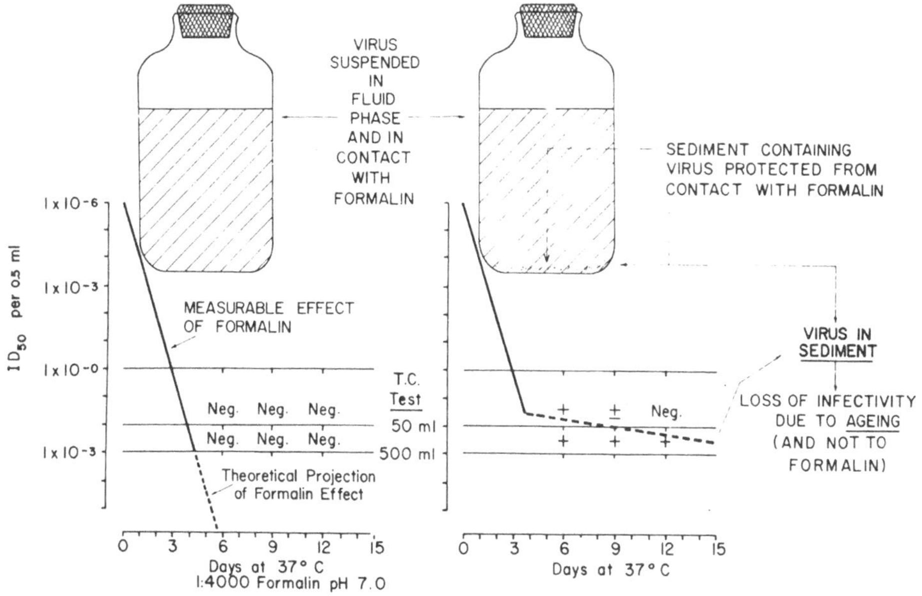

Figure 23 Effect of virus-formaldehyde contact upon the rate of destruction of virus infectivity. (From Salk[82]; courtesy of the *American Journal of Public Health.*)

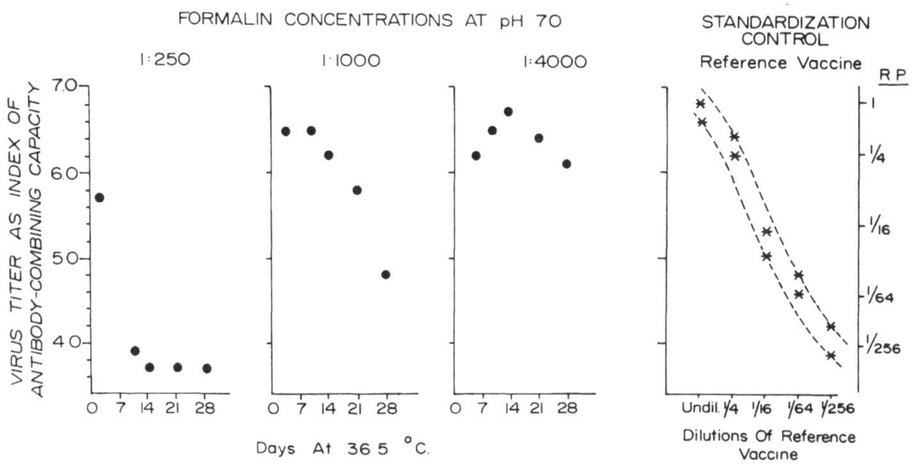

Figure 24 Rate of loss of antibody-combining capacity as a function of formalin concentration (Mahoney strain of type I poliovirus). R. P. is the relative potency as compared with the reference vaccine. (From Salk[83]; courtesy of the New York Academy of Science.)

Antigenicity of poliovirus is also affected by high concentrations of formalin (Figure 24), but there is a wide margin between the effects of formalin on antigenicity and on infectivity. Under conditions of vaccine manufacture, antigenicity is reliably maintained while infectivity is destroyed (Figure 25).

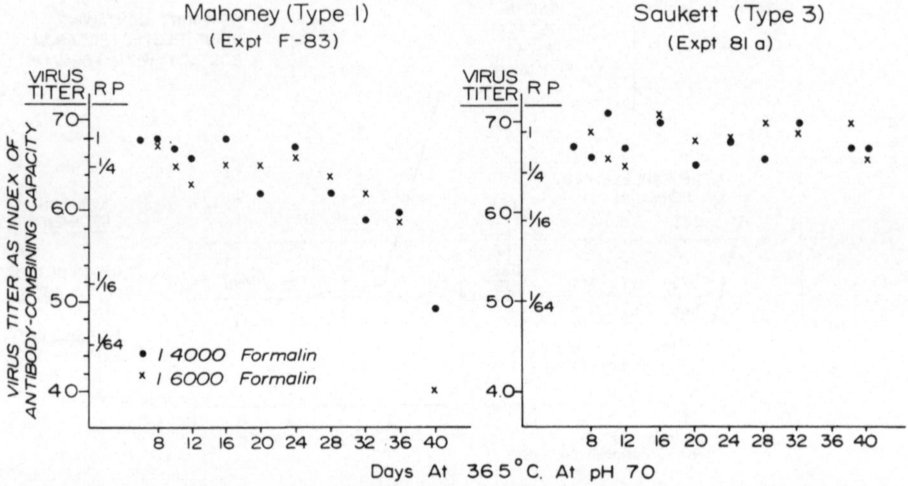

Figure 25 Degree of retention of antibody-combining capacity at intervals after the initiation of formalin treatment; infectivity is no longer demonstrable after 3 or 4 days. R. P. represents relative potency as compared with the reference standard as shown in the standardization in Figure 24. (From Salk [83]; courtesy of the New York Academy of Science.)

VACCINOLOGY

Immunization against infectious disease, like many other scientific endeavours, was initially developed by trial and error. Now that the relevant biological phenomena are better understood, we can approach the development and use of immunizing agents more rationally.

The study and application of the requirements for effective immunization might be called 'vaccinology'. This body of knowledge would include an understanding of the fundamental properties of the immune system and of specific immunogens. Each disease presents different problems, and these require solutions based on an understanding of the *aetiological agents*, the *pathogenic mechanisms*, and the *epidemiology* peculiar to each disease. Applied vaccinology would involve the combined application of basic knowledge and practical solutions to the development of effective vaccination programmes suitable for particular population groups.

In order for vaccination to protect against the pathological consequences of infection, it must induce an *appropriate* immune response. Differences in the pathogenic mechanisms of different diseases must be considered. In the case of influenza, for example, it is necessary to protect against infection itself; whereas in the case of diphtheria or tetanus, it is necessary only to protect against the toxin produced subsequent to infection. Similarly for polio, in order to protect against paralysis it is necessary only to prevent secondary localization of poliovirus in the central nervous system; primary intestinal infection does not produce significant pathology in this disease.

Stimulation of the immune system with a *sufficient quantity* of antigen will result in a response which is *specific* for that antigen. The humoral immune system reacts initially with both a *primary antibody response* and the induction of *immunologic memory*. Immunologic memory is revealed by a *secondary antibody response* following restimulation. This 'hyper-reactive' response occurs more rapidly and produces more antibody than that following primary stimulation. There is a direct dose–response relationship between the quantity of antigen used for primary stimulation, and the level of both the primary and secondary antibody responses[10]. These relationships can be utilized in establishing the optimal dose of antigen required to induce an appropriate immune response against a specific pathogenic organism.

Protection of non-vaccinated members of a population by the herd effect can be maximized by appropriate vaccination programmes, and eradication of a pathogenic organism from a population is possible under certain circumstances. The social, political, and cultural characteristics of the population, as well as the epidemiological characteristics of the disease in those particular circumstances, must be considered in developing effective vaccination programmes. Periodic re-evaluation of programmes is necessary so as to adjust to changing circumstances.

Before the development of tissue culture techniques which could provide large quantities of virus, antiviral vaccines depended on the uncontrollable multiplication of attenuated virus in the vaccinated person in order to provide a sufficient *quantity* of a suitably *specific antigen* for stimulation of the immune system. However, improved technology now allows for the production of large quantities of concentrates of virus particles, which can be rendered non-infectious in a variety of ways, and can even be split into sub-units which retain specific antigenicity appropriate for protection against the pathological consequences of infection. Controllable chemical and biological phenomena can be exploited on a large scale in the development and preparation of non-infectious vaccines.

SUMMARY

Application of basic knowledge about the manipulation of viral antigens, the immune response of individuals, and the response of populations to programmes of vaccination can help solve the residual problems in the control of paralytic poliomyelitis in the world today. In areas of the world where polio is well controlled, and live virus vaccine-associated paralytic poliomyelitis is recognized, routine use of killed poliovirus vaccine will prevent the occurrence of vaccine virus-associated disease, and will maintain control of the wild virus disease. This will lead to eradication of both the attenuated and wild polioviruses circulating in a population. In areas of the world where poliomyelitis is endemic, killed poliovirus vaccine administered parenterally can effectively control the disease, and avoids the problem of intestinal inhibitors which interfere with the establishment of immunity following vaccination with the live poliovirus vaccine. In addition, killed poliovirus vaccine potency can be adjusted, and the most appropriate immunization schedule for any particular set of circumstances can be reliably achieved: it is possible to use a combined DTP–polio vaccine, or a polio vaccine which will provide effective immunity following a single dose. Although it will be many decades before worldwide eradication of poliovirus is achieved, it may some day be possible to contemplate eliminating routine immunization against paralytic poliomyelitis, just as we have eliminated routine immunization against smallpox in many parts of the world today.

References

1. John, J. (1977). Christian Medical College and Hospital, Vellore, India personal communication
2. Goldblum, N. (1977). Hebrew University, Jerusalem, Israel, personal communication
3. Beale, A. J. (1969). Immunization against poliomyelitis. *Br. Med. Bull.*, **25** (2), 148
4. Ghosh, S., Kumari, S., Balaya, S. and Bhargava, S. K. (1970). Antibody response to oral polio vaccine in infancy. *Indian Pediatr.*, **7**(11), 1
5. Fillastre, C., N'da, K., Orssaud, E., Chippaux, A., Dutertre, J. and Gurin, N. (1976). Un Essai Controle de Vaccination Antipoliomyelitque en Cote D'Ivoire. A report presented before Onzieme Conference Technique de Organization de Coordination pour la Lutte Contres les Endemies en Afrique Centrale, Yaounde, 25–27 March
6. Cohen, H., Hofman, B., Brouwer, R., van Wezel, A. L. and Hannik, C. A. (1973). In F. T. Perkins (acting ed.,). *International Symposium on Vaccination Against Communicable Disease*, pp. 131–141 (Basel: Karger)
7 Wilson, R. J. (1976). Connaught Laboratories Limited, Willowdale, Ontario, Canada, personal communication concerning data on 12 lots of vaccine produced in 1974 and 1975
8. Bijkerk, H. (1973). In F. T. Perkins (acting ed.). *International Symposium on Vaccination Against Communicable Diseases*, pp. 271–276 .(Basel: Karger)
9. Salk, J. and Salk, D. (1977). Control of influenza and poliomyelitis with killed virus vaccines. *Science*, **195**, 834
10. Salk, J. and Salk, D. In E. Kurstak (ed.). *Viruses and Environment: Proceedings of the Third International Conference on Comparative Virology*, (New York, Academic Press). (In press)
11. Bottiger, M. (1969). Sero-immunity to poliomyelitis virus in Sweden 10 years after introduction of vaccinations with inactivated poliovirus vaccine. A pilot study, *Acta Pathol. Microbiol. Scand.*, **76**, 106
12. Brown, G. C. (1961). In *Poliomyelitis: Papers and Discussions Presented at the Fifth International Poliomyelitis Conference*, pp. 146–154 (Philadelphia: J. B. Lippincott)
13. Salk, J. (1960). Persistence of immunity after administration of formalin-treated poliovirus vaccine, *Lancet*, **ii**, 715
14. Bottiger, M. (1973). Antibody stimulation in individuals without demonstrable poliovirus antibodies following a fifth injection of inactivated poliovirus vaccine, *Acta Pathol. Microbiol. Scand. B*, **81**, 795
15. Lundbeck, H. (1973). In F. T. Perkins, (acting ed.). *International Symposium on Vaccination Against Communicable Diseases*, pp. 279–286. (Basel: Karger)

16. Noro, L. In F. T. Perkins (acting ed.). *International Symposium on Vaccination Against Communicable Diseases*, pp. 279–286. (Basel: Karger)
17. Salk, J., 'A concept of the mechanism of immunity for preventing paralysis in poliomyelitis,' *Ann. N. Y. Acad. Sci.* **61**: 1023 (1955).
17. Salk, J., A concept of the mechanism of immunity for preventing paralysis in poliomyelitis, *Ann. N. Y. Acad. Sci.*, **61**, 1023 (1955).
18. Salk, J. (1955). Vaccination against paralytic poliomyelitis – performance and prospects, *Am. J. Public Health*, **45**, 575
19. Salk, J. (1956). Requirements for persistent immunity to poliomyelitis, *Trans. Assoc. Am. Physicians*, **69**, 105
20. Wehrle, P. F., Reichert, R., Carbonaro, O. and Portnoy, B. (1958). Influence of prior active immunization on the presence of poliomyelitis virus in the pharynx and stools of family contacts of patients with paralytic poliomyelitis, *Pediatrics*, **21**, 353
21. Bodian, D. (1961). Poliomyelitis immunization, *Science*, **134**, 819
22. Marine, W. M., Chin, T. D. Y. and Gravelle, G. R. (1962). Limitation of fecal and pharyngeal poliovirus excretion in Salk-vaccinated children: A family study during a type I poliomyelitis epidemic, *Am. J. Hyg.*, **76**, 173
23. Henry, J. L., Jaikarau, E. S., Davies, J. R., Tomlinson, A. J. H., Mason, P. J., Barnes, J. M. and Beale, A. J. (1966). A study of poliovaccination in infancy: excretion following challenge with live virus by children given killed or living poliovaccine. *J. Hyg., Camb.*, **64**, 105
24. Dane, D. S. (1964). The future of inactivated poliomyelitis vaccines. *Proc. R. Soc. Med.*, **57**, 462
25. Report to the American Medical Association House of Delegates, 'The present status of poliomyelitis vaccination in the United States – summary statement of the Council on Drugs' (20 June, 1961).
26. Stickle, G. (1964). Observed and expected poliomyelitis in the United States, 1958–1961. *Am. J. Public Health*, **54**, 1222
27. Salk, J. (1963). Polio immunization and the herd effect. *Zentrabl. Bakteriol.*, **191**, 68 (Abstr. 1 Orig.)
28. Hofman, B. (1972). Poliomyelitis in the Netherlands 1958–69: the influence of a vaccination programme with inactivated poliovaccine. *Bull. W.H.O.*, **45**, 735
29. Sirken, M. G. (1962). National participation trends, 1955–61 in the poliomyelitis vaccination program. *Public Health Repts.*, **77**, 661
30. Hofman, B. (1967). Poliomyelitis in the Netherlands before and after vaccination with inactivated poliovaccine. *J. Hyg.*, **65**, 547
31. Lundbeck, H., Halonen, P. and Griffith, A. H. (1973). In F. T. Perkins (acting ed.). *International Symposium on Vaccination Against Communicable Diseases*, pp. 319–320. (Basel: Karger) General discussion
32. Bottiger, M. (1977). In *Institute of Medicine Evaluation of Poliomyelitis Vaccines: Report of the Committee for the Study of Poliomyelitis Vaccines*, Vol. II, Appendix C – Contributed Papers, pp. 107–118. (Washington, DC: National Academy of Sciences)
33. Lapinleimu, K. (1976). Central Public Health Laboratory, State Serum Institute, Helsinki, Finland, personal communication
34. Casey, A. E. (1942). The incubation period in epidemic poliomyelitis. *J. Am. Med. Assoc.*, **120**, 805
35. Aycock, W. L. and Kessel, J. F. (1943). The infectious period of poliomyelitis and virus detection. *Am. J. Med. Sci.*, **205**, 454
36. Howe, H. A., Bodian, D. and Wenner, H. A. (1945). Further observations on the presence of poliomyelitis virus in the human boro-pharynx. *Bull. Johns Hopkins Hosp.*, **76**, 19
37. Horstmann, D. M., Melnick, J. L. and Wenner, H. A. (1946). The isolation of poliomyelitis virus from human extra-neural sources. I. Comparison of virus content of pharyngeal swabs, oropharyngeal washings, and stools of patients. *J. Clin. Invest.*, **25**, 270
37a. Horstman, D. M., Ward, R. and Melnick, J. L. (1946). The isolation of poliomyelitis virus from human extra-neural sources. III. Persistence of virus in stools after acute infection. *J. Clin. Invest.*, **25**, 278
38. Wenner, H. A. and Tanner, W. A. (1947). Widespread distribution of poliomyelitis in households attacked by the disease. *Proc. Soc. Exp. Biol. Med.*, **66**, 92

39. Sabin, A. B. (1959). Present position of immunization against poliomyelitis with live virus vaccines. *Br. Med. J.*, **1**, 663
40. Center for Disease Control (Atlanta) (Feb. 1974). *Neurotropic Diseases Surveillance: Poliomyelitis, Annual Summary 1972.* (Washington, DC: Printing Office)
41. National Communicable Disease Center (July 1967). *Neurotropic Viral Diseases Surveillance: Poliomyelitis, Annual Summary 1966.* (Washington, DC: Government Printing Office)
42. National Communicable Disease Center (June 1968). *Neurotropic Viral Disease Surveillance: Poliomyelitis, Annual Summary 1967.* (Washington, DC: Government Printing Office)
43. National Communicable Disease Center (June 1969). *Neurotropic Viral Disease Surveillance: Poliomyelitis, Annual Summary 1968.* (Washington, DC: Government Printing Office)
44. National Communicable Disease Center (June 1970). *Neurotropic Viral Diseases Surveillance: Poliomyelitis, Annual Summary 1969.* (Washington, DC, Government Printing Office)
45. Center for Disease Control (Atlanta). (Sept. 1971). *Neurotropic Diseases Surveillance Poliomyelitis, Annual Summary 1970.* (Washington, DC: Government Printing Office)
46. Center for Disease Control (Atlanta). (Mar. 1973). *Neurotropic Diseases Surveillance: Poliomyelitis, Annual Summary 1971*
47. Davis, L. E., Bodian, D., Price, D., Butler, I. J. and Vickers, J. H. (1977). Chronic progressive poliomyelitis secondary to vaccination of an immunodeficient child. *N. Engl. J. Med.*, **297**(5), 241
48. Sencer, D. J. (1975). Center for Disease Control, Atlanta, Georgia, USA (personal communication)
49. Center for Disease Control (Atlanta) (Feb. 1975). *Neurotropic Diseases Surveillance: Poliomyelitis, Annual Summary 1973.* (Washington, DC: Government Printing Office)
50. Center for Disease Control (Atlanta) (1977). personal communication
51. Nakano, J. H., Gelfand, H. M. and Cole, J. T. (1963). The use of a modified Wecker technique for serodifferentiation of type I polioviruses related and unrelated to Sabin's vaccine strain. II. Antigenic segregation of isolates from specimens collected in field studies. *Am. J. Hyg.*, **78**, 214
52. Cossart, Y. E. (1977). Evolution of poliovirus since introduction of attenuated vaccine. *Br. Med. J.*, **1**, 1621
53. Polio vaccines and polioviruses (editorial) (1977). *Br. Med. J.*, **1**, 1617
54. Center for Disease Control (Atlanta) (Oct. 1977). *Neurotropic Diseases Surveillance: Poliomyelitis, Annual Summary 1974–76.* (Washington, DC: Government Printing Office)
55. Salk, J. (1965). Mechanisms of immunity in virus infections. *Recent Prog. Microbiol.*, **8**, 388
56. Langmuir, A. D. and Alexander, E. R. (1960). Present vaccination status of United States population and effectiveness of Salk vaccine. *Bull. Acad. Med. New Jersey*, **6**(3), 91
57. The National Foundation for Infantile Paralysis, New York (1958). (The National Foundation-March of Dimes, White Plains, NY), *Poliomyelitis Annual Statistical Review*
58. Langmuir, A. D. (1961). In *Poliomyelitis: Papers and Discussions Presented at the Fifth International Poliomyelitis Conference*, pp. 105–113. (Philadelphia: J. B. Lippincott)
59. Langmuir, A. D. (1959). Effectiveness of the vaccine. A report on the surveillance of poliomyelitis in the United States, 1955 to 1958. *J. Am. Osteopathic Assoc.*, **58**, 583
60. Salk, J. and Gori, J. B. (1960). A review of theoretical, experimental, and practical considerations in the use of formaldehyde for the inactivation of poliovirus. *Ann. N.Y. Acad. Sci.*, **83**, 609
61. Charney, J., Fischer, W. P. M., Sagin, J. F. and Tytell, A. A. (1960). Inactivation of concentrated purified poliovirus suspensions. *Ann. N.Y. Acad. Sci.*, **83**, 649
62. Zacarias, F. Z. (1977). In *Institute of Medicine Evaluation of Poliomyelitis Vaccines: Report of the Committee for the Study of Poliomyelitis Vaccines*, Vol. II, Appendix C – Contributed Papers, pp. 223–234. (Washington, DC: National Academy of Sciences)

63. Oduntan, S. O., Lucas, A. O. and Wennen, E. M. (1976). Department of Preventive and Social Medicine, University of Ibadan, Ibadan, Nigeria; personal communication of abstract, 'The immunological response of Nigerian babies to live and attenuated poliovaccines', presented before the Women's Medical Association Congress, Toyko
64. Center for Disease Control (Atlanta) (1975). *Immunization Against Disease*—1974. (Washington, DC: Government Printing Office)
65. Salk, J. (1955). Considerations in the preparation and use of poliomyelitis virus vaccine. *J. Am. Med. Assoc.*, **158**, 1239
66. Salk, J. (1956). Antigenic potency of poliomyelitis vaccine—influence on degree and duration of vaccine effect. *J. Am. Med. Assoc.*, **162**, 1451
67. Salk, J. (1958). How many injections of poliomyelitis vaccine for effective and durable immunity? *J. Am. Med. Assoc.*, **167**, 1
68. Halonen, P. (1976). Department of Virology, University of Turku, Turku Kiinamyl-lvnkatu, Finland (personal communication)
69. Cohen, H. (1975). Rijks Instituut voor de Volksgezondheid, Bilthoven, The Netherlands (personal communication)
70. Communicable Disease Center (June 1965). *Poliomyelitis Surveillance Report*, No. 287 (Washington, DC: Government Printing Office)
71. Salk, J. (1959). Preconceptions about vaccination against paralytic poliomyelitis. *Ann. Intern. Med.*, **50**, 843
72. Ogra, P. L., Karzon, D. T., Righthand, F. and MacGillivrany, M. (1968). Immunoglobulin response in serum and secretions after immunization with live and inactivated poliovaccine and natural infection. *N. Engl. J. Med.*, **279**, 898
73. Center for Disease Control (Atlanta) (1973). *Immunization against Disease—1972*. (Washington, DC: Government Printing Office)
74. Cohen, H. (1977). In *Institute of Medicine Evaluation of Poliomyelitis Vaccines: Report of the Committee for the Study of Poliomyelitis Vaccines*, Vol. II, Appendix C - Contributed Papers, pp. 119–152. (Washington, DC: National Academy of Sciences)
75. Oker-Blom, N. and Halonen, P. (1977). In *Institute of Medicine Evaluation of Poliomyelitis Vaccines: Report of the Committee for the Study of Poliomyelitis Vaccines*, Vol. II, Appendix C - Contributed Papers, pp. 187–190
76. Stuart-Harris, C. (1977). In *Institute of Medicine Evaluation of Poliomyelitis Vaccines: Report of the Committee for the Study of Poliomyelitis Vaccines*, Vol. II, Appendix C - Contributed Papers, pp. 191–206
77. Communicable Disease Center (Sept. 1964). *Poliomyelitis Surveillance Report*, No. 285 (Washington, DC: Government Printing Office)
78. Communicable Disease Center (June 1966). *Poliomyelitis Surveillance Report*, No. 288. (Washington, DC: Government Printing Office)
79. Salk, D. and Salk, J., Prospects for the eradication of poliomyelitis in the United States. (in preparation)
80. Schoenberger, L. (1978). (personal communication)
81. Salk, J. (1959). Vaccination against poliomyelitis—an ounce of prevention. *R. Soc. Health J.*, **79**, 310
82. Salk, J. (1956). Poliomyelitis vaccine in the fall of 1955. *Am. J. Public Health*, **46**, 1
83. Salk, J. (1957). Viral and cellular factors pertinent to the control of paralytic poliomyelitis with a non-infectious vaccine. *N. Y. Acad. Sci.*, Special Publication, **5**, 77
84. Ravenholt, R. T. (1961). Poliomyelitis in an immunized country. *Public Health Reports*, **76**, 166
85. Gregg, M. B. (1977). In *Institute of Medicine Evaluation of Poliomyelitis Vaccines: Report of the Committee for the Study of Poliomyelitis Vaccines*, Vol. II, Appendix C - Contributed Papers, pp. 77–106. (Washington, DC: National Academy of Sciences)
86. Parry, W. H. (1969). Recent trends in immunization and vaccination. (Abst.), *World Med.*, **43**, 545

11
Hepatitis viruses and vaccines

M. R. HILLEMAN, V. M. VILLAREJOS, E. B. BUYNAK, O. L. ITTENSOHN, W. J. McALEER, A. A. McLEAN, W. J. MILLER, P. J. PROVOST, A. A. TYTELL AND B. S. WOLANSKI

Viral hepatitis continues to merit the rank of 'greatest importance' among the unconquered diseases of mankind. The general term, viral hepatitis, refers principally to hepatitis A (infectious hepatitis) and to hepatitis B (serum hepatitis), although other known viruses such as yellow fever virus, Epstein–Barr virus, and cytomegalovirus can also cause hepatitis in man. Most recently, with the development of means for identifying hepatitis A and B in the laboratory, it has become evident that a third major but hypothetical agent of hepatitis may exist for which the name hepatitis C has already been suggested.

Both hepatitis A and B have stubbornly resisted all attempts at meaningful and reliable propagation *in vitro* in the laboratory and it was not until very recently that non-human primates replaced the human volunteer as the means for studying these diseases. Interestingly, these viruses found their animal hosts on opposite sides of the world – hepatitis B in the Old World chimpanzee and hepatitis A in the New World marmoset.

With such a background, I would like to discuss today the two most recent events in hepatitis research. The one is the development of a highly promising vaccine against hepatitis B; the other is the identification of human hepatitis A virus and the development of laboratory serologic tests by which the disease can be studied.

HEPATITIS B VACCINE

As already noted, the virus of hepatitis B does not multiply significantly in cell culture and there is no source of laboratory propagated virus for vaccine preparation. About 10 years ago, however, Dr B. Blumberg and associates[1,2] discovered an antigen circulating in the blood of certain human beings. This

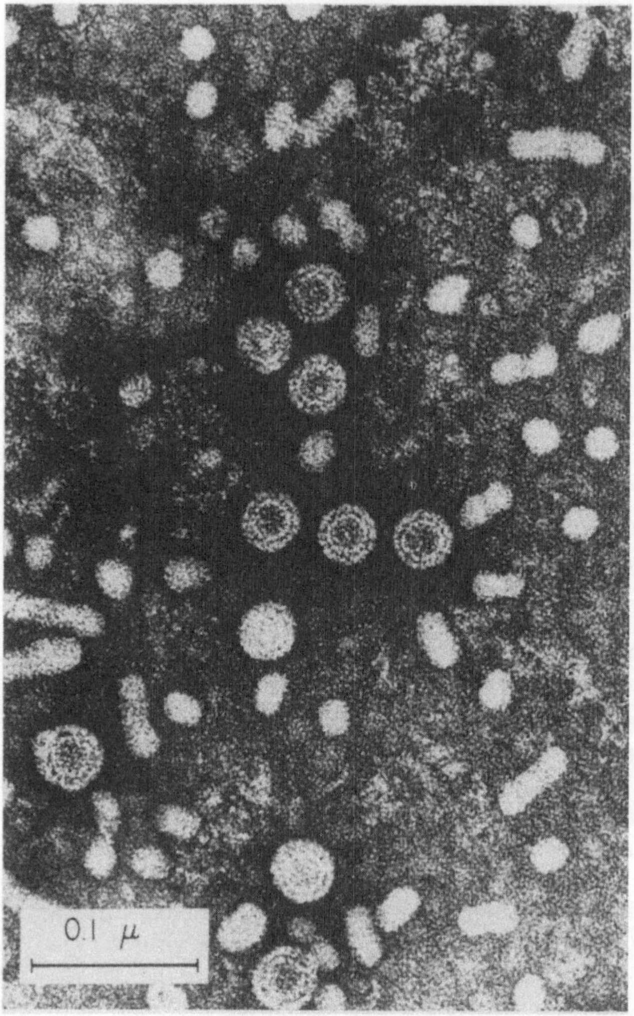

Figure 1 Purified Australia antigen, filamentous and Dane particles prepared from sera from a human hepatitis B carrier

substance, named Australia antigen because it was first found in the blood of an Australian aboriginee, was subsequently found by Dr A. Prince[3] to be the surface antigen of hepatitis B virus that is produced in abundance by certain persons who are chronically infected with the agent. Figure 1 presents an electron micrograph showing Australia antigen (20 mμ) now called hepatitis

B surface antigen or HB_sAg and also the Dane particle (42 mμ) that is believed to be the whole virus. In 1971, Dr Saul Krugman and associates[4] reported the development of a crude vaccine that consisted of boiled plasma from a carrier of Australia antigen. The vaccine, when given to susceptible human subjects, stimulated antibody against the virus of hepatitis B and afforded protection against the disease.

Since that time, we have prepared a far more refined vaccine using highly purified Australia antigen from infected human carriers[5–7]. To prepare vaccine, plasma pools were collected from overtly healthy human donors with hepatitis B antigenaemia. The Australia antigen was purified from the plasma by isopycnic banding and rate zonal separation to yield a partially purified material. Further chemical procedures yielded highly purified hepatitis B antigen for vaccine. The purified antigen was adjusted to a concentration of 20 μg/ml protein and was treated for 72 h at 36 °C with 1:4000 formalin. The treated material was the vaccine.

A great variety of tests were carried out on the plasma pools and on the final product by conventional animal, chick embryo, and cell culture procedures to insure microbial sterility and absence of extraneous viruses. Most importantly, the vaccine was tested for live hepatitis A virus in marmosets and for live hepatitis B virus in chimpanzees. In the tests for hepatitis B virus, none of the chimpanzees developed hepatitis B antigenaemia, elevated transaminase levels, or antibody against the core antigen of the virus (anti-HB_c). The conditions used to purify the hepatitis viral antigen, even before addition of formalin, sufficed to destroy the infectivity of all of nine representatives of different virus families, thereby giving added assurance of viral inactivation. The antigen was so highly purified that all the tests for blood proteins and for blood group substances were negative. Hepatitis virus consists of different subtypes, primarily type ad and ay and this is expressed in the Australia antigen. The vaccine we made was composed mainly of type ad antigen. Evidence to date suggests that there is a substantial sharing of common antigen between the various subtypes and that a single subtype vaccine will afford broad-spectrum protection against hepatitis B viruses. Although several lots of vaccine have been made, the data reported here refer to a single vaccine lot number 559.

Tests to measure antigenic potency of lot 559 vaccine were carried out in guinea pigs. In the tests, groups of 14 initially seronegative animals weighing 350–400 g were given graded doses of vaccine in 1.0 ml volume by the subcutaneous route initially and 2 and 8 weeks later. The animals were bled just prior to each dose of vaccine and 28 days after the third injection, and the sera were tested for antibody against hepatitis B surface antigen by the passive haemagglutination test (Ausure). The findings given in Figure 2 show a dose–response curve in the 0.5–20 μg antigen/dose range, both in terms of seroconversion rate and also in geometric mean antibody titre. Importantly, nearly all animals developed antibody after the third dose of vaccine and although the height of antibody was proportional to antigen dose, the range was small, viz., 20–75.

To measure antibody responses in chimpanzees, six initially seronegative animals weighing 20–40 lb were each given three doses subcutaneously of vaccine containing 20 μg per dose in 1 ml volume. The findings summarized

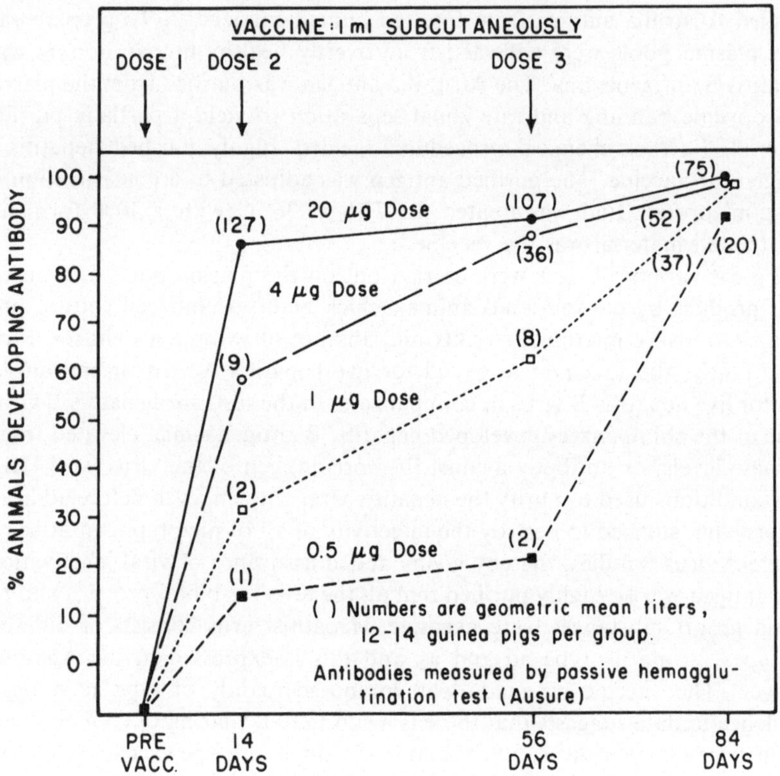

Figure 2 Antibody responses, according to time, in guinea pigs given graded doses of hepatitis B vaccine, Lot 559

in Figure 3 showed that all butone of the six animals developed antibody after only two doses of vaccine. The third dose of vaccine sufficed to boost antibody titres, but the sixth animal still failed to develop detectable antibody.

Tests to measure the protective efficacy of the vaccine were carried out in chimpanzees given three 20 μg doses of vaccine subcutaneously 1 month apart. The vaccinated animals, together with the seronegative control animals, were challenged intravenously with approximately 1000 chimpanzee infectious doses of live hepatitis B virus 2 months after the last dose of vaccine was given.

The findings in a single vaccinated chimpanzee (No. 834) and an unvaccinated control (No. 769) are shown in Figure 4. The vaccinated animal developed antibody against hepatitis B surface antigen (anti-Hb_s) after the first vaccine

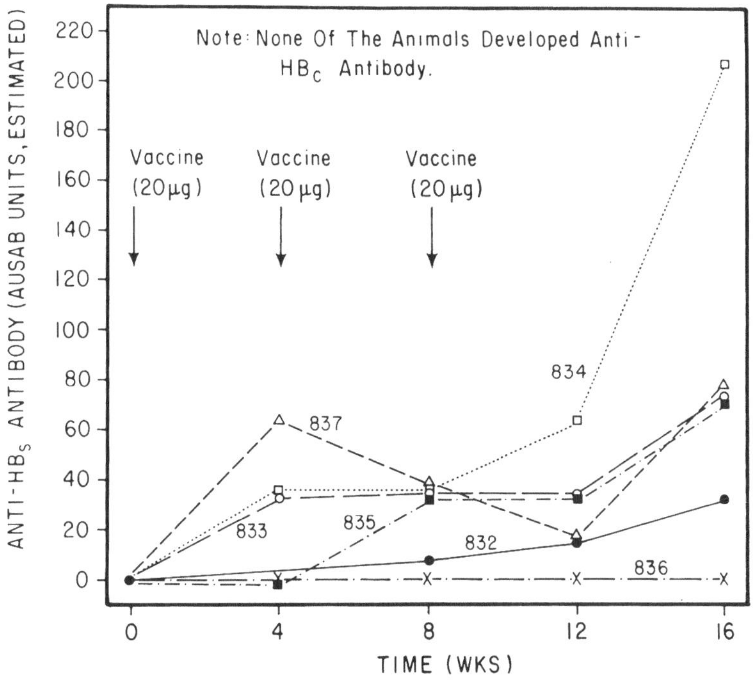

Figure 3 Hepatitis B antibody response, according to time, in six chimpanzees given three doses, subcutaneously, of 20 μg each (1 ml) of Lot 559 vaccine at monthly intervals

dose and there was further increase in antibody when additional doses were given. The vaccine was safe and did not cause hepatitis in this animal, as indicated by lack of hepatitis B antigenaemia, retention of normal levels of serum transaminase, by retention of normal liver histopathology, and by failure to develop antibody against the core antigen (anti-HB_c) of the virus. Following challenge with life hepatitis B virus, this animal was protected against the disease. By contrast, the unvaccinated control chimpanzee developed hepatitis with antigenaemia, transaminase elevation, positive liver histopathologic findings, and the appearance of antibody against core antigen which is a sensitive assay for hepatitis B virus infection.

The experimental findings in all the eleven animals in the tests to measure protective efficacy are summarized in Table 1. All of the six unvaccinated control animals developed hepatitis on challenge. All five of the vaccinated chimpanzees were protected, including one animal that had failed to develop detectable antibody after vaccination.

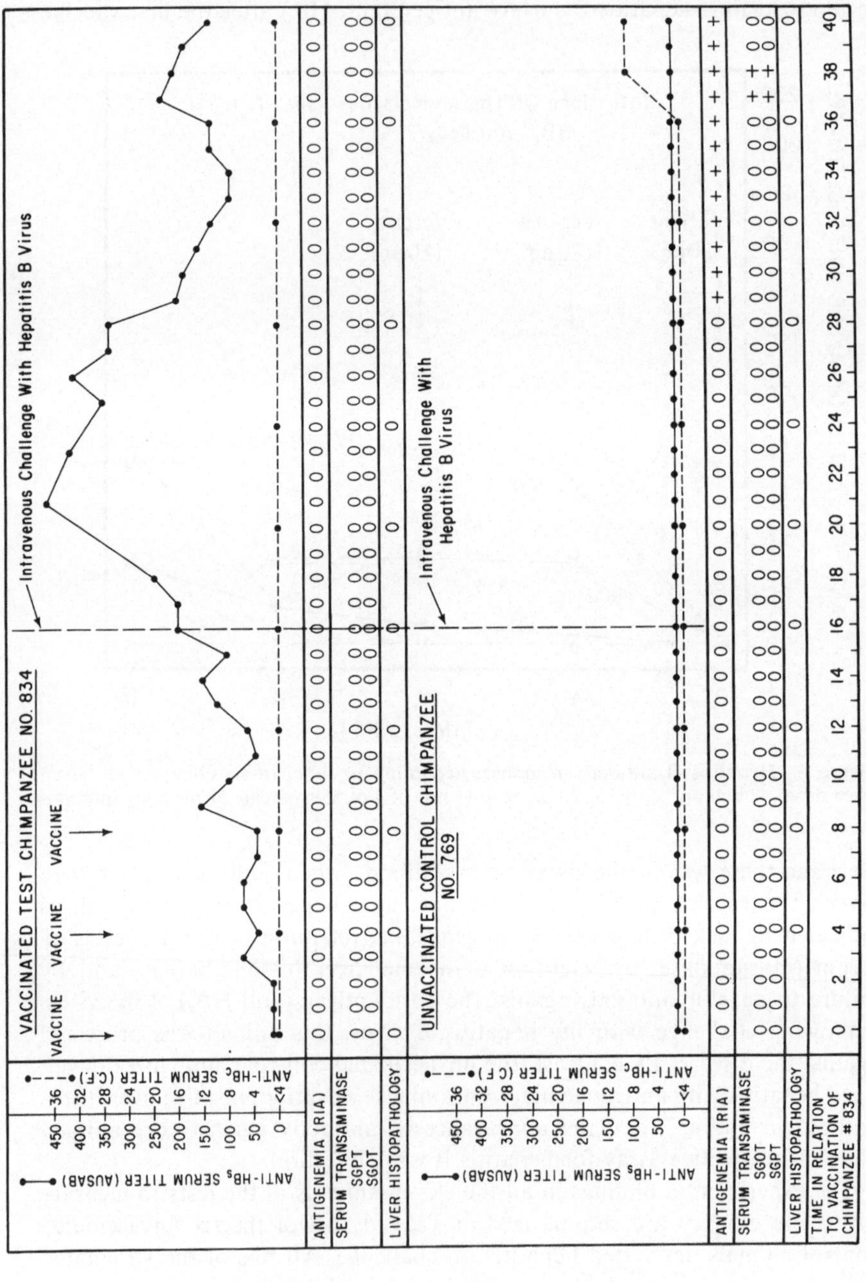

Figure 4 Chart showing dynamics of viral, pathogenic and serological responses in a vaccinated and non-vaccinated control chimpanzee prior to, and following, intravenous, challenge with human hepatitis B virus

Table 1 Tests for protective efficacy of lot 559 hepatitis B vaccine in chimpanzees on challenge with human hepatitis B virus and observation for 24 weeks

Group	*Results* No. becoming infected* / Total in group	Protection (%)
Vaccinated animals	0/5	100
Controls	6/6	

* Measured by development of antigenaemia, serum enzyme elevation, and development of antibody against virus core antigen.

The demonstration of protection in chimpanzees against hepatitis B virus by administering purified formalin-treated hepatitis B surface antigen is consistent with the protection afforded human subjects given crude boiled human plasma in the early experiments carried out by Krugman *et al.*[4]. The findings in these studies show promise for practical control of hepatitis B by a highly purified viral antigen vaccine. Tests in human volunteers to date have established safety for man and tests to measure immunizing potency are in progress. Animal studies of purified hepatitis B vaccines along similar lines are being carried out by Purcell and Gerin[8]. Maupas *et al.*[9] are testing a purified hepatitis B vaccine for protective efficacy in man. An effective vaccine against hepatitis B should find very important application initially in high-risk populations such as patients and personnel in renal dialysis centres, in laboratory workers who test bloods, and in susceptible recipients of blood transfusions. With established safety and efficacy, and with continued high world incidence of hepatitis, the disease may be judged so important as to warrant general immunization.

HEPATITIS A

The lack, until recently, of an animal host and the absence of a specific *in vitro* test for hepatitis A virus infection all but precluded significant progress toward the understanding of hepatitis A virus infections. This picture was changed quite dramatically when Deinhardt and co-workers[10–12] demonstrated serum enzyme elevations and liver pathology in marmosets of the genus *Saguinus* inoculated with sera from patients with hepatitis A, but not when sera from normal persons were given.

Studies in our laboratories[13–25] led to the recovery of agents in *Saguinus mystax* marmosets from cases of hepatitis A that occurred in Costa Rica. These agents caused elevations in serum transaminases and liver pathology in marmosets. Hepatitis A strain CR326 was chosen for further detailed study. This strain was shown to be human hepatitis A virus by serum neutralization tests with paired sera from human hepatitis A cases.

The finding of a susceptible host species, and the discovery that the livers of infected marmosets contained large quantities of virus, made possible rapid progress towards defining the properties of hepatitis A virus. It also aided in the development of serological test procedures that have proved most useful in the diagnosis of cases of hepatitis A and in studies of the epidemiology of the disease.

Figure 5 shows an electron micrograph of hepatitis A virus purified by

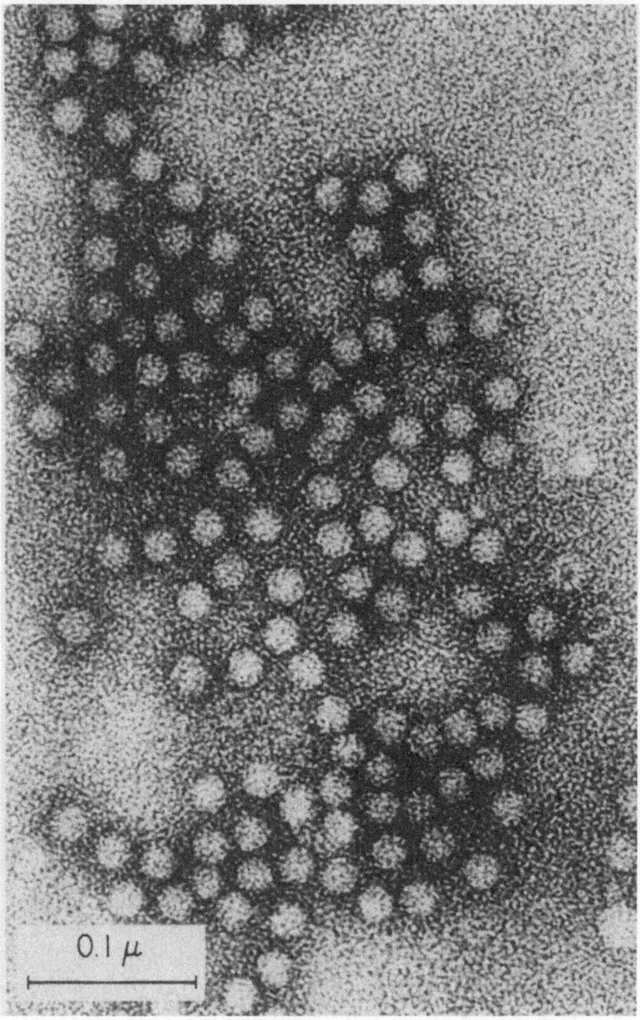

Figure 5 Purified CR32 6 strain human hepatitis A virus prepared by CsCI density gradient separation from injected marmoset serum

isopycnic banding from infected marmoset serum. The particles are spheres of 27 mμ diameter and have been identified as hepatitis A virus based on tests for infectivity in marmosets and in specific serological tests employing acute and convalescent sera from human cases of hepatitis A. The virus was found to have a density in caesium chloride of 1.34 g/cm^3 and was heat- (60 °C), ether- and acid-stable but was destroyed by heating at 100 °C or by treating with 1:4000 formalin or ultraviolet light. Presumptive findings for RNA together with intracytoplasmic location (see Figure 6) suggests that the

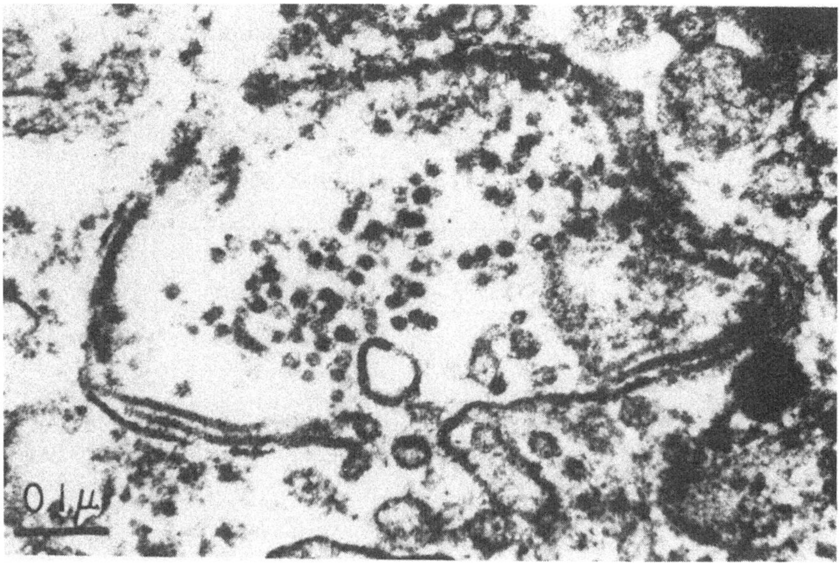

Figure 6 Portion of a hepatocyte cytoplasm showing a group of virions in a vesicle-like structure. Both full and empty particles are present. Thin section

virus is of RNA type. These attributes of the virus indicate that it is a likely member of, or closely related to, the enterovirus family.

Using virus purified from infected marmoset liver, we devised three tests for hepatitis A antibody that can be used in serodiagnosis or in epidemiological investigations of the disease. These were the serum neutralization test, the complement-fixation or CF test, and the immune adherence (IA) assay. The findings in tests of sera from a typical case of human hepatitis A are shown in Figure 7. It is seen that the patient developed all three kinds of antibody in the course of convalescence from his disease. The findings in five cases of hepatitis A and B are shown in Table 2. All of the cases of hepatitis A and none of those of hepatitis B developed hepatitis A antibody. The neutralization test is far too costly for routine use since it requires the use of marmosets.

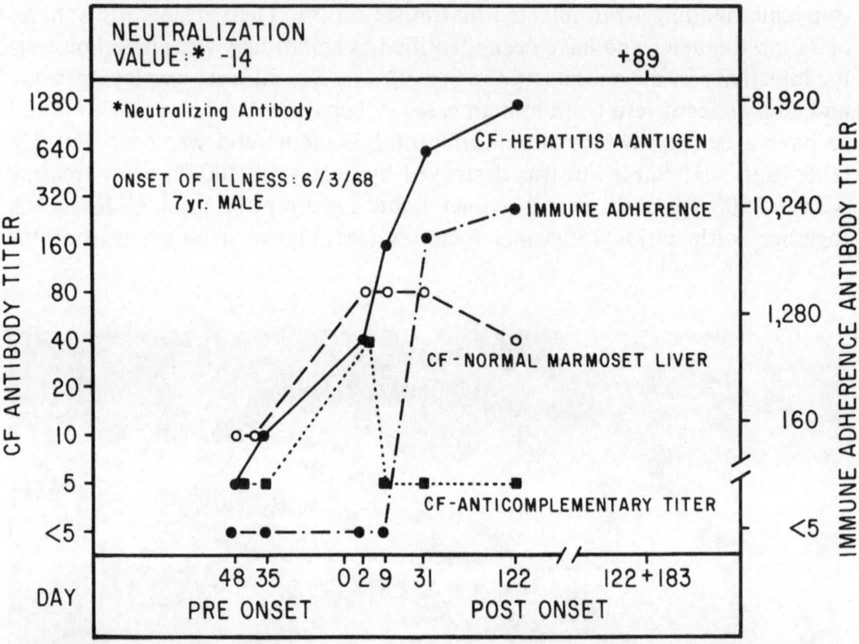

Figure 7 Hepatitis A CF and IA antibody titres and neutralizing antibody values, Costa Rica hepatitis A case No. 068-330-08

Table 2 Immune adherence, complement-fixation, and serum neutralization test findings in hepatitis A and B cases

		Hepatitis A antibody titres		
Case No.	*Serum specimen*	*Immune adherence*	*Complement-fixation*	*Neutralization value*
Hepatitis A cases				
08	Pre-onset	<5	5 or <	−14
	Post-onset	10 240	1280	89
11	Pre-onset	<5	20 or <	0
	Post-onset	81 960	640	78
07	Pre-onset	<5	10 or <	18
	Post-onset	25 600	640	89
*Hepatitis B cases**				
01	Pre-onset	<5	20 or <	
	Post-onset	<5	20 or <	
05	Pre-onset	640	40	50
	Post-onset	640	40	67

These findings are typical of tests of sixteen hepatitis cases.

* Australia antigen was detected in all hepatitis B cases.

The CF test is simple and useful but is somewhat technical to interpret since patients may also develop antibody against normal marmoset liver and the sera may be anticomplementary. The immune adherence assay has none of these disadvantages and is the most economical, sensitive, and specific assay for routine use at this time. Use of purified antigen in radioimmune assays is possible and this provides an alternative choice for assay[26].

The immune adherence assay is of very great value in epidemiological investigations of hepatitis infections such as is illustrated in Table 3 in an

Table 3 Family outbreak, hepatitis A and B, Costa Rica, 1967

Age of subject (years)	*Date of hepatitis onset*	*Hepatitis A serology*		*Hepatitis B antigenaemia*	*Diagnosis*
		Immune adherence	*Complent-fixation*		
9	March 2	Immune	Immune	+	Hepatitis B
4*	April 20	Rise	Rise	0	Hepatitis A
5*	May 2	Rise	Rise	0	Hepatitis A
2†	Well	Susceptible	Susceptible	0	Well
37†	Well	Susceptible	Susceptible	0	Well
40	Well	Immune	(?)	0	Well
14	Well	Immune	Immune	0	Well
13	Well	Immune	Immune	0	Well
10	Well	Immune	Immune	0	Well
7	Well	Immune	Immune	0	Well

* Subject age 4 was anicteric and subject age 5 was subclinical. All had diagnostic enzyme elevations.

† These subjects had developed hepatitis A CF and IA antibody when tested 7 years later.

outbreak of hepatitis A and B in a family in Costa Rica. Five members of the family were already immune to hepatitis A and two of the four initially susceptible persons developed hepatitis A in the outbreak. These individuals, an infant and his mother, had developed hepatitis A antibody by the time that serological tests were performed again 7 years later. Hepatitis A has been found in our studies to be subclinical in about half the persons infected with the virus, indicating that individuals may become immune to the virus without ever knowing they were infected.

The findings in serological surveys of normal persons of various ages in open populations in the USA and Costa Rica are shown in Table 4. Hepatitis A is typically a disease of children in Costa Rica and this explains the evolution at early age of antibody in the human population. By contrast, few persons in the high socioeconomic group in the USA had acquired infection before adulthood. Table 5 shows, however, that persons of lower socioeconomic standing in the USA, especially those in institutions or persons in close contact with such individuals, may show a high incidence of antibody against hepatitis A virus.

Table 4 Age distribution, hepatitis A IA antibody in persons in open populations, Pennsylvania and Costa Rica

Age (years)	Proportion seropositive			
	Pennsylvania		Costa Rica	
1	0/18	0%	4/20	20%
2	0/17	0%	10/20	50%
3	0/16	0%	8/20	40%
4–6	0/22	0%	38/60	63%
7–9	0/16	0%	48/60	80%
10–14	0/18	0%	19/20	95%
15–19	0/20	0%	19/20	95%
20–29	2/20	10%	18/20	90%
30–39	6/21	29%	18/20	90%
40–49	10/17	59%	18/20	90%
50+	5/12	42%	16/20	80%

Table 5 Occurrence of hepatitis A IA antibody among persons from selected populations, Pennsylvania

Population	Age (years)	Serostatus: Positive/Total	Serostatus: Percentage positive
Adult residents at Hamburg State School and Hospital	21–51	9/10	90
Employees at Laurelton State School and Hospital	19–63	19/30	63
Plasma donors, Philadelphia	⩾18	29/50	58
Child residents at St Joseph's Home, Scranton, and Hamburg State School and Hospital	1–8	0/20	0

Human immune globulin has been employed for many years for routine prophylaxis of hepatitis A in persons exposed or likely to be exposed to the infection. The recent elimination of hepatitis B virus carriers as blood donors in the USA and the increasing trend towards the use of volunteer donors, rather than paid donors, as a blood source has tended to reduce the proportion of individual plasmas in which hepatitis A antibody of high titre is found. Marked individual variation of hepatitis A antibody titre in human immune globulin lots has been demonstrated as shown in Table 6. Fortunately, the development of the immune adherence assay makes it possible to assay for hepatitis A antibody in immune globulins and to prepare lots in which a minimum standard of potency can be achieved.

Table 6 Distribution, hepatitis A immune adherence titres, twenty-four commercial lots of human immune globulin

IA titre	*No. lots*
1 000	1
2 000	2
4 000	11
8 000	9
16 000	1

COMMENT

In closing, I believe it fair to conclude that the developments of the past several years have permitted remarkable progress towards our understanding of human hepatitis A and B. The occurrence of a heavy viral antigenaemia in a proportion of persons persistently infected with hepatitis B virus has made possible the development of practical systems for testing for hepatitis B antigen and antibody and, in addition, has permitted the evolution of a promising vaccine for protection against hepatitis B in the world population. Hepatitis A virus is very unlike the hepatitis B agent, and there is no human source for the antigen to prepare vaccine. However, the reliable propagation of the virus in marmosets and the evolution of simple *in vitro* assays for virus and antibody have permitted great progress in our understanding of this disease. The embargo placed on the export of marmosets from the Amazon region in South America has greatly hampered any widespread research programme employing the new tests and has precluded to date the development of a commercial source of antigen. It is hoped that this may be changed in the future.

The progress of research with hepatitis A and B, employing antigen from human plasma and studies in New World and Old World primates, must be considered precarious, indeed, until some means for reliable *in vitro* propagation of these agents are found. Further, the development of hepatitis A vaccine must, indeed, depend upon growth of the virus in cell culture.

References

1. Blumberg, B. S., Alter, H. J. and Visnich, S. (1965). A 'new' antigen in leukemia sera. *J. Am. Med. Assoc.*, **191,** 541
2. Blumberg, B. S., Gerstley, B. J. S., Hungerford, D. A., London, W. T. and Sutnick, A. I. (1967). A serum antigen (Australia antigen) in Down's syndrome, leukemia, and hepatitis. *Ann. Int. Med.*, **66**, 924
3. Prince, A. M. (1968). An antigen detected in the blood during the incubation period of serum hepatitis. *Proc. Nat. Acad. Sci.* (USA), **60**, 814
4. Krugman, S., Giles, J. P. and Hammond, J. (1971). Viral hepatitis, type B (MS-2 strain). Studies on active immunization. *J. Am. Med. Assoc.*, **217**, 41
5. Hilleman, M. R., Buynak, E. B., Roehm, R. R., Tytell, A. A., Bertland, A. U. and Lampson, G. P. (1975). Purified and inactivated human hepatitis B vaccine: progress report. *Amer. J. Med. Sci.*, **270**, 401

6. Buynak, E. B., Roehm, R. R., Tytell, A. A., Bertland, A. U., II, Lampson, G. P. and Hilleman, M. R. (1976). Development and chimpanzee testing of a vaccine against human hepatitis B. *Proc. Soc. Exp. Biol. Med.*, **151**, 694
7. Buynak, E. B., Roehm, R. R., Tytell, A. A., Bertland, A. U., II, Lampson, G. P. and Hilleman, M. R. (1976). Vaccine against human hepatitis B. *J. Am. Med. Assoc.*, **235**, 2832
8. Purcell, R. H. and Gerin, J. L. (1975). Hepatitis B subunit vaccine: a preliminary report of safety and efficacy tests in chimpanzees. *Amer. J. Med. Sci.*, **270**, 395
9. Maupas, P., Goudeau, A., Coursaget, P., Drucker, J. and Bagros, P. (1976). Immunisation against hepatitis B in man. *The Lancet*, **1**, 1367
10. Deinhardt, F., Holmes, A. W., Capps, R. B. and Popper, H. (1967). Studies on the transmission of human viral hepatitis to marmoset monkeys. I. Transmission of disease, serial passages, and description of liver lesions. *J. Exp. Med.*, **125**, 673
11. Holmes, A. W., Wolfe, L., Rosenblate, H. and Deinhardt, F. (1969). Hepatitis in marmosets: induction of disease with coded specimens from a human volunteer study. *Science*, **165**, 816
12. Holmes, A. W., Wolfe, L., Deinhardt, F. and Conrad, M. E. (1971). Transmission of human hepatitis to marmosets: further coded studies. *J. Infect. Dis.*, **124**, 520
13. Mascoli, C. C., Ittensohn, O. L., Villarejos, V. M., Arguedas, G. J. A., Provost, P. J. and Hilleman, M. R. (1973). Recovery of hepatitis agents in the marmoset from human cases occurring in Costa Rica. *Proc. Soc. Exp. Biol. Med.*, **142**, 276
14. Provost, P. J., Ittensohn, O. L., Villarejos, V. M., Arguedas, G. J. A. and Hilleman, M. R. (1973). Etiologic relationship of marmoset-propagated CR326 hepatitis A virus to hepatitis in man. *Proc. Soc. Exp. Biol. Med.*, **142**, 1257
15. Provost, P. J., Wolanski, B. S., Miller, W. J., Ittensohn, O. L., McAleer, W. J. and Hilleman, M. R. (1975). Physical, chemical and morphologic dimensions of human hepatitis A virus strain CR326. *Proc. Soc. Exp. Biol. Med.*, **148**, 532
16. Provost, P. J., Ittensohn, O. L., Villarejos, V. M. and Hilleman, M. R. (1975). A specific complement-fixation test for human hepatitis A employing CR326 virus antigen. Diagnosis and epidemiology. *Proc. Soc. Exp. Biol. Med.*, **148**, 962
17. Miller, W. J., Provost, P. J., McAleer, W. J., Ittensohn, O. L., Villarejos, V. M. and Hilleman, M. R. (1975). Specific immune adherence assay for human hepatitis A antibody. Application to diagnostic and epidemiologic investigations. *Proc. Soc. Exp. Biol. Med.*, **149**, 254
18. Hilleman, M. R., Provost, P. J., Miller, W. J., Villarejos, V. M., Ittensohn, O. L. and McAleer, W. J. (1975). Immune adherence and complement-fixation tests for human hepatitis A. Diagnostic and epidemiologic investigations. *Develop. Biol. Standard.*, **30**, 383
19. Hilleman, M. R., Provost, P. J., Wolanski, B. S., Miller, W. J., Ittensohn, O. L. and McAleer, W. J. (1975). Characterization of CR326 human hepatitis A virus, a probable enterovirus. *Develop. Biol. Standard.*, **30**, 418
20. Hilleman, M. R., Provost, P. J., Miller, W. J., Villarejos, V. M., Ittensohn, O. L. and McAleer, W. J. (1975). Development and utilization of complement-fixation and immune adherence tests for human hepatitis A virus and antibody. *Amer. J. Med. Sci.*, **270**, 93
21. Provost, P. J., Wolanski, B. S., Miller, W. J., Ittensohn, O. L., McAleer, W. J. and Hilleman, M. R. (1975). Biophysical and biochemical properties of CR326 human hepatitis A virus. *Amer. J. Med. Sci.*, **270**, 87
22. Villarejos, V. M., Visona, K. A., Eduarte, A. C. A., Provost, P. J. and Hilleman, M. R. (1975). Evidence for viral hepatitis other than type A or type B among persons in Costa Rica. *N. Engl. J. Med.*, **293**, 1350
23. Hilleman, M. R., Provost, P. J., Villarejos, V. M., Buynak, E. B., Miller, W. J., Ittensohn, O. L., Wolanski, B. S. and McAleer, W. J. (1976). Infectious hepatitis (hepatitis A) research in nonhuman primates. Pan American Health Organization Scientific Publication No. 317, WHO, pp. 110–124
24. Villarejos, V. M., Gutierrez-Diermissen, A., Anderson-Visona, K., Rodriguez-Aragones, A., Provost, P. J. and Hilleman, M. R. (1976). Development of immunity against hepatitis A virus by subclinical infection. *Proc. Soc. Exp. Biol. Med.* (In press)

25. Villarejos, V. M., Provost, P. J., Ittensohn, O. L., McLean, A. A. and Hilleman, M. R. (1976). Seroepidemiologic investigations of human hepatitis caused by A, B and a possible third virus. *Proc. Soc. Exp. Biol. Med.* (In press)
26. Purcell, R. H., Wong, D. C., Moritsugu, Y., Dienstag, J. L., Routenberg, J. A. and Boggs, J. D. (1976). A microtiter solid-phase radioimmunoassay for hepatitis A antigen and antibody. *J. Immunol.*, **116**, 349

12
Developments with hepatitis B vaccines

A. J. ZUCKERMAN

INTRODUCTION

There is an urgent need for a hepatitis B vaccine for groups which are at an increased risk of acquiring this infection. These groups include health care and laboratory personnel, and staff and residents of institutions for the mentally retarded and other large semi-closed institutions. Other groups at high risk include patients on maintenance haemodialysis, patients requiring repeated blood transfusions or the administration of blood products, patients undergoing treatment with immunosuppressive or cytotoxic drugs, patients with malignant diseases, and disorders associated with depression of the immune response. Consideration will also have to be given to persons living in certain tropical areas where present socioeconomic conditions are poor and the prevalence of hepatitis B infection is high. Some authors also include military personnel, and women of childbearing age in areas of the world where the carrier rate in this group is excessive.

The repeated failure to passage hepatitis B virus serially in tissue or organ cultures has hampered progress towards the development of a conventional vaccine[1,2]. Attention has therefore been directed towards the use of other preparations for active immunization. The foundations for such hepatitis B immunogens were laid by the demonstration of the relative efficacy of heated diluted serum containing hepatitis B virus in preventing or modifying the infection in susceptible persons[3–5]: in other studies serum containing hepatitis B surface antigen obtained from a healthy carrier was heated at 60 °C for 10 h, but the virus was not completely inactivated as was shown by the acquisition of antigen and elevated serum transaminase levels in a proportion of the recipients[6]. The use of heated whole serum is a crude way of inducing immunity and it is unlikely to be accepted for general use. Nevertheless, the studies carried out in human volunteers at the Willowbrook State School laid the foundations for the development of hepatitis B immunogens that could be used as vaccines.

SUBUNIT VACCINES

Since the isolated viral coat protein, in this instance hepatitis B surface antigen, leads to the production of protective surface antibody as shown in serological surveys and experimental studies, the possibility of using purified 22 nm spherical hepatitis B surface antigen particles seems attractive[7]. Such experimental vaccines have been prepared from the plasma of apparently healthy carriers of this antigen. Human hepatitis B infection has been successfully transmitted to chimpanzees, and although the infection is mild the biochemical, histological and serological responses in these primates is very similar to that in man. The relative susceptibility of man compared with chimpanzees for developing hepatitis B infection is not known, and it cannot be measured for obvious reasons. Sensitive tests for surface antigen, surface antibody, core antibody, DNA polymerase, and techniques for *e*-antigen and *e*-antibody are available[8] and thus provide a means of monitoring vaccines. A limited number of susceptible chimpanzees have so far been shown to be protected by the 22 nm particle immunogens that had been treated by heat or with formalin[9–11]. A trial had also been conducted in man[12]. However, the formulation of the requisite safety criteria for limited evaluation of this unique type of vaccine in man is still under consideration[13].

Although it is generally accepted that the viral subunit preparations, when pure, are free of nucleic acid and therefore non-infectious, the fact that the starting material for their preparation is human plasma obtained from persons infected with hepatitis B virus means that extreme caution must be exercised to ensure their freedom from all harmful contaminating material[7]. Indeed the plasma is collected from individuals who are persistent carriers of hepatitis B surface antigen, which is a marker associated with hepatitis B virus. In addition, some concern has been expressed on the possible induction of harmful immunological reactions to host components, including pre-existing structures of the liver cells, which may be present in such vaccine preparations[14]. The argument that blood products had been transfused for many years without such apparent adverse immunological reactions is difficult to accept since these products had been prepared from healthy blood donors selected for the absence of any evidence of infection of the liver.

Furthermore, it has been reported that antigenic determinants related to human plasma proteins are constituents of hepatitis B surface antigen. These determinants appear to be related to antigenic specificities of prealbumin, albumin, apolipoproteins C and D, and the γ chain of immunoglobulin G. Other studies indicated that the larger polypeptides of purified surface antigen are probably adsorbed serum proteins which are necessary for the preservation of antigenic activity. In addition, the close association of the surface antigen with normal serum components has been an acknowledged difficulty in developing purification techniques for separation of the antigen, and a number of host proteins may be tightly bound to the surface antigen during purification procedures. Demonstrable and significant levels of carbohydrate in purified fractions of the surface antigen have also been found. The total carbohydrate content of purified small antigen particles is reported as 3.6–6.5%. Three glycoproteins were also found as well as a glycolipid and three major phospholipids. The carbohydrate may be necessary for maintaining the structure and functional integrity of the antigenic determinants, or the carbohydrate itself may constitute a major antigenic determinant. The carbohydrate might have a novel haptenic specificity which is either virus-coded or virus-induced host cell coded. Alternatively, the carbohydrate, and some lipoprotein components, might simply be derived from the host cell membranes as the mature virus particles are released. There may be some similarity between such a carbohydrate hapten, or the lipoprotein components, and those carbohydrate and lipoprotein antigens of normal cell surfaces, leading to a degree of tolerance because of a close antigenic resemblance between hepatitis B surface antigen and 'self' antigens. Alternatively, an autoimmune reaction may be initiated. Such an autoimmune reaction may be induced by hepatitis B infection because of a change in antigenicity of the hepatocyte cell membranes, due to alteration of existing antigens or the appearance of viral determinants. T-lymphocytes responsive to such new antigenic determinants could promote a B-cell response to unaltered 'self' antigens. The synthesis and release of the resulting autoantibody is subject in turn to control by suppressor T-cells. These complex interactions between T- and B-cells, could be of fundamental importance in the pathogenesis of chronic liver damage. These topics have been discussed and reviewed extensively[7,8,13–19].

In summary, purified preparations of hepatitis B surface antigen are known to contain significant amounts of complex protein, carbohydrate, phospholipid and glycolipid. The molecular weight of DNA extracted from the core of the Dane particle is only up to 2.3×10^6 and it appears unlikely that all the components of the surface antigen are coded by the viral genome. It is quite conceivable, therefore, that certain components are simply derived from the host cell membranes or from the plasma. In addition, the possibility has been discussed that hepatitis B cores derived from infected liver nuclei contain short segments of host cell double-stranded DNA[20]. It may therefore be undesirable to use preparations of hepatitis B surface antigen which contain host cell components or host proteins for immunization against this infection. Careful preliminary studies in experimental animal models are thus required.

POLYPEPTIDE VACCINES

The potential use of antigenic polypeptides derived from hepatitis B surface antigen is under investigation in several laboratories[21–23]. A number of these polypeptides are immunogenic and have been found to contain the group-specific antigenic determinant *a*, and certain of the polypeptides have induced a cell-mediated immune response in experimental animals. It should be noted that although there was no response to normal human serum, immunization with a low molecular weight component did elicit a cell-mediated response to normal human serum, suggesting that at least one integral component may contain an antigenic determinant related to a human serum protein[24,25].

Another aspect for consideration in formulating a suitable immunogen is the possible need for stimulating an anti-*e* response[26]. This antibody might be related to protection against infection, perhaps by aggregating hepatitis B virus. Such studies have yet to be carried out in susceptible animal models.

SAFETY CRITERIA FOR HEPATITIS B VACCINES IN RELATION TO OTHER HUMAN HEPATITIS VIRUSES

With the availability of certain species of marmosets and chimpanzees as animal models for the other recognized major cause of hepatitis in man, hepatitis A virus, it became feasible to monitor, at least on a limited scale, candidate vaccines for evidence of possible contamination with this virus. Furthermore, sensitive serological techniques for hepatitis A antigen and antibody are now available. The more recent serological and epidemiological evidence for the existence of yet other hepatitis viruses, hepatitis virus C or non-A:non-B hepatitis now poses another difficulty to the monitoring and safety testing of the unique experimental hepatitis B vaccines.

It has also become apparent as a result of a number of studies of post-transfusion hepatitis that despite the application of sensitive techniques for screening blood for hepatitis B surface antigen, hepatitis remains a major problem[7]. Only relatively few patients were found to have serological evidence of exposure to hepatitis B virus. Epidemiological evidence, a lengthy incubation period and serological evidence that hepatitis A, EB virus or CMV were not implicated clearly suggest the existence of an additional hepatitis virus or viruses which are transmissible by blood[27–32].

Additional evidence that an agent other than type B hepatitis may be transmitted by blood was provided by the report of an outbreak of short-incubation non-B hepatitis and hepatitis B in southern England associated with the use of three out of four batches of a commercial Factor VIII concentrate[33]. Details of a non-B acute hepatitis outbreak in a haemodialysis unit in London have also been published[34]. And in studies of hepatitis in an endemic zone in Costa Rica, evidence was provided for vital hepatitis other than type A or type B which was not associated with blood transfusion. In this study EB virus and CMV infection were excluded in all but one of the patients[35].

It is evident from these studies that there is a third and possibly other types of human hepatitis viruses, but there are as yet no precise criteria or specific tests for these agents. The question which must now be asked is how to ensure that the current candidate hepatitis vaccines are free of these viruses? It should be noted that although the conditions employed for the purification of the 22 nm hepatitis B surface antigen particles, apart from treatment with formalin, were found in at least one published study to destroy the infectivity of a number of viruses representing a wide range of virus families[36], cautious extrapolation is required in view of the known stability of the hepatitis viruses.

VACCINES OF THE FUTURE

Perhaps one of the most interesting prospects for the future is the development of a synthetic vaccine. An immunochemical study of purified hepatitis B surface antigen is essential for this project. Knowledge of the primary sequence of the haptenic peptide of hepatitis B antigen would be required for developing a synthetic peptide, which, when coupled to a macromolecular carrier, could serve as a suitable immunogen. Once detailed data are available on the protein, peptide and amino-acid composition of this antigen, it should be possible to define by animal immunization the moiety responsible for the antigenic activity. Provided a sufficiently small fragment of the molecule would be immunogenic, then a synthetic vaccine may be feasible.

Acknowledgements

The work in progress at the London School of Hygiene and Tropical Medicine is supported by generous grants from the Medical Research Council, the World Health Organization, the Wellcome Trust and the Wolfson Foundation.

References

1. Zuckerman, A. J. (1970). Attempts to isolate the hepatitis virus by tissue culture methods. In: *Virus Diseases of the Liver*, pp. 46–58 (London: Butterworths)
2. Zuckerman, A. J. (1975). Tissue and organ culture studies of hepatitis B virus. *Amer. J. Med. Sci.*, **270**, 205
3. Krugman, S., Giles, J. P. and Hammond, J. (1970). Hepatitis virus: effect of heat on the infectivity and antigenicity of the MS-1 and MS-2 strains. *J. Infect. Dis.*, **122**, 432
4. Krugman, S., Giles, J. P. and Hammond, J. (1971). Viral hepatitis type B (MS-2 strain). Studies on active immunization. *J. Am. Med. Assoc.*, **217**
5. Krugman, S. and Giles, J. P. (1973). Viral hepatitis type B (MS-2) strain: further observations on natural history and prevention. *N. Engl. J. Med.*, **288**, 755
6. Soulier, J. P., Blatix, C., Courouce, A. M., Benamon, D., Amouch, P. and Drouet, J. (1972). Prevention of virus B hepatitis (SH hepatitis). *Am. J. Dis. Child.*, **123**, 429
7. World Health Organization (1975). Technical Report Series, No. 570. *Viral Hepatitis.* Report of a WHO Meeting. (Geneva)
8. Zuckerman, A. J. (1975). *Human Viral Hepatitis.* 2nd Ed., pp. 155–189 (Amsterdam: North Holland–American Elsevier)
9. Purcell, R. H. and Gerin, J. L. (1975). Hepatitis B subunit vaccine: a preliminary report of safety and efficacy tests in chimpanzees. *Amer. J. Med. Sci.*, **270**, 395

10. Hilleman, M. R., Buynak, E. B., Roehm, R. R., Tytell, A. A., Bertland, A. U. and Lampson, G. P. (1975). Purified and inactivated human hepatitis B vaccine. *Amer. J. Med. Sci.*, **270**, 401
11. Buynak, E. B., Roehm, R. R., Tytell, A. A., Bertland, A. U., Lampson, G. P. and Hilleman, M. R. (1976). Vaccine against human hepatitis B. *J. Am. Med. Assoc.*, **235**, 2832
12. Maupas, P., Goudeau, A., Coursaget, P., Drucker, J. and Bagros, P. (1976). Immunisation against hepatitis B in man. *Lancet*, **1**, 1367
13. Zuckerman, A. J. (1976). Hepatitis B vaccine: safety criteria and non-B infection. *Lancet*, **1**, 1396
14. Zuckerman, A. J. (1975). Hepatitis vaccine: a note of caution. *Nature*, **255**, 104
15. Melnick, J. L., Dreesman, G. R. and Hollinger, F. B. (1976). Approaching the control of viral hepatitis type B. *J. Infect. Dis.*, **133**, 210
16. Zuckerman, A. J. and Howard, C. R. (1976). Hepatitis B vaccine: tests in humans. *Science*, **191**, 1126
17. Eddleston, A. L. W. F. and Williams, R. (1974). Inadequate antibody response to HB Ag or suppressor T cell defect in development of active chronic hepatitis. *Lancet*, **2**, 1543
18. Lee, W. M., Reed, W. D., Mitchell, C. G., Galbraith, R. M., Eddleston, A. L. W. F., Zuckerman, A. J. and Williams, R. (1975). Cellular and humoral immunity to the hepatitis B surface antigen in active chronic hepatitis. *Brit. Med. J.*, **1**, 705
19. Eddleston, A. L. W. F. (1976). Aetiological factors in immune-mediated liver disease. In A. Ferguson and R. N. M. Mac Sween (eds.). *Immunological Aspects of the Liver and Gastrointestinal Tract*, pp. 291–317 (Lancaster: MTP Press)
20. Hirschman, S. Z. (1975). Integration enzyme hypothesis for replication of hepatitis B virus. *Lancet*, **2**, 436
21. Rao, K. R. and Vyas, G. N. (1973). Hepatitis B antigen activity in protein subunits produced by sonication. *Nature New Biol.*, **241**, 240
22. Howard, C. R. and Zuckerman, A. J. (1974). Characterization of hepatitis B antigen polypeptides. *Intervirology*, **4**, 31
23. Zuckerman, A. J. and Howard, C. R. (1975). Toward hepatitis B vaccines. *Bull. NY Acad. Med.*, **51**, 491
24. Dreesman, G. R., Hollinger, F. B. and Melnick, J. L. (1975). Biophysical and biochemical properties of purified preparations of hepatitis B surface antigen (HB_sAg). *Amer. J. Med. Sci.*, **270**, 123
25. Cabral, G. A., Chairez, R., Marciano-Cabral, F., Suarez, M., Dreesman, G. R., Melnick, J. L. and Hollinger, F. B. (1975). Cell-mediated immunity in guinea pigs to subunits derived from hepatitis B surface antigen. *Infect. Immun.*, **12**, 564
26. Neurath, A. R., Trepo, C., Chen, M. and Prince, A. M. (1976). Identification of additional antigenic sites on Dane particles and the tubular forms of hepatitis B surface antigen. *J. Gen. Virol.*, **30**, 277
27. Prince, A. M., Brotman, B., Grady, G. F., Kuhns, W. J., Hazzi, C., Levine, R. W. and Millian, S. J. (1974). Long-incubation post-transfusion hepatitis without serological evidence of exposure to hepatitis B virus. *Lancet*, **2**, 241
28. Prince, A. M. (1975). Post-transfusion hepatitis: etiology and prevention. In E. Ikkala and A. Nykanen (eds.). *Transfusion and Immunology*, pp. 81–96 (Finland: Vammala)
29. Alter, H. J., Purcell, R. H., Holland, P. V., Feinstone, S. M., Morrow, A. G. and Moritsugu, Y. (1975). Clinical and serological analysis of transfusion-associated hepatitis. *Lancet*, **2**, 838
30. Feinstone, S. M., Kapikian, A. Z., Purcell, R. H., Alter, H. J. and Holland, P. V. (1975). Transfusion-associated hepatitis not due to viral hepatitis type A or B. *N. Engl. J. Med.*, **292**, 767
31. Knodell, R. G., Conrad, M. E., Dienstag, J. L. and Bell, C. J. (1975). Etiological spectrum of post-transfusion hepatitis. *Gastroenterology*, **69**, 1278
32. Seeff, L. B., Wright, E. C., Zimmerman, H. J. and McCollum, R. W. (1975). VA cooperative study of post-transfusion hepatitis, 1969–1974: incidence and characteristics of hepatitis and responsible risk factors. *Amer. J. Med. Sci.*, **270**, 355
33. Craske, J., Dilling, N. and Stern, D. (1975). An outbreak of hepatitis associated with intravenous injection of Factor-VIII concentrate. *Lancet*, **2**, 221

34. Galbraith, R. M., Portmann, B., Eddleston, A. L. W. F., Williams, R. and Gower, P. E. (1975). Chronic liver disease developing after outbreak of HBsAg-negative hepatitis in haemodialysis unit. *Lancet*, **2**, 886
35. Villarejos, V. M., Visona, K. A., Eduarte, C. A., Provost, P. J. and Hilleman, M. R. (1975). Evidence for viral hepatitis other than type A or type B among persons in Costa Rica. *N. Engl. J. Med.*, **293**, 1350
36. Buynak, E. B., Roehm, R. R., Tytell, A. A., Bertland, A. U., Lampson, G. P. and Hilleman, M. R. (1976). Development and chimpanzee testing of a vaccine against human hepatitis B. *Proc. Soc. Exp. Biol. Med.*, **151**, 694

13

Herpesvirus vaccine development: studies of virus morphological components

S. K. VERNON, W. C. LAWRENCE, CAROLE A. LONG, G. H. COHEN AND B. A. RUBIN

INTRODUCTION

Interest in the development of herpesvirus vaccines for humans has been intensified by recent evidence linking members of this virus group to human cancer. Of the five human herpesviruses (herpes simplex virus type 1 and 2 [HSV-1, HSV-2], Epstein-Barr virus [EBV], human cytomegalovirus [CMV], varicella-zoster virus [VZV]), EBV and HSV-2 have been associated with neoplastic disease[1–14] and all but VZV have been shown to possess *in vitro* cell transforming capability[12,13,15–18].

Characteristics of herpesvirus–host relationships, which include the establishment of both persistent and latent infections[3,16,19–30], indicate that live homologous or heterologous virus or inactivated virus may be unacceptable, from the standpoint of safety, for use in human vaccines. Thus, for the foreseeable future, a reasonable approach to immunoprophylaxis against herpesvirus diseases of man is the development of subunit vaccines free of viral genetic material.

As part of an effort to discover the immunogenic characteristics of herpesvirus constituents, we have begun to investigate methods of removing and isolating morphological components from purified virus particles. This paper briefly reviews recent progress towards the development of herpesvirus subunit vaccines, and describes some preliminary results of our investigations within that context.

HERPESVIRUS VACCINES

A number of herpesvirus diseases of domestic animals can be prevented by vaccination. Chickens have been successfully protected from Marek's disease by vaccination with live, cell-associated Marek's disease virus (MDV) or antigenically related turkey herpesvirus and with live, cell-free turkey herpesvirus[31-33]. Efficacy of the live MDV vaccines is somewhat dependent on the degree of attenuation of the virus, which varies among field isolates and with the extent of virus passage in tissue culture.[34-36]. Most of the other commercial vaccines for animals contain live, attenuated viruses; inactivated virus vaccines generally have been ineffective in preventing disease[37].

Humans also have been inoculated with experimental herpesvirus vaccines. Inactivated virus vaccines were employed to afford protection of susceptible subjects to simian B virus[38,39] and as therapeutic treatment for patients with recurrent HSV infections[39-43]. More recently, a live CMV vaccine was developed for possible use in preventing *in utero* infection and subsequent mental retardation[44]. Although virus-neutralizing antibodies were detected in immunized subjects, the protective effects of these vaccines were not established definitively. A recent live (VZV) vaccine appears to have protected children against both primary infections and development of herpes zoster[45].

Recent investigations have provided evidence that neoplastic disease of animals can be prevented with inactivated virus vaccines and with virus-free vaccines. Chickens were protected from Marek's disease by inoculation with glutaraldehyde-fixed Marek's disease lymphoblastoid cell lines[46] and with purified plasma membranes from cultured cells infected with turkey herpesvirus[47]. Subunit vaccines prepared by detergent extraction of MDV-infected cells also were effective[48]. Marmosets failed to develop malignant lymphomas[49,50] upon challenge following vaccination with heat and formaldehyde-inactivated *Herpesvirus saimiri* or *Herpesvirus ateles*[51,52]. Thus live virus, inactivated virus, and virus-free vaccines have provided protection against herpesvirus-associated neoplasias. Other studies have shown that virus-free vaccines can elicit production of virus-neutralizing antibodies and protect laboratory animals from lethal herpesvirus challenge[53-55].

CHARACTERIZATION OF VIRUS-SPECIFIC ANTIGENS

Development of a subunit vaccine will require the thorough immunological characterization of virus-specific antigens. During herpesvirus infection, a wide variety of virus-determined cell membrane and cell nuclear antigens, as well as virus structural antigens, are detectable *in vivo* and *in vitro*[1,3,4,9,10,24,55-60]. For example, ten to twelve virus-specific antigens have been detected in HSV-1-infected BHK 21 cells[61,62]. At least 47 virus-specific polypeptides have been detected both in HSV-1 and HSV-2-infected HEp-2 cells, and as many as 24 of those were tentatively identified as viral structural proteins[63,64]. The most direct approach towards determining the requisite antigens for a subunit vaccine would entail characterization of highly purified virus-specific proteins alone, in combination, and under varying conditions of association. This approach will require the use of suitable animal models for the relevant viral infection and can provide insight as to a suitable source for the requisite antigen(s), whether cellular or viral.

Because of the difficulties encountered in preparing purified herpesvirus antigens, progress in this area has been slow. Nevertheless, a number of investigators have demonstrated the elicitation of human herpesvirus neutralizing antibodies in animals inoculated with solubilized antigens from infected cell cultures or partially purified virus preparations[53,54,65,66]. In other studies of isolated antigens, Watson and his colleagues have characterized an antigen ('Band II') from HSV-1-infected BHK cells which elicited neutralizing antibodies in rabbits both to HSV-1 and HSV-2 and appeared to be a virus structural component. Antiserum to Band II possessed both type-specific and type-common neutralizing activities[61,67–70].

A more direct approach consisted of the isolation of an antigen from disrupted virions, by polyacrylamide gel electrophoresis (PAGE), which elicited type-specific neutralizing activity; the antigen included one of the major viral glycoproteins[71,72]. In other studies, an antigen associated with squamous cervical tumours has been tentatively identified as a minor component of HSV-2, which apparently did not elicit virus neutralizing antibody in rabbits[73,74]. Cohen and his colleagues isolated a virus-induced, soluble cellular antigen from HSV-1-infected BHK cells by chromatographic methods. The antigen, which was also detectable on the surfaces of cells transformed with inactivated HSV-1, appeared to comprise a viral structural component which contained glycoprotein and elicited neutralizing antibody in rabbits[75–77].

At this time, however, little can be said of the protection that purified subunit preparations can provide *in vivo*. It remains to be seen whether such vaccines, derived from infected or transformed cells or culture fluids or from disrupted virus, can provide protection against disease associated with not only primary, but chronic and recurrent infections.

CHARACTERIZATION OF VIRAL STRUCTURAL COMPONENTS

It is appropriate here to review briefly the current knowledge of herpesvirus structure, much of which has been gained using recent technical improvements in purification methods and PAGE. Since the first description of herpesvirus morphology was published by Wildy, Russell, and Horne[78], the structure has been investigated in great detail, and the results have been reviewed more comprehensively elsewhere[59,60,79–84,147].

The herpesviruses consist of icosahedral nucleocapsids, which are synthesized in host cell nuclei, surrounded by flexible, trilaminar lipid-containing envelopes which are acquired as the capsids pass through the nuclear membrane into the cytoplasm[85–87]. The envelopes are studded with projections morphologically similar to the haemagglutinin 'spikes' of influenza virus[78,88].

The viral genome, comprising a linear, double-stranded DNA with a molecular weight of P approximately 100 x 10^6 daltons, is associated with a core[86] structure within the capsid[78,89,90].

Intact virions of HSV, CMV, EBV, and equine herpesvirus type 1 (EHV-1) have been reported to contain 28 to 33 polypeptides[91–94], although somewhat lower figures (20 to 24) have been obtained[95–99]. Although at least eight glycopeptides were associated with CMV[100], HSV, EBV, and EHV-1 contain several more[91,94,101]. Comparisons of the constituents of de-enveloped nucleocapsids and non-enveloped intracellular nucleocapsids have established that most of the virus polypeptides are extrinsic to the capsid. The assignment of the outermost proteins to the envelope *per se* or to the underlying tegument, a descriptive term for the amorphous material between the envelope and capsid[78,80], has not been established definitively, although the radial distribution of some HSV-1 proteins has been described[80,81].

The icosahedral herpesvirus capsid consists of twelve vertex pentamers and 150 hollow, columnar hexamers, which are connected by inter-capsomeric fibrils[78,88,102]. Hollow ('light') capsids extracted from nuclei of cells infected with HSV-1 or EHV-1[103,104] contain only four major polypeptides; one of these, with a molecular weight of approximately 150 000 daltons[103,104], probably is a structural subunit of the hexamer, which appears to contain three morphological subunits[88]. 'Heavy' capsids, which contain core structures and at least some of the viral DNA, contain five or six major, and several minor, polypeptides[103–105]. De-enveloped capsids of HSV and EBV reportedly contain at least seven major polypeptides[91,103,106]. 'Heavy' intranuclear capsids are thought to be precursors of mature virions, whereas it is not certain whether light capsids become enveloped or are defective products[103,107]. All of the polypeptides of HSV-1 heavy (B) capsids were present in de-enveloped capsids with one exception—a phosphorylated 39 000 MW protein (no. 22a), bound to B capsids, appeared to be cleaved or more extensively phosphorylated during envelopment. The alleged product (no. 22) had a slightly higher electrophoretic mobility and could be extracted from virions by treatment with NP-40, DOC, and BRIJ-58[103,108].

The virus cores seem to be somewhat variable in structure. The HSV-1 core apparently consists of a DNA-containing torus wrapped around a proteinaceous cylindrical structure[109], and several other herpesviruses contain morphologically similar cores[107,110–113] In some cases, a DNA-containing thread appears to be wound helically around the central cylinder[111,114].

None of the antigens described above as having afforded protection to laboratory animals or eliciting production of neutralizing antibodies have been shown to consist of only a single polypeptide. However, all the subunit vaccines thus far described have contained glycoprotein and have included infected cell membrane or virus envelope polypeptides. Thus, the immunogenic characteristics of individual viral proteins remain unknown.

STRUCTURAL STUDIES OF EHV-1 COMPONENTS

HSV-1 and EHV-1 have been the most thoroughly studied members of the herpesvirus group; O'Callaghan and Randall[115] have pointed out the basic similarities between these two viruses. Using EHV-1 as a model herpesvirus we have undertaken two lines of investigation: one consists of the development of methods to remove and characterize envelope components from virions in a controlled manner; the other is a search for means of isolating nucleocapsid components. The results described here are only preliminary, but useful knowledge has been obtained concerning the structure and stability of viral and subviral particles.

De-envelopment of EHV-1 virions

Methods

Highly purified EHV-1 virions, appropriately labelled with [^{3}H]-amino acids, [^{3}H]-glucosamine, or [^{35}S]-methionine, were obtained by the method of Lawrence[116], which, briefly, employs ammonium sulphate precipitation of concentrated extracellular virus from infected LM strain mouse fibroblast cultures and two or three cycles of flotation in CsCR density gradients. Virus-containing bands were stored in CsCl until used; no significant losses of infectivity or morphological changes were detected after storage for at least 2 weeks.

Samples were prepared for electron microscopy by fixation with OsO_4 or glutaraldehyde, application to carbon-coated specimen grids and staining with 1.0% uranyl acetate (UAc), 1.0% sodium zirconium glycollate (NZG), pH 7.0, or 1.0% sodium phosphotungstate (PTA), ph 7.0, before virus particles were permitted to dry. The usefulness of these procedures has been described[117]. Specimen grids were shadow-cast with platinum-carbon evaporated from angles of 10–15°.

Virions in CsCl or after dialysis against 0.02 M phosphate-buffered saline (PBS) were incubated at ambient temperature or 4° with the following lipid solvents: 0.5% or 1% Nonidet-P40 (NP40), 1% NP40 and 1% sodium deoxycholate, 0.8% Triton X-100, or 0.3% tri(*n*-butyl) phosphate (TNBP) and 0.1% Tween 80[118], all in PBS. Treated virus particles were recovered by sedimentation or flotation in preformed gradients of Renografin-76 (35% to 55% [w/v]) at 90 000 *g* in Beckman SW-40 or SW-65 rotors[94]. Flotation gradients were spun for 18 h; sedimentation gradients for 3.5 h. Occasionally, virus was centrifuged in CsCl gradients as described previously[116] or was pelleted by centrifugation and resuspended in PBS before being applied to Renografin gradients.

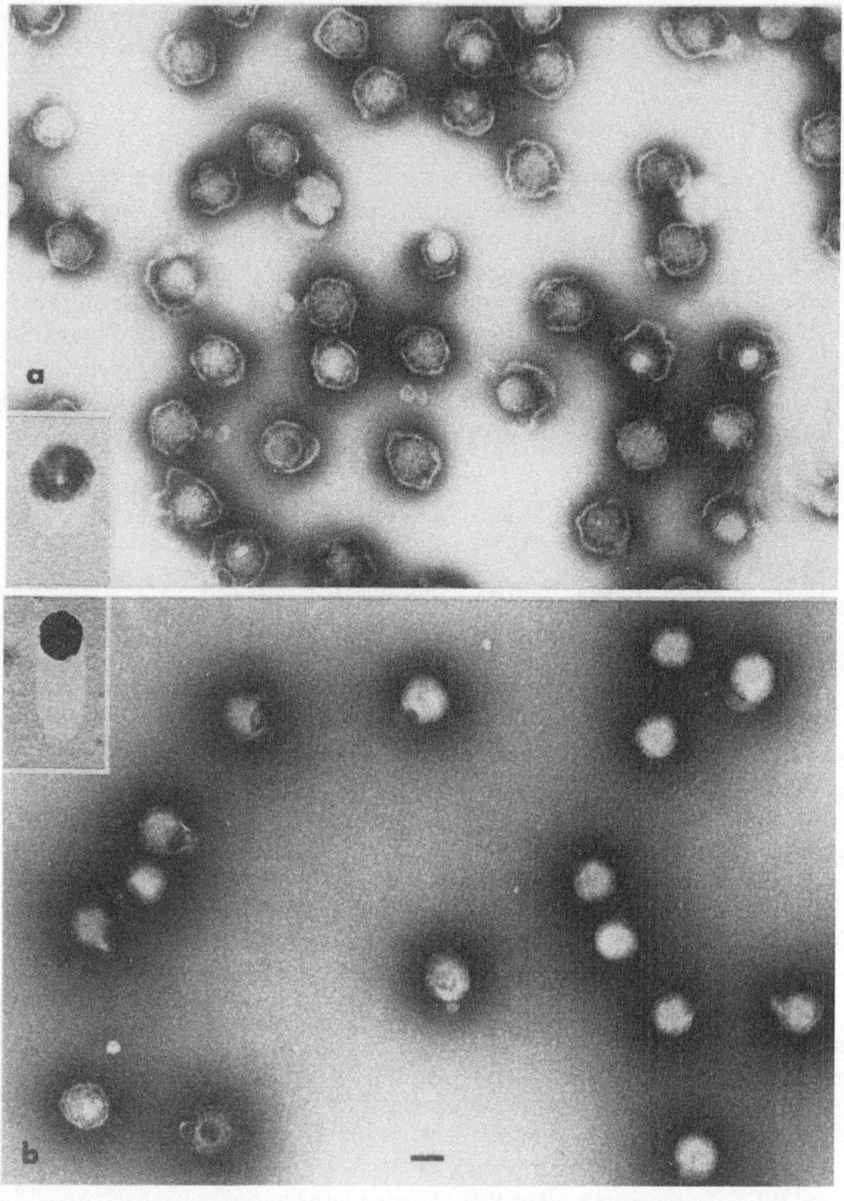

Figure 1 Effect of fixation on EHV-1 virions negatively stained with 1% NZG. (a) Unfixed viruses, exhibiting envelope disruption and exposure of capsids. The inset shows a typical unfixed shadowed particle, whose shadow indicates particle flattening. (b) Viruses fixed with 1% OsO_4, then stained. The particles are relatively homogeneous in size and shape, and most envelopes have not ruptured. Envelope surface projections are more easily seen on unfixed particles. The inset shows an unflattened, shadowed particle whose electron density has been increased by fixation. ×50 000. This and subsequent scale markers represent 100 nm

Treated virus recovered from gradients was dialysed against PBS, incubated at 37 °C with 250–400 μg TPCK-trypsin (Worthington)/ml for up to 20 h, and then subjected to centrifugation in Renografin gradients as above. Gradient fractions were assayed for radioactivity, and labelled peaks were dialysed against water for analysis by SDS-polyacrylamide gel electrophoresis (SDS-PAGE) using Laemmli's procedure[119].

Morphology

Electron microscopic observations of disrupted envelopes and fragmented capsids in purified preparations of virions which exhibited stable levels of infectivity prompted an investigation of the effects of negative staining on virus components. A comparison of unfixed virions with particles fixed with OsO_4 indicated that visible envelope disruption was caused primarily by

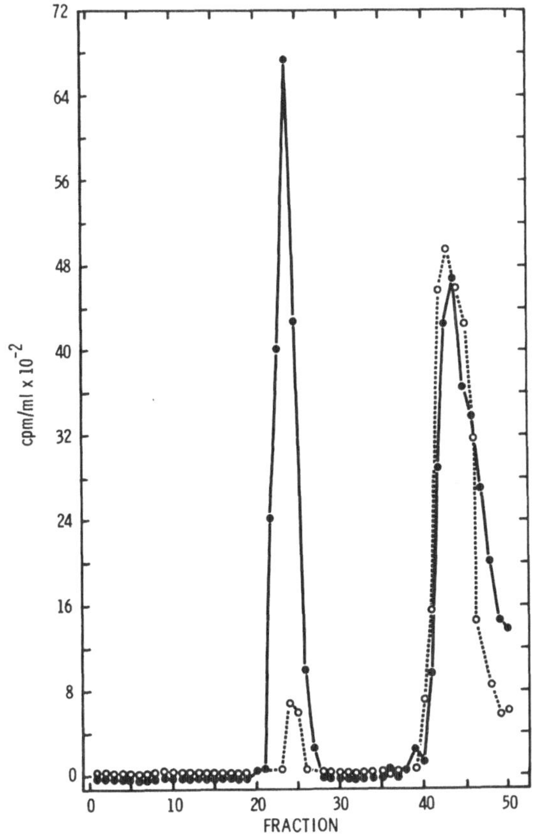

Figure 2 Distribution of [^{3}H]-amino acid labelled proteins (●—●) and [^{3}H]-glucosamine-labelled glycoproteins (o - - - o) after sedimentation, in 35–55% (w/v) Renografin-76 gradients, of EHV-1 following incubation for 18 h with NP40 and sodium deoxycholate; sedimentation was from right to left. No recognizable virus constituents were observed in any fractions but those within the virus peak at the middle of the gradient

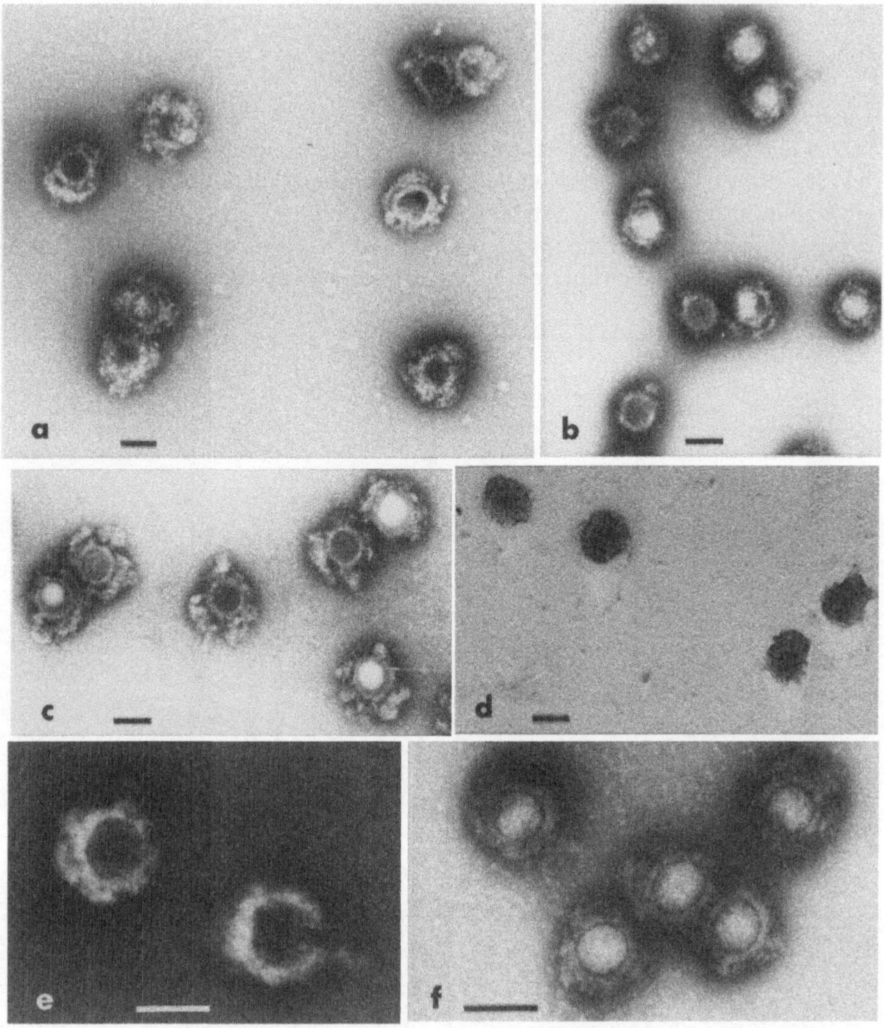

Figure 3 EHV-1 treated with lipid solvents, recovered from Renografin-76 or CsCl gradients, and stained with UAc. (a) Treated with NP40 and sodium deoxycholate. (b) NP40 only. (c) TNBP and Tween 80. (d,e) Same as (a). The particles in (d) were shadow-cast after being stained. The width of the shadows indicates that the capsids are covered with residual envelope material. The particles in (e) lie in densely-pooled stain. Virtually all such particles are smooth-surfaced, but the boundaries of the partially-flattened viruses are poorly contrasted. (f) Treated with 0.8% Triton X-100. The appearance of the material adhering to the capsids varies with the stain and its deposition thickness. All treatments produced similar morphological effects. (a–d) ×50 000; (e,f) ×105 000

dehydration, on specimen grids, of viruses insufficiently protected by fixation and relatively thick deposits of negative stain. Viruses which were dehydrated before being stained almost always exhibited broken envelopes; these often virtually 'exploded' from capsids, and flattened sheets of capsomers[88,117]. The necessity for protection from such premature dehydration was confirmed by shadow-casting (Figure 1). We concluded that these precautions were of great importance for accurate electron microscopic evaluation of virus samples[117].

The distribution of radioactive viral proteins in a Renografin gradient following a detergent treatment and sedimentation is shown in Figure 2. The only subviral particles recognizable by electron microscopy were contained in the peak at the middle of the gradient, which consistently appeared at a buoyant density of 1.235–1.245 g/cm^3.

Electron microscopy of treated virus, both before and after recovery in Renografin gradients, detected populations of capsids retaining tegument; naked capsids were seen, occasionally, only after CsCl centrifugation. By shadow-casting negatively stained viruses or in areas of unusually heavy stain deposition, it could be observed that all capsids remained enclosed within spikeless, amorphous material. Usually, negative staining alone resulted in the observation of varying amounts of residual material adhering to the capsids (Figure 3). We concluded that the outermost components of the 'envelope' had been removed, and the remaining envelope–tegument complex was obscured after staining procedures alone. No significant differences in the effects of any of the solvent treatments were detected by centrifugation or electron microscopy. However, only NP40-treated viruses have so far been subjected to PAGE analysis.

Polypeptide composition of NP40-treated virus

Intact virions were compared to virus particles treated with NP40 by SDS-PAGE. As shown in Figure 4, the virion polypeptide content was similar to that previously described for EHV-1[94,120], with only minor differences; for convenience, therefore, the bands have been numbered in accordance with the system summarized by O'Callaghan and Randall[115]. The effect of NP40 on EHV-1 was remarkably similar to that described for HSV-1 by Spear and Roizman[99]. The most significant effects were:

1. Treated viruses contained markedly decreased levels of polypeptides 10, 13–15, 17–19, and 22A and B. In addition, the content of high molecular weight proteins (nos. 1–8) was reduced.
2. The poorly separated bands in the 13–15 peak were resolved into five clearly separated bands.
3. The no. 18, 19 peak, which usually appeared as two overlapping bands, was resolved as a single band corresponding to no. 18.
4. A new band, (d), appeared, which migrated slightly behind band 21.

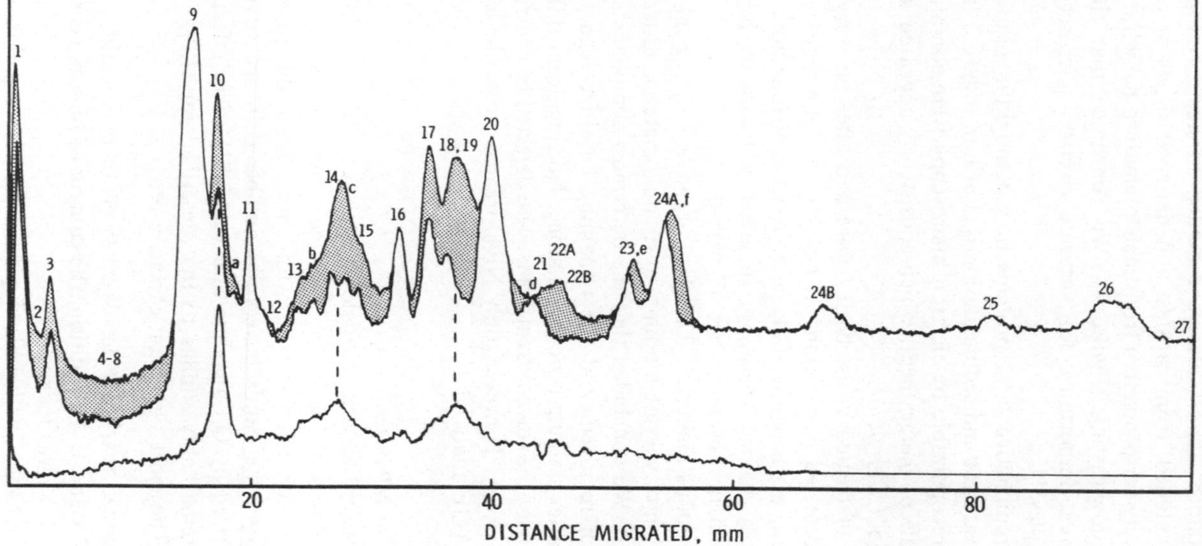

Figure 4 Electrophoretic analysis, in a 10% slab gel, of products obtained by incubation of EHV-1 virions with 1.0% NP40 for 4 h at room temperature. A Joyce–Loebl micro-densitometer was used to scan photographic negatives of gels stained with Coomassie brilliant blue. The curves obtained for intact virions (top) and NP40-treated virus (middle were superimposed; normalization of the curves was unnecessary as the areas under the polypeptide 9 peaks (the major capsid polypeptide) were similar for both curves. Thus, the shaded areas between the curves indicate material removed by NP40. Intact virions contained five bands which could not be correlated with the numbered polypeptides described by O'Callaghan and Randall[115]; their positions are indicated by letters. Polypeptide *d* was observed only in NP40-treated virus, which was recovered in Renografin gradients. Polypeptides solubilized by NP40 (bottom curve) were recovered in supernatent fluids after treated virus was pelleted by centrifugation at 90 000 *g* for 2 h. The dashed lines indicate the positions of the major solubilized polypeptides relative to virus bands

It is not yet known whether or not some of these changes were simply migration rate alterations resulting from the removal of carbohydrate moieties from glycoproteins. The NP40-soluble material consisted mostly of polypeptide 10 and lesser amounts of polypeptides 13–15 and 17–19. It could not be determined whether polypeptide 19 had been completely solubilized or merely shifted in position. Analyses using other gel concentrations (6–14%) did not clarify the result described.

Effect of trypsin

When NP40-treated particles were incubated with trypsin, electron microscopy, both before and after recovery in Renografin gradients, indicated that capsids were not disrupted by the enzyme, in contrast to previously

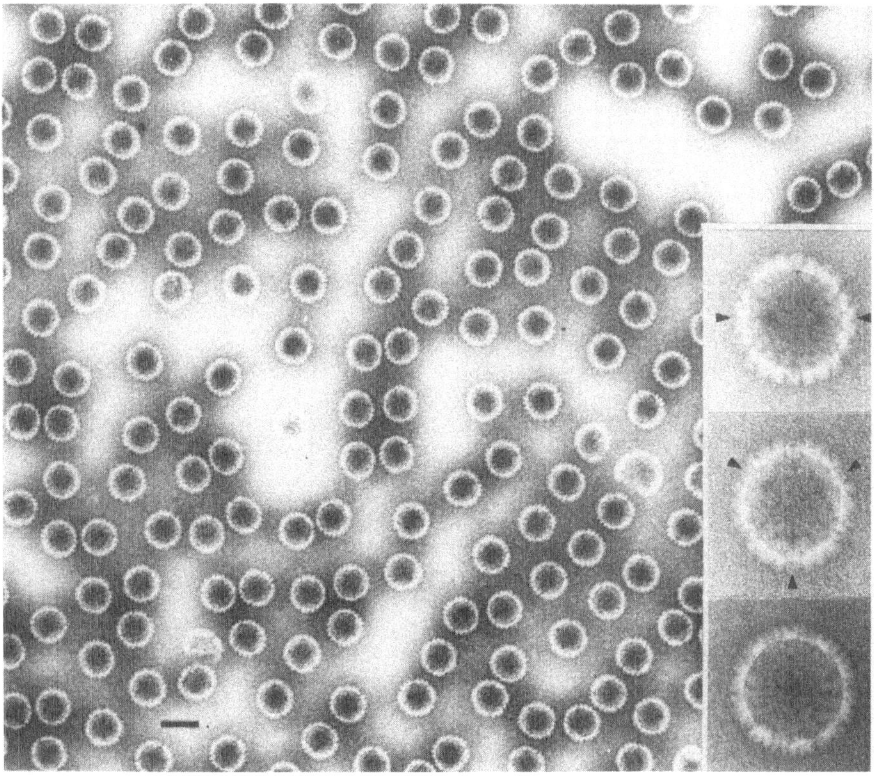

Figure 5 Removal of envelope–tegument complex from capsids previously treated with NP40. De-enveloped virus particles, as shown in Figure 3, were incubated overnight at 37 °C with 300 μg TPCK-trypsin per ml and recovered in a Renografin-76 gradient at a buoyant density of 1.26 g/cm^3. The presence of vertex holes becomes more easily detectable at higher magnifications. (Inset) De-enveloped capsids exhibiting vertex holes and viewed along 2-fold, 3-fold, and 5-fold rotational axes. Penetration of such particles by negative stain decreases the contrast of the capsid surface image. Stained with NZG. ×50 000; inset, ca. ×160 000

reported results with HSV and VZV[102]. Furthermore, the nucleocapsids lacked residual envelope–tegument complex, and at least some pentamers were missing (Figure 5). As shown in Figure 6, trypsinized nucleocapsids could be recovered by centrifugation in Renografin gradients.

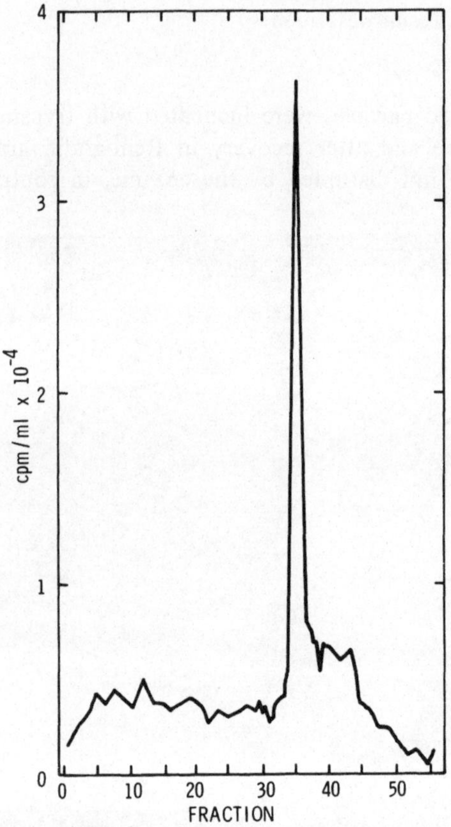

Figure 6 Distribution of radioactivity after flotation, in a Renografin-76 gradient, of [^{35}S]-methionine-labelled EHV-1 treated with NP40 and then incubated with trypsin at 37 °C for 18 h. Capsids lacking tegument and pentamers, as shown in Figure 5, were recovered in the sharp peak contained in Fractions 34–37. Fraction 35 had a buoyant density of 1.26 g/cm^3. No viral constituents were recognized in other fractions. Fraction 1 was the bottom of the gradient

Only five bands were observed when trypsinized, de-enveloped particles were subjected to PAGE. As shown in Figure 9, only one of these—polypeptide B—migrated at the same rate as a virion band (polypeptide 20). Identical results were obtained when nucleocapsids extracted from infected cell lysates were incubated with trypsin (see following section).

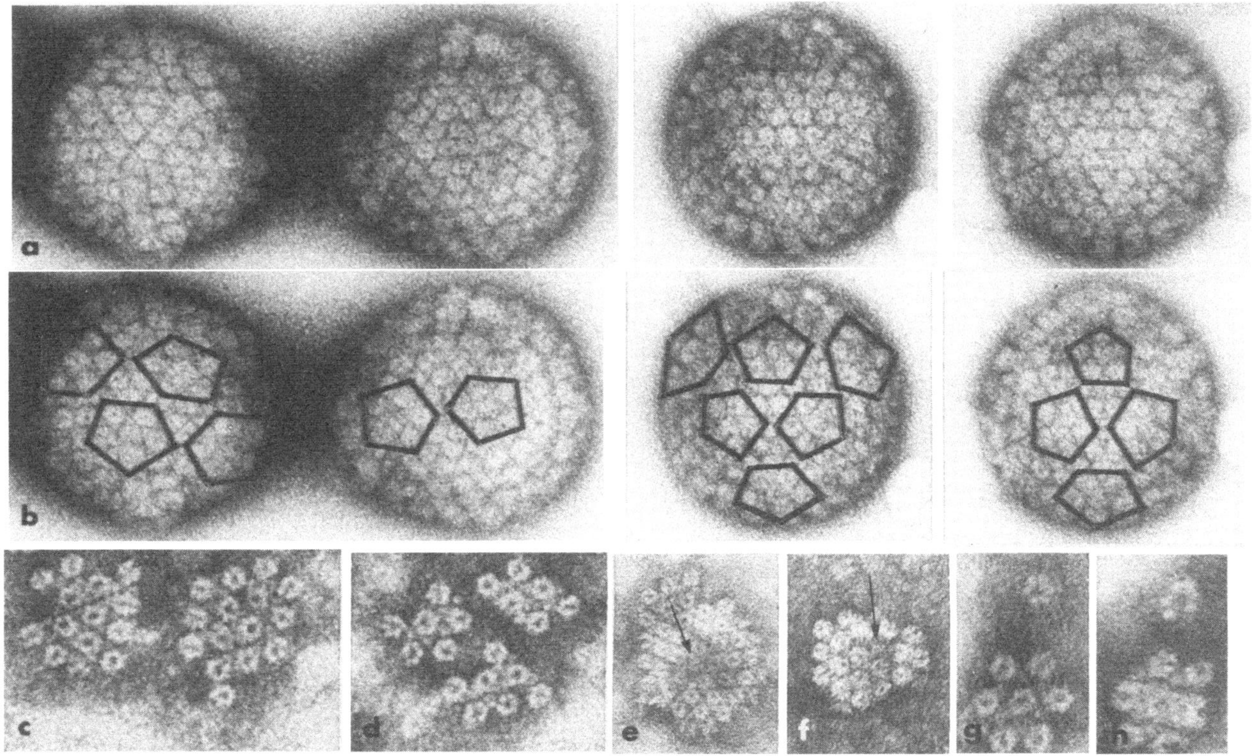

Figure 7 EHV-1 capsids and subunits negatively stained with 1% UAc, shown at various magnifications. (a) Unfixed capsids. (b) The same particles with peripentameric hexamers outlined so that visible pentamers can be located easily. The visibility of pentamers often is obscured by the angle of view or by axial or radial displacement. They appear to be held loosely within the capsid structure. Although the spaces they fill often have a pentagonal shape, the shape of the pentamers themselves is difficult to determine because of varying negative stain depth and the presence of intercapsomeric fibrils. (c–h) Sheets of capsomers from virus particles fragmented *in situ*. Intercapsomeric fibrils usually can be seen. The arrows in (e) and (f) indicate pentamers. The individual hexamer in (g) has a tripartite structure. In (h), the single hexamer appears to be separating into three dumbbell-like subunits

Disruption of purified EHV-1 nucleocapsids

These experiments involved a search for methods of disrupting nucleocapsids into morphologically-identifiable components.

Methods

Nucleocapsids of EHV-1 were purified from lysates of infected LM strain mouse fibroblasts (W. C. Lawrence, unpublished procedure). The purified virus consisted of a mixture of heavy, intermediate, and light nucleocapsids[104] with a predominance of light particles. They were recovered from CsCl density gradients and dialysed against PBS or the buffers described below. For degradativ estudies, they were treated at 37 °C with various concentrations of TPCK-trypsin or formamide, either on specimen grids or in suspension. Trypsinized nucleocapsids were recovered in Renografin density gradients as described above; particles treated with formamide were centrifuged at 90 000 *g* for 1 h on to CsCl cushions (buoyant density = 1.6 g/cm^3. Specimens were examined both before and after centrifugation by negative staining with 1% UAc, unbuffered, and neutral 1% NZG or 1% PTA. The effects of treatments were assessed using fixed and unfixed samples and at least two negative stains.

Morphology

Purified nucleocapsids were found to be as susceptible to dehydration during negative staining as were virions. Particles unprotected by glutaraldehyde and/or thick stain deposits were flattened and fragmented; capsomers, individually and in sheets, were seen in dehydrated samples, whereas they rarely were found in protected samples[117]. Capsids were protected from such destruction better by negative staining with UAc or NZG than with several other stains, including sodium phosphotungstate. It became clear that capsomer sheets seen in unfixed samples could not be considered as indicators of capsid disruption in suspension.

Examination of capsomer sheets seen when virus particles were dehydrated before staining led to the discovery of a matrix of intercapsomeric fibrils connecting the hexamers[88]; other investigators have found similar structures in trypsin-digested HSV capsids[102]. As reported previous[88], micrographs of individual hexamers were subjected to rotational image enhancement[122], and each of these capsomers appeared to consist of three structural subunits arranged similarly to those of the adenovirus hexon[121]. Several examples of capsid subunits are shown in Figure 7.

Electron microscopic examination indicated that capsids were stable after storage for at least 1 week in CsCl or PBS. Similarly, no morphological evidence of disruption was seen in samples stored after dialysis against water; 0.02 M tris buffer, pH 7.4; 0.1 M sodium acetate–acetic acid buffer, ph 4.9; or 0.2 sodium carbonate–sodium bicarbonate buffer, pH 10.

Effects of trypsin

Incubation of purified nucleocapsids with trypsin produced particles which lacked pentamers and which could be recovered in Renografin gradients. No differences between trypsinized nucleocapsids and trypsinized de-enveloped nucleocapsids were detected by electron microscopy or PAGE (Figures 8 and 9). The polypeptides of undigested nucleocapsids were numbered according to the system of O'Callaghan and Randall[115]. Of the five bands detected in trypsinized particles, only polypeptide B migrated at the same rate as a nucleocapsid polypeptide. This band was located at the same position as nucleocapsid Band II and virion band 20; the latter had not been removed by NP40. The four major nucleocapsid polypeptides corresponded in position to virion bands 9, 20, 24A and 26, respectively.

Effects of formamide

Structural similarities between herpesvirus capsids and adenoviruses prompted the use of methods which have been successful in disrupting the latter viruses. Attempts to remove EHV-1 pentamers using methods which remove adenovirus pentons[123–125] have so far been unsuccessful. However, formamide, which cleaves intercapsomeric bonds of adenoviruses and causes the exposure of virus cores after the release of capsomers[126,127], appeared more promising. When formamide, in concentrations as high as 50%, was applied to EHV-1 nucleocapsids adsorbed to specimen grids, no widespread effect was discernible by electron microscopy. However, within 5 min of the application of 100% formamide, the capsomers lost their structural integrity and the capsids collapsed into amorphous, stringy particles (Figure 10). Occasionally, densely-stained spherical particles were seen associated with collapsed capsids; these retained UAc internally after stained grids were rinsed with water to remove negative stain. The particles, which we refer to as virus cores, appeared to have limiting boundaries which often were obscured by stain or were ruptured (Figure 11). Positively-stained fibrous material, possibly nucleoprotein, often was associated with ruptured cores, which were seen more frequently when grids were dried before staining. Many particles contained internal components which usually appeared as electron-transparent oval or rod-like structures (Figure 11). Other particles lacking dense stain and usually oval or spherical in shape were also seen occasionally; these were somewhat smaller than dense particles and had diameters of about 50 to 80 nm (Figure 12). Diameters of both types of particles varied considerably, possibly as a result of variable flattening during the staining procedure.

Nucleocapsids were treated in suspension by the addition of formamide to a final concentration of 90% (v/v). After incubation for 2 h at 37°C, they were dialysed against PBS and centrifuged on to CsCl cushions. The resultant flocculent bands were collected and examined by electron microscopy. As shown in Figure 13, denatured capsids were recovered as discrete particles.

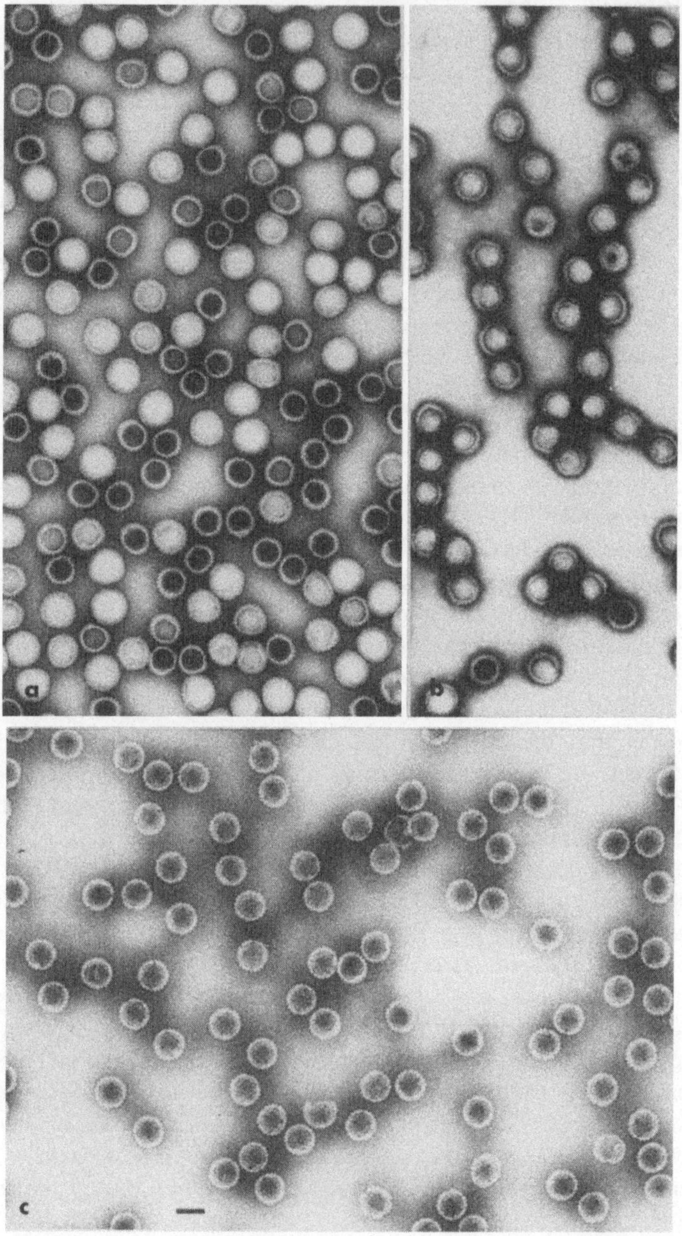

Figure 8 Effect of trypsin on purified capsids. (a,b) Purified capsids fixed with glutaraldehyde and stained with NZG and UAc, respectively. (c) Capsids adsorbed to specimen grids, incubated with 300 μg trypsin/ml for 4 h at 37 °C, rinsed and stained with NZG. Vertex holes are visible on most particles. The occasional evidence of disruption could be almost eliminated by fixation after digestion, but the holes on fixed capsids were more difficult to observe. ×50 000

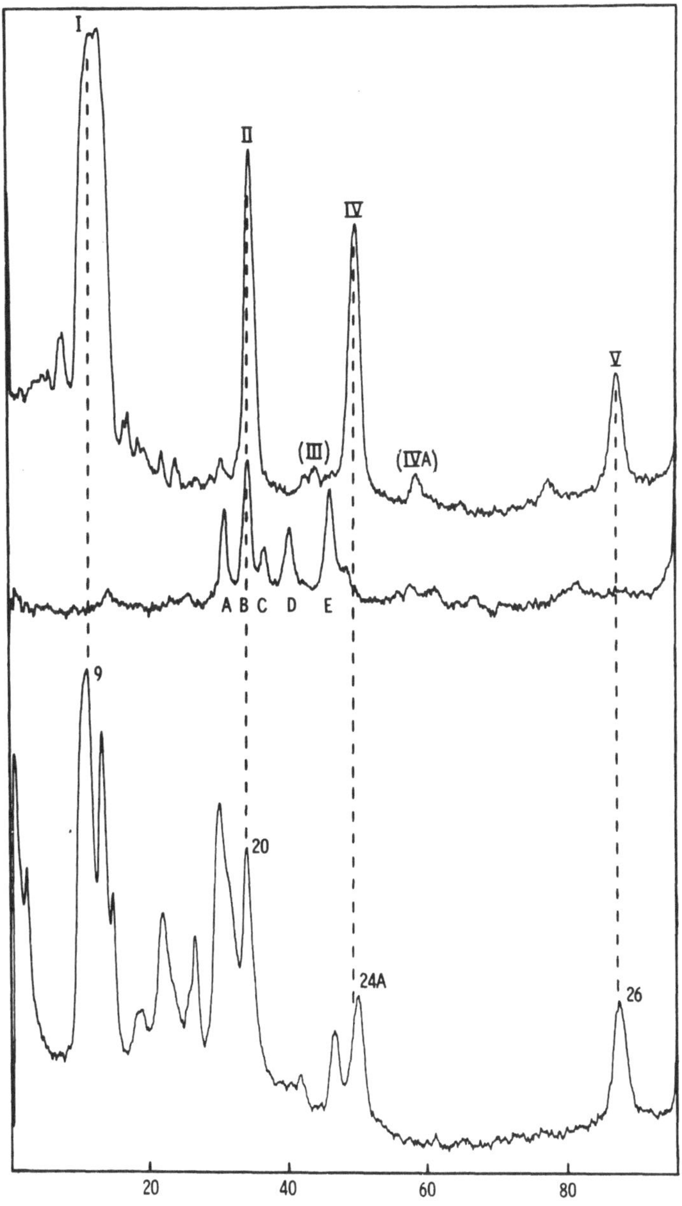

Figure 9 Electrophoretic analysis, in a 10% slab gel, of trypsinized nucleocapsids. The polypeptide content of trypsinized, de-enveloped particles (middle curve) was identical to that of trypsinized intracellular nucleocapsids (not shown). The polypeptides of purified, undigested nucleocapsids are shown in the top curve; peak I probably represents the hexamer protein. Parentheses indicate tentative identifications. Proteins III and IVA are not present in light nucleocapsids[104]. Correspondence of nucleocapsid polypeptides with numbered virion polypeptides (bottom curve) is indicated by the dashed lines

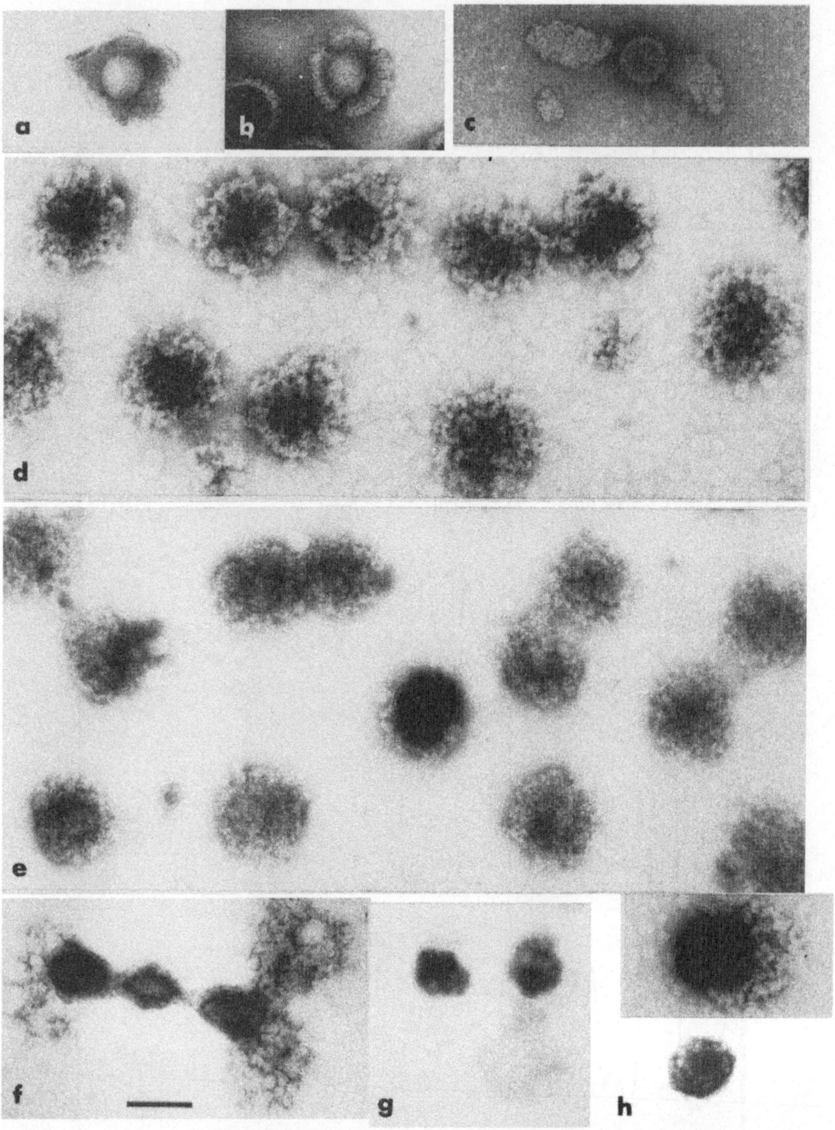

Figure 10 Effect of formamide on EHV-1 nucleocapsids treated on specimen grids, stained with UAc except as noted. (a) A virion with a spherical, 70 nm core. (b) Spontaneously broken capsid treated with 10% formamide for 5 min. A 70 nm core has been exposed. Capsomere sheets were rarely seen in formamide-treated samples, and their frequency did not increase with increasing treatment times. Therefore, we concluded that their appearance was a result of the staining procedure. (d–h) Capsids treated on grids with undiluted formamide for 5–30 min. The capsids have collapsed into amorphous, stringy structures. Occasionally, densely stained particles were present, as shown in (e), which was stained with PTA. These always were associated with denatured capsids. In (f), three such particles are connected by fibrous material and are printed to show internal components. The particle in (h) has been printed twice to show the heavy electron density (upper) and particle detail. The easiest method for distinguishing the particles, as shown in (g), was to stain with UAc and rinse off negative stain with water. With this method, the particles stand out clearly against unstained backgrounds, and the particle borders are easily distinguished

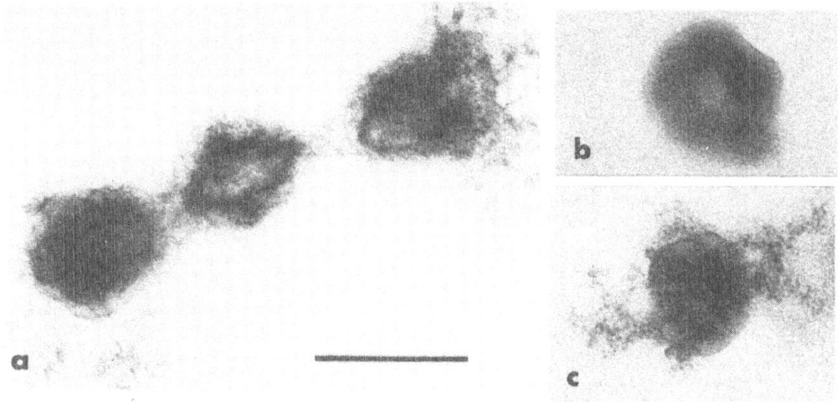

Figure 11 Electron-dense particles exposed by formamide treatment of EHV-1 capsids. (a) Figure 10(f) at higher magnification. Note the rod-like internal components. (b,c) Rinsed with water after UAc staining. In (b) an internal component is visible. The particle in (c) apparently has ruptured, and positively stained fibrous material, probably nucleoprotein, has been extruded. The unstained denatured capsid lies to the right of the particle. ×225 000

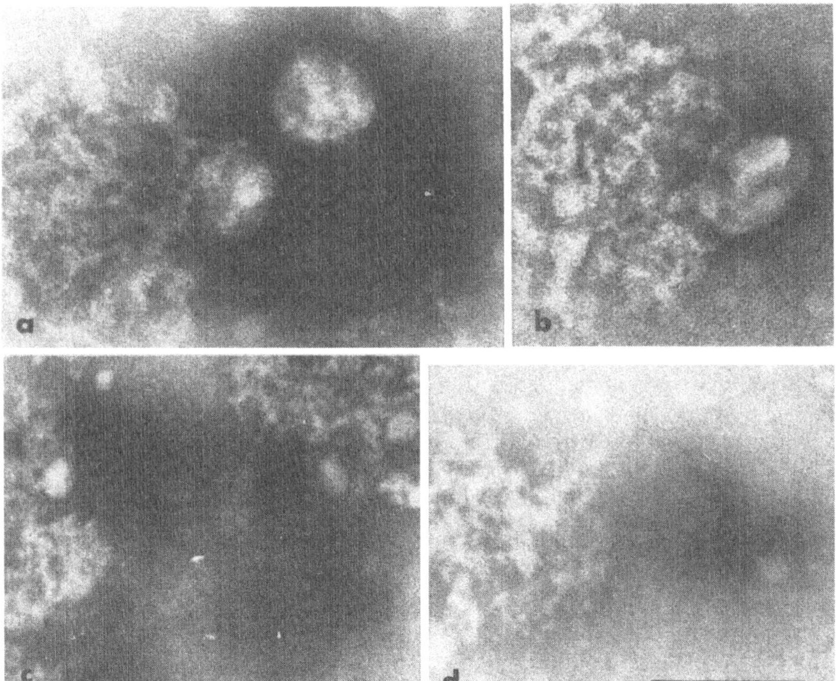

Figure 12 Other material exposed by formamide treatment, (a,b) Electron-lucent particles associated with denatured capsids. These sometimes appear to consist of coiled strands. (c,d) Masses of positively stained fibrous material frequently observed when treated capsids were dried on grids before being stained. ×225 000

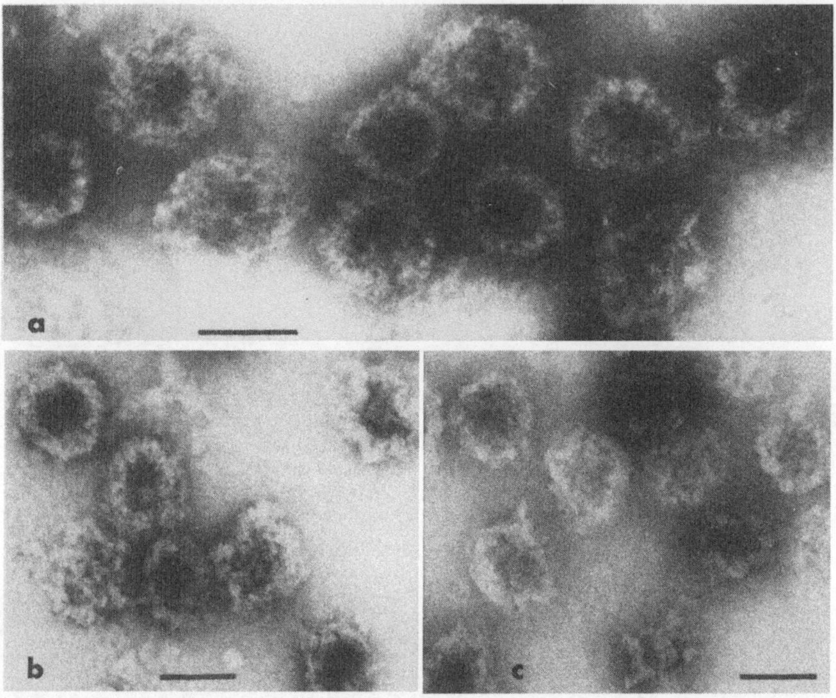

Figure 13 Denatured capsids recovered by centrifugation of formamide-treated capsids on to CsCl cushions. Stained with (a) PTA, (b) UAc, and (c) NZG. Most of the particles were seen in large aggregates. Although intra-capsomeric bonds have been disrupted, the capsids retain a particulate structure and consist mostly of hexamer polypeptide (see Figure 14). A few internal components also were observed

However, most material observed was highly aggregated, and the micrographs shown represent exceptional fields. Some core particles of both high and low electron density were also present, but they usually were ruptured and they remained associated with denatured capsids.

The cushioned, denatured material was compared to undenatured nucleocapsids by PAGE. As shown in Figure 14, the recoverable formamide-treated particles were enriched with regard to the concentration of polypeptide 1.

The other major polypeptides apparently had been at least partially solubilized.

SUMMARY

Stabilization of viral particles

The affinity of the herpesviruses for host cell membranes and their relatively low extracellular concentrations in tissue cultures have caused difficulties in

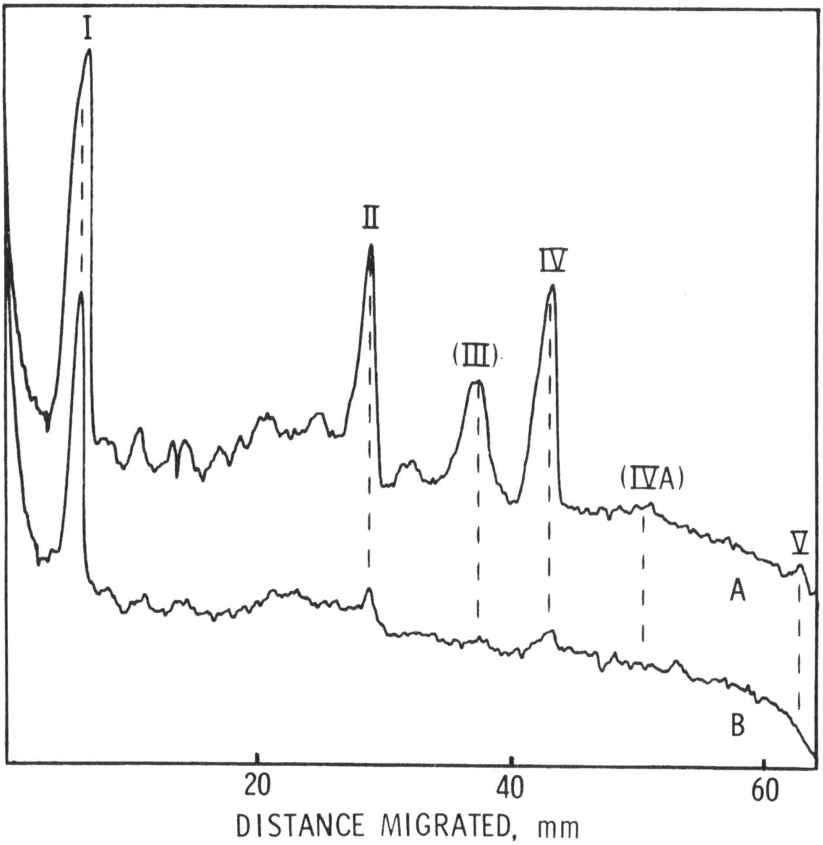

Figure 14 Polyacrylamide gel electrophoresis of formamide-treated EHV-1 capsids. Nucleocapsids were made up to 90% (v/v) with formamide and incubated for 2 h at 37 °C, then dialysed and centrifuged on to CsCl cushions. The resultant flocculent band was dialysed and subjected to PAGE in 10% cylindrical gels. Curve A represents untreated nucleocapsids. Curve B represents material cushioned after formamide treatment. The recovery of polypeptide I after treatment is approximately 55% of that in the control. The concentrations of the other nucleocapsid polypeptides, whose positions are indicated by dashed lines, have been decreased relative to the concentration of the major polypeptide

their purification. Since Spear and Roizman[99] first reported a successful method for the purification of HSV-1, several laboratories have described methods for the purification of human herpesviruses both from cell lysates[64,96,128] and extracellular fluids[71,91,92,94,97,98,100,116,129].

Several recent papers have described the use of CsCl[72,116] or iodinated salts[94,128,130] for density gradient centrifugation of herpesviruses. During the development of the purification method used in the studies described here, it was noted that about 90% of infectivity was lost when virions were sedimented into CsCl gradients; in contrast, about 50% of infectivity was recovered after flotation[116]. This difference may be attributable to hydrodynamic shearing of the relatively light lipoprotein viral envelope from the dense nucleocapsid during sedimentation. In addition, it has been shown that herpesvirions are sensitive to osmotic shock, particularly when virions in concentrated salt solutions are diluted rapidly with water[131]. In the purification method employed here, virions concentrated by sedimentation were maintained in solutions of high osmolarity. The purified virions were stored routinely in CsCl; when they were diluted rapidly, significant losses of infectivity occurred, and labelled proteins were released which did not sediment with virus particles at 50 000 *g*. These phenomena can largely be avoided by slow stepwise dilution. Therefore, it seems possible that some of the losses of infectivity reported by other investigators using CsCl[100,132–134] may reflect the effect of osmotic shock on herpesvirions. However, these hypotheses have not been systematically investigated.

The sensitivity of herpesvirus envelopes and capsids to dehydration and osmotic changes is a critical factor in the electron microscopic evaluation of virus preparations. Dehydration before staining can result in negative stain penetration of envelopes[135,136], fragmentation of capsids and degradation of envelopes[117], and the extrusion of DNA-containing strands on to specimen grids[117,137]. Therefore, it is possible that the frequent occurrence of naked capsids in published descriptions of purified herpesvirions may be a result of envelope disruption during preparation for electron microscopy. The use of measures to preserve and support virus particles by fixation and dense negative-staining can facilitate the differentiation of virion or capsid disruption *in situ* from experimentally-induced disruption.

Products of de-envelopment

The morphological effects on EHV-1 virions of each of the lipid solvents used in these experiments were similar, as determined by electron microscopy. However, in order to show clearly that virtually all nucleocapsids remained enclosed within residual envelope–tegument complex, a combination of shadow casting and negative staining was required. Negative staining alone resulted in an underestimation of the amount of residual material, probably reflecting the accumulation of dense stain around capsids which obscured flattened, dehydrated tegument. When particles were supported by thick stain deposits, they appeared to possess smooth surfaces lacking surface projections. Naked capsids were observed only in preparations recovered from CsCl gradients.

The difficulties in observing tegument by electron microscopy may account for the varying published descriptions of detergent-treated herpesvirus particles. Although residual tegument has been noted frequently, it is difficult to determine what effects detergent-treatment alone or additional procedures, such as treatment with urea, centrifugation, or sonication, have produced[91,95,99,138–143].

A total of 32 virion polypeptides were detected by analytical SDS-PAGE. This figure includes four more polypeptides than were detected in EHV-1 by Perdue *et al.* [94] and Kemp *et al.*[120]; it is close to the 33 virion polypeptides detected in HSV-1 by Heine *et al.*[112]. The actual number of herpesvirion polypeptides is not known with certainty, and it is not clear whether differences observed result from variations in virus purification methods or in PAGE procedures or represent real structural differences. However, as discussed by O'Callaghan and Randall[115], the polypeptide compositions of these viruses are strikingly similar.

The effects of NP40 on HSV-1 were described by Spear and Roizman[99]. Treatment of HSV-1 with NP40 removed glycoproteins without entirely removing the envelope. Glycoproteins nos. 7–8, later reported, along with nos. 17–18, to represent the outermost virion proteins[80,81], were almost quantitatively removed[99].

The results described here for EHV-1 were similar: polypeptide 10 (and perhaps *a*), apparently analogous to HSV-1 polypeptide 7–8[115], was the major protein found in NP40-soluble material. Polypeptides 17 and 18, apparently analogous to HSV-1 nos. 17–18, and EHV-1 nos. 13–15 comprised most of the remaining solubilized material. Correlation of these PAGE analyses and the lack of surface projections on NP40-treated particles suggests that EHV-1 polypeptide 10 may be a constituent of the envelope spikes. Finally, the proteins removed by this treatment constitute a subset of virion proteins from which individual polypeptides may be isolated.

Products of trypsinization

It is remarkable that trypsinized capsids, whether derived from intracellular populations or from extracellular virions, appeared to retain their characteristic morphology with the exception that vertex pentamers frequently were missing. The appearance of only five polypeptides after PAGE of these particles indicated that the various components had been nicked *in situ* and separated into tryptic peptides only after being heated with SDS and mercaptoethanol. The bulk of the nucleocapsid protein and the entire residual envelope–tegument complex apparently were cleaved into low molecular weight products. Of the products retained in gels, only one could represent an uncleaved nucleocapsid constituent. The other bands would, by elimination, be derived from Band I, probably the hexamer protein. If the similar migration rates of Bands II and B are merely coincidental, then the tryptic peptides could be derived from, at the most, Bands I and II. It is also possible that polypeptide B represents polypeptide II, which may be an internal component not accessible to tryptic digestion. Experiments designed to identify the origins of the tryptic peptides are in progress.

The correspondence between nucleocapsid Bands II and IV and virion polypeptides 20 and 24, respectively, is the only significant difference between our results and the polypeptide analysis reviewed by O'Callaghan and Randall[115]. These discrepancies may reflect differences in the methods for PAGE.

Denaturation of capsids

At least two morphologically-distinct particles were exposed when nucleocapsids were treated with formamide. The electron-dense particles may represent the 'middle capsid' proposed by Roizman *et al.*[144] for HSV-1, within which the viral DNA and associated structures are located. These particles, to which we refer as 'M-cores', frequently appeared to be ruptured, permeated by negative stain, and bounded by a smooth surface visible when particles were flattened on grids.

The electron-transparent particles may represent the cylindrical structures of the core model proposed by Furlong *et al.*[109], the internal cylindrical structures within immature intermediate nucleocapsids described by Perdue *et al.*[107], or both. Alternatively, all such particles may constitute a single population, some particles of which had been exposed by degradation of surrounding M-cores. The sensitivity of M-cores to osmotic shock and trypsin is suggested by the extrusion of DNA-containing strands from dehydrated virions[117] and by uniform stain penetration into trypsinized nucleocapsids, respectively.

The amorphous products of capsid degradation by formamide were similar to those obtained when HSV-1 nucleocapsids were disrupted with guanidine-HCl, mercaptoethanol, or lithium iodide[145]. Similar morphological effects were observed when EHV-1 nucleocapsids were treated on specimen grids with 35–70% lithium thiocyanate (unpublished results), which has been used to disrupt other icosahedral viruses[146]. We are not aware of any procedure, except dehydration, which has disrupted herpesvirus intercapsomeric bonds before disrupting intracapsomeric bonds, which are responsible for the characteristic morphology of the hexamer. The relative weakness of the intracapsomeric bonds, and our ability to virtually eliminate the appearance of sheets of capsomers during negative staining, prompt us to postulate that such sheets always have been a result of *in situ* fragmentation. It is not surprising that intact herpesvirus capsomers have not yet been isolated.

The particles recovered by centrifugation of formamide-treated nucleocapsids retain a remarkable degree of structural integrity in suspension and appear to consist mostly of nucleocapsid polypeptide I. This result provides further evidence that polypeptide I represents a hexamer protein. Whether the reduced concentrations of residual polypeptides represent adherent structural components, or reflect the presence of sedimented internal components, has not yet been determined.

Epilogue

Although the immunogenic value of external proteins of herpes and other enveloped viruses has been well established, it would be premature to discount *a priori* the possible value of internal herpesvirus antigens, as well, in affecting the course of latent and persistent infections. These investigations seek means of purifying each of the components released during the procedures described and also alternative degradative methods which may facilitate the isolation of other components. The results described, though incomplete, illustrate the potential value of combining biochemical and morphological approaches to better understand immunological studies of herpesviruses.

The immunological value of any purified herpesvirus subunit preparations will be difficult to determine. Some of the problems inherent in the development of herpesvirus vaccines have been discussed[147–149].

Because of both the complexity of immune responses to virus-associated antigens and the ubiquity, in human and animal populations, of antigenically cross-reactive herpesviruses[1,2,9,10,20–23,27,30,57,150–152], the effects of introducing particular antigens into susceptible hosts are difficult to estimate. There is general agreement that the protective roles of humoral and cell-mediated immune responses must be elucidated; interactions of these mechanisms during herpesvirus infections can, at times, be detrimental to the host by inducing the suppression of protective responses. Moreover, vaccine efficacy may be critically dependent upon other factors such as the subject's pre-exposure to homologous or heterologous herpesviruses, age, physiological status, and genetic susceptibility to infection[153].

Perhaps the one factor common to the employment of all the herpesvirus vaccines has been the lack of understanding as to how they induce protection. The efficacy of a vaccine will depend on its ability, not only to protect against primary infection, but to elicit only those immune responses necessary to prevent or attenuate disease while leaving dormant those responses which may render the subject more susceptible to other consequences of herpesvirus infection.

Acknowledgments

We are grateful for the continuing support and contributions of Manuel Ponce de Leon. We thank Mario Durso and Richard Hartzell for expert technical assistance and Terry Schaffer for typing.

References

1. Aurelian, L. and Strand, B. C. (1976). Herpesvirus-virus type 2-related antigens and their relevance to humoral and cell-mediated immunity in patients with cervical cancer. *Cancer Res.*, **36**, 810

2. Epstein, M.A. and Achong, B. G. (1973). The EB Virus. *Ann. Rev. Microbiol.*, **27**, 413
3. Glaser, R. and Rapp, F. (1975). Biological properties of the Epstein-Barr virus and its possible role in human malignancy. *Progr. Med. Virol.*, **21**, 43
4. Goldberg, R. J. and Gravell, M. (1976). A search for herpes simplex virus type 2 markers in cervical carcinoma. *Cancer Res.*, **36**, 795
5. Henle, W. and Henle, G. (1974). Epstein-Barr virus and human malignancies. *Cancer*, **34**, 1368
6. Klein, G. (1972). Herpesviruses and onogenesis. *Proc. Nat. Acad. Sci. USA*, **69**, 1056
7. Klein, G. (1974). Studies on the Epstein-Barr virus genome and the EBV-determined nuclear antigen in human malignant disease. *Cold Spring Harbor Symp. Quant. Biol.*, **XXXIX**, 783
8. Melnick, J. L., Adam, E. and Rawls, W. E. (1974). The causative role of herpesvirus type 2 in cervical cancer. *Cancer*, **34**, 1375
9. Melnick, J. L., Courtney, R. J., Powell, K. L., Schaffer, P. A., Benyesh-Melnick, M., Dreesman, G. R., Anzai, T. and Adam, E. (1976). Studies on herpes simplex virus and cancer. *Cancer Res.*, **36**, 845
10. Nahmias, A. J., Shore, S. L., Kohl, S., Starr, S. E. and Ashman, R. B. (1976). Immunology of herpes simplex virus infection: relevance to herpes simplex virus vaccines and cervical cancer. *Cancer Res.*, **36**, 836
11. Pagano, J. S. (1974). The Epstein-Barr virus and malignancy: molecular evidence. *Cold Spring Harbor Symp. Quant. Biol.*, **XXXIX**, 797
12. Rapp, F. (1974). Herpesviruses and cancer. *Adv. Cancer Res.*, **19**, 265
13. Rapp, F. and Li, J.-L. H. (1974). Demonstration of the oncogenic potential of herpes simplex viruses and human cytomegalouirus. *Cold Spring Harbor Symp. Quant. Biol.*, **XXXIX,** 747
14. Rapp, R. and Reed, C. (1976). Experimental evidence for the oncogenic potential of hermes simplex viruses. *Cancer Res.*, **36,** 800
15. Duff, R. and Rapp, F. (1973). The induction of oncogenic potential by herpes simplex viruses. In M. Pollard (ed.). *Persistent Virus Infections, Perspectives in Virology* VIII, Chapter 10, pp. 189–210. (New York and London: Academic Press)
16. Pagano, J. S. (1975). Diseases and mechanisms of persistent DNA virus infection: latency and cellular transformation. *J. Infect. Dis.*, **132**, 209
17. Pope, J. H. (1975). Transformation *in vitro* by herpesviruses—a review. In G. de-Thé, M. A. Epstein, and H. zur Hausen (eds.). *Oncogenesis and Herpesviruses.* **li**, Part 1, pp. 367–378. (Lyon: International Agency for Research on Cancer)
18. Rapp, F. and Duff, R. (1974). Oncogenic conversion of normal cells by inactivated herpes simplex viruses. *Cancer*, **34**, 1353
19. Baringer, J. R. (1975). Herpes simplex virus infection of nervous tissue in animals and man. *Prog. Med. Virol.*, **20**, 1
20. Epstein, M. A. (1975). Transformation *in vivo*—a review. In G. de-Thé, M. A. Epstein and H. zur Hausen (eds.). *Oncogenesis and Herpesviruses*, II, Part 2, pp. 141–151. (Lyon: International Agency for Research on Cancer)
21. Gold, E. and Nankervis, G. A. (1973). Varicella-zoster viruses. In A. S. Kaplan (ed.). *The Herpesviruses*, Chapter 11, pp. 327–351. (New York and London: Academic Press)
22. Henle, W. and Henle, G. (1975). Host responses to herpesviruses—a review. In G. de-Thé, M. A. Epstein, and H. zur Hausen (eds.). *Oncogenesis and Herpesviruses*, II, Part 2, pp. 215–224. (Lyon: International Agency for Research on Cancer)
23. Klein, G. (1973). The Epstein-Barr virus. In A. S. Kaplan (ed.). Chapter 16, pp. 521–555. (New York and London: Academic Press)
24. Miller, G. (1975). Epstein-Barr herpesvirus and infectious mononucleosis. *Prog. Med. Virol.*, **20**, 84
25. Plummer, G. (1973). Cytomegaloviruses of man and animals. *Prog. Med. Virol.*, **15**, 92
26. Rapp, F. and Jerkofsky, M. A. (1973). Persistent and latent infections. In A. S. Kaplan (ed.). *The Herpesviruses*, Chapter 9, pp. 271–289. (New York and London: Academic Press)
27. Rawls, W. E. (1973). Herpes simplex virus. In A. S. Kaplan, (ed.). *The Herpesviruses*, Chapter 10, pp. 291–325. (New York and London: Academic Press)

28. Stevens, J. G. (1975). Herpes simplex viral latency—a review. In G. de-Thé, M. A. Epstein, and H. zur Hausen (eds.). *Oncogenesis and Herpesvirus*, II, Part 2, pp. 67–72. (Lyon; International Agency for Research on Cancer)
29. Stevens, J. G. and Cook, M. L. (1974). Maintenance of latent herpetic infection: an apparent role for anti-viral IgG. *J. Immunol.*, **113**, 1685
30. Wright, H. T., Jr. (1973). Cytomegaloviruses. In A. S. Kaplan (ed.). *The Herpesviruses*, Chapter 12, pp. 353–388. (New York and London: Academic Press)
31. Biggs, P. M. (1973). Marek's disease. In A. S. Kaplan (ed.). *The Herpesviruses*, Chapter 17, pp. 557–594, (New York and London: Academic Press)
32. Biggs, P. M. (1975). Marek's disease—the disease and its prevention by vaccination. *Br. J. Cancer*, **31**, (Suppl. 11), 152
33. Purchase, H. G. (1976). Prevention of Marek's disease: a review. *Cancer Res.*, **36**, 696
34. Churchill, A. E., Chubb, R. C. and Baxendale, W. (1969). The attenuation, with loss of oncogenicity, of the herpes-type virus of Marek's disease (strain HPRS-16) on passage in cell culture. *J. Gen. Virol.*, **4**, 557
35. Churchill, A. E., Payne, L. N. and Chubb, R. C. (1969). Immunization against Marek's disease using a live attenuated virus. *Nature* (*Lond.*), **221**, 744
36. Purchase, H. G., Burmester, B. R. and Cunningham, C. H. (1971). Response of cell cultures from various avian species to Marek's disease virus and herpesvirus of turkeys. *Am. J. Vet. Res.*, **32**, 1811
37. McKercher, D. G. (1973). In A. S. Kaplan (ed.). *The Herpesviruses*, Chapter 14, pp. 427–493. (New York and London: Academic Press)
38. Hull, R. N. (1971). B virus vaccine. *Lab. Animal Sci.*, **21**, 1068
39. Hull, R. N. and Peck, F. B., Jr. (1967). *Vaccination against Herpesvirus Infections.* Pan American Health Organization Scientific Publication No. 147, 266–275
40. Chapin, H. B., Wong, S. C. and Reapsome, J. (1962). The value of tissue culture vaccine in the prophylaxis of recurrent attacks of herpetic keratitis. *Am. J. Ophthal.*, **54**, 255
41. Kasparov, A. A. and Maievskaya, T. M. (1972). Experience with diagnostic and therapeutic employment of herpetic polyvaccine. *Oftalmol. Zh.*, **27**, 119
42. Kern, A. B. and Schiff, B. L. (1964). Vaccine therapy in recurrent herpes simplex. *Arch. Dermatol.*, **89**, 844
43. Lazar, M. P. (1956). Vaccination for recurrent herpes simplex infection. Initiation of a new disease site following the use of unmodified material containing the live virus. *Arch. Derm.*, **73**, 70
44. Elek, S. D. and Stern, H. (1974). Development of a vaccine against mental retardation caused by cytomegalovirus infection *in utero*. *Lancet*, **1**, 1
45. Takahashi, M. and Asano, Y. (1977). A live varicella vaccine used for children in hospital. In *Oncogenesis and Herpesvirus*. III. (in press)
46. Powell, P. C. (1975). Immunity to Marek's disease induced by glutaraldehyde-treated cells of Marek's disease lymphoblastoid cell lines. *Nature* (*Lond.*), **257**, 684
47. Kaaden, O. R. and Dietzschold, B. (1974). Alterations of the immunological specificity of plasma membranes from cells infected with Marek's disease and turkey herpes viruses. *J. Gen. Virol.*, **25**, 1
48. Lesnik, F. and Ross, L. J. N. (1975). Immunization against Marek's disease using Marek's disease virus-specific antigens free from infectious virus. *Int. J. Cancer*, **16**, 153
49. Deinhardt, F. W., Falk, L. A. and Wolfe, L. G. (1974). Simian herpesviruses and neoplasia. *Adv. Cancer Res.*, **19**, 167
50. Melandez, L. V., Daniel, M. D., Barahona, H. H., Fraser, C. E. O., Hunt, R. D. and Garcia, F. G. (1971). New herpesviruses from South American monkeys. Preliminary report. *Lab. Animal Sci.*, **21**, 1050
51. Laufs, R. and Steinke, H. (1975). Vaccination of non-human primates against malignant lymphoma. *Nature* (*Lond.*), **253**, 71
52. Laufs, R. and Steinke, H. (1975). A killed vaccine derived from the oncogenic *Herpesvirus ateles*. *J. Natl Cancer Inst.*, **55**, 649
53. Cappel, R. (1976). Comparison of the humoral and cellular immune responses after immunization with live, UV inactivated herpes simplex virus and a subunit vaccine and efficacy of these immunizations. *Arch. Virol.*, **52**, 29

54. Kitces, E. N., Morahan, P. S., Tew, J. G. and Murray, B. K. (1977). Protection from oral herpes simplex virus infection by a nucleic acid-free virus vaccine. *Infect. Immun.*, **16**, 955
55. Pearson, G. R. and Scott, R. E. (1977). Isolation of virus-free *Herpesvirus saimiri* antigen-positive plasma membrane vesicles. *Proc. Natl Acad. Sci. USA*, 74, 2546
56. Clements, J. B. and Hay, J. (1977). RNA and protein synthesis in herpesvirus-infected cells. *J. Gen. Virol.*, **35**, 1
57. Klein, E., Klein, G. and Levine, P. H. (1976). Immunological control of human lymphoma: discussion. *Cancer Res.*, **36**, 724
58. Klein, G. (1975). Virus induced antigens—a review. In G. de-Thé, M. A. Epstein and H. zur Hausen (eds.). *Oncogenesis and Herpesviruses.* II, Part 1, pp. 293–308. (Lyon: International Agency for Research on Cancer)
59. Roizman, B., Kozak, M., Honess, R. W. and Hayward, G. (1974). Regulation of herpesvirus macromolecular synthesis: evidence for multilevel regulation of herpes simplex 1 RNA and protein synthesis. *Cold Spring Harbor Symp. Quant. Biol.*, **XXXIX**, 687
60. Roizman, B., Spear, P. G. and Kieff, E. D. (1973). Herpes simplex viruses I and II: a biochemical definition. In M. Pollard (ed.). *Persistent Virus Infections. Perspectives in Virology*, VIII, Chapter 8, pp. 129–169. (New York and London: Academic Press)
61. Honess, R. W., Powell, K. L., Robinson, D. J., Sim, C. and Watson, D. H. (1974). Type specific and type common antigens in cells infected with herpes simplex virus type 1 and on the surfaces of naked and enveloped particles of the virus. *J. Gen. Virol.*, **22** 159
62. Watson, D. H., Shedden, W. I. H., Elliot, A., Tetsuka, T., Wildy, P., Bourgaux-Ramoisy, D. and Gold, E. (1966). Virus specific antigens in mammalian cells infected with herpes simplex virus. *Immunology*, **11**, 399
63. Honess, R. W. and Roizman, B. (1973). Proteins specified by simplex virus. XI. Identification and relative molar rates of synthesis of structural and nonstructural herpes virus polypeptides in the infected cell. *J. Virol.*, **12**, 1347
64. Strand, B. C. and Aurelian, L. (1976). Proteins of herpesvirus type 2: 1. Virion, non-virion, and antigenic polypeptides in infected cells. *Virology*, **69**, 438
65. Tokumaru, T. (1970). Further analysis of physicochemical and immunologic properties of herpes simplex virus precipitating antigens. *Arch. Ges. Virusforsch.*, **29**, 295
66. Zaia, J. A., Palmer, E. L. and Feorino, P. M. (1975). Humoral and cellular immune responses to an envelope-associated antigen of herpes simplex virus. *J. Infect. Dis.*, **132**, 660
67. Honess, R. W. and Watson, D. H. (1974). Herpes simplex virus-specific polypeptides studied by polyacrylamide gel electrophoresis of immune precipitates. *J. Gen. Virol.*, **22**, 171
68. Sim, C. and Watson, D. H. (1973). The role of type-specific and cross-reacting structural antigens in the neutralization of herpes simplex virus types 1 and 2. *J. Gen. Virol.*, **19**, 217
69. Watson, D. H. (1969). The separation of herpes virus-specific antigens by polyacrylamide gel electrophoresis. *J. Gen. Virol.*, **4**, 151
70. Watson, D. H. and Wildy, P. (1969). The preparation of 'monoprecipitin' antisera to herpes virus specific antigens. *J. Gen. Virol.*, **4**, 163
71. Powell, K. L., Buchan, A., Sim, C. and Watson, D. H. (1974). Type-specific protein in herpes simplex virus envelope reacts with neutralizing antibody. *Nature* (*Lond.*), **29**, 360
72. Powell, K. L. and Watson, D. H. (1975). Some structural antigens of herpes simplex virus type 1. *J. Gen. Virol.*, **29**, 167
73. Aurelian, L., Davis, H. J. and Julian, C. G. (1973). Herpesvirus type 2 induced tumor specific antigen in cervical carcinoma. *Am. J. Epidemiol.*, **98**, 1
74. Strand, B. C. and Aurelian, L. (1976). Proteins of herpesvirus type 2. II. Studies demonstrating a correlation between a tumor-associated antigen (AG-4) and a virion protein. *Virology*, **73**, 244
75. Cohen, G. H., Ponce de Leon, M. and Nichols, C. (1972). Isolation of a herpes simplex virus-specific antigenic fraction which stimulates the production of neutralizing antibody. *J. Virol.*, **10**, 1021

76. Ponce de Leon, M., Hessle, H. and Cohen, G. H. (1973). Separation of herpes simplex virus-induced antigens by Concanavalin A affinity chromatography. *J. Virol.*, **12**, 766
77. Reed, C. L., Cohen, G. H. and Rapp, F. (1975). Detection of a virus-specific antigen on the surface of herpes simplex virus-transformed cells. *J. Virol.*, **15**, 668
78. Wildy, P., Russell, W. C. and Horne, R. W. (1960). The morphology of herpes virus. *Virology*, **12**, 204
79. Gentry, G. A. and Randall, C. C. (1973). The physical and chemical properties of the herpesviruses. In A. S. Kaplan (ed.). *The Herpesviruses*, Chapter 3, pp. 45–92. (New York and London: Academic Press)
80. Roizman, B. and Furlong, D. (1974). The replication of herpesviruses. In H. Fraenkel-Conrat and R. R. Wagner (eds.). *Comprehensive Virology 3, Reproduction: DNA Animal Viruses,*, Chapter 4, pp. 229–403. (New York and London: Plenum Press)
81. Roizman, B., Hayward, G., Jacob, R., Wadsworth, S., Frenkel, N., Honess, R. W. and Kozak, M. (1975). Human herpesviruses I: a model for molecular organization and regulation of herpesviruses—a review. In G. de-Thé, M. A. Epstein and H. zur Hausen (eds.). Oncogenesis and Herpesviruses II. Part I, pp. 3–38. (Lyon; International Agency for Research on Cancer)
82. Roizman, B. and Spear, P. G. (1973). Herpesviruses. In A. J. Dalton and F. Haguenau (eds.). *Ultrastructure of Animal Viruses and Bacteriophages: An Atlas.* Chapter 5, pp. 83–107. (New York and London: Academic Press)
83. Watson, D. H. (1973). Morphology. In A. S. Kaplan (ed.). *The Herpesviruses*, Chapter 2, pp. 27–43. (New York and London: Academic Press)
84. Watson, D. H. (1973). Replication of the viruses–morphological aspects. In A. S. Kaplan (ed.). *The Herpesviruses*, Chapter 5, pp. 133–161. (New York and London: Academic Press)
85. Darlington, R. W. and Moss, L. H., III (1968). Herpesvirus envelopment. *J. Virol.*, **2**, 48
86. Epstein, M. A. (1962). Observations on the fine structure of mature herpes simplex virus and on the composition of its nucleoid. *J. Exp. Med.*, **115**, 1
87. Nii, S., Morgan, C. and Rose, H. M. (1968). Electron microscopy of herpes simplex virus II. Sequence of development. *J. Virol.*, **2**, 517
88. Vernon, S. K., Lawrence, W. C. and Cohen, G. H. (1974). Morphological components of herpesvirus. I. Intercapsomeric fibrils and the geometry of the capsid. *Intervirology*, **4**, 237
89. Fenner, F. (1976). Classification and nomenclature of viruses. Second report of the International Committee on Taxonomy of Viruses. *Intervirology*, **7**, 1
90. Goodheart, C. R. and Plummer, G. (1975). The densities of herpesviral DNAs. *Prog. Med. Virol.*, **19**, 324
91. Dolyniuk, M., Wolff, E. and Kieff, E. (1976). Proteins of Epstein-Barr virus. II. Electrophoretic analysis of the polypeptides of the nucleocapsid and the glucosamine- and polysaccharide-containing components of enveloped virus. *J. Virol.*, **18**, 289
92. Gupta, P., St. Jeor, S. and Rapp, F. (1977). Comparison of the polypeptides of several strains of human cytomegalovirus. *J. Gen. Virol.*, **34**, 447
93. Heine, J. W., Honess, R. W., Cassai, E. and Roizman, B. (1974). Proteins specified by herpes simplex virus. XII. The virion polypeptides of type 1 strains. *J. Virol.*, **14**, 640
94. Perdue, M. L., Kemp, M. C., Randall, C. C. and O'Callaghan, D. J. (1974). Studies of the molecular anatomy of the L-M cell strain of equine herpes virus type 1: proteins of the nucleocapsid and intact virion. *Virology*, **59**, 201
95. Abodeely, R. A., Palmer, E., Lawson, L. A. and Randall, C. C. (1971). The proteins of enveloped and de-enveloped equine abortion (herpes) virus and the separated envelope. *Virology*, **44**, 146
96. Cassai, E. N., Sarmiento, M. and Spear, P. G. (1975). Comparison of the virion proteins specified by herpes simplex virus types 1 and 2. *J. Virol.*, **16**, 1327
97. Fiala, M., Honess, R. W., Heiner, D. C., Heine, J. W., Jr., Murnane, J., Wallace, R. and Guze, L. B. (1976). Cytomegalovirus proteins. I. Polypeptides of virions and dense bodies. *J. Virol.*, **19**, 243
98. Sarov, I. and Abody, I. (1975). The morphogenesis of human cytomegalovirus. Isolation and polypeptide characterization of cytomegalovirions and dense bodies. *Virology*, **66**, 464

99. Spear, P. G. and Roizman, B. (1972). Proteins specified by herpes simplex virus. V. Purification and structural proteins of the herpesvirion. *J. Virol.*, **2**, 143
100. Stinski, M. (1976). Human cytomegalovirus: glycoproteins associated with virions and dense bodies. *J. Virol.*, **19**, 594
101. Savage, T., Roizman, B., and Heine, J. W. (1972). Immunological specificity of the glycoproteins of herpes simplex virus subtypes 1 and 2. *J. Gen. Virol.*, **17**, 31
102. Palmer, E. L., Martin, M. L. and Gary, G. W., Jr. (1975). The ultrastructure of disrupted herpesvirus nucleocapsids. *Virology*, **65**, 260
103. Gibson, W. and Roizman, B. (1972). Proteins specified by herpes simplex virus. VIII. Characterization and composition of multiple capsid forms of subtypes 1 and 2. *J. Virology*, **10**, 1044
104. Perdue, M. L., Cohen, J. C., Kemp, M. C., Randall, C. C. and O'Callaghan, D. J. (1975). Characterization of three species of nucleocapsids of equine herpesvirus type 1 (EHV-1). *Virology*, **64**, 187
105. Allen, G. P. and Bryans, J. T. (1976). Cell-free synthesis of equine herpesvirus type 3 nucleocapsid polypeptides. *Virology*, **69**, 751
106. McCombs, R. M. (1974). Antigens specified by herpesviruses. III. Viral-induced nuclear polypeptides. *Virology*, **57**, 448
107. Perdue, M. L., Cohen, J. C., Randall, C. C. and O'Callaghan, D. J. (1976). Biochemical studies of the maturation of herpesvirus nucleocapsid species. *Virology*, **74**, 194
108. Gibson, W. and Roizman, B. (1974). Proteins specified by herpes simplex virus. X. Staining and radiolabeling properties of B capsid and virion proteins in polyacrylamide gels. *J. Virol.*, **13**, 155
109. Furlong, D., Swift, H. and Roizman, B. (1972). Arrangement of herpesivirus deoxyribonucleic acid in the core. *J. Virol.*, **10**, 107
110. Chai, L. S. (1971). Architecture of the DNA molecule within Epstein-Barr virus (EBV). *Proc. Amer. Assoc. Cancer Res.*, **12** 18(abst.)
111. Heine, U. and Cottler-Fox, M. (1975). Electron microscopic observations on the composition of herpes-type virions. In G. de-Thé, M. A. Epstein, and H. zur Hansen. (eds.). *Oncogenesis and Herpesviruses*. II, Part 1, pp 103–110. (Lyon; International Agency for Research on Cancer)
112. Nazerian, K. (1974). DNA configuration in the core of Marek's disease virus. *J. Virology*, **13**, 1148
113. Nii, S. and Yasuda, I. (1975). Detection of viral cores having toroid structures in eight herpesviruses. *Biken J.*, **18**, 41
114. Strandberg, J. D. and Carmichael, L. E. (1965). Electron microscopy of a canine herpesvirus. *J. Bacteriol.*, **90**, 1790
115. O'Callaghan, D. J. and Randall, C. C. (1976). Molecular anatomy of herpesviruses: recent studies. *Progr. Med. Virol.*, **22**, 152
116. Lawrence, W. C. (1976). Purification of equine herpesvirus type 1. *J. Gen. Virol.*, **31**, 81
117. Vernon, S. K., Lawrence, W. C., Cohen, G. H., Durso, M. and Rubin, B. (1976). Morphological components of herpesvirus. II. Preservation of virus during negative staining procedures. *J. Gen. Virol.*, **31**, 183
118. Neurath, A. R., Stasny, J. T., Rubin, B. A., Fontes, A. K., Pierzchala, W. A., Wiener, F. P. and Hartzell, R. W. (1970). The effect of non-aqueous solvents on the quaternary structure of viruses: properties of haemagglutinins obtained by disruption of influenza viruses with tri(*n*-buty 1)phosphate. *Microbios*, **2**, 209
119. Laemmli, U.K. (1970). Cleavage of structural proteins during the assembly of the head of bacteriophage T4. *Nature* (*Lond.*) **227**, 680
120. Kemp, M. C., Perdue, M. L., Rogers, H. W. O'Callaghan, D. J. and Randall, C. C. (1974). Structural polypeptides of the hamster strain of equine herpesvirus type 1: products associated with purification. *Virology*, **61**, 361
121. Crowther, R. A. and Franklin, R. M. (1972). The structure of the groups of nine hexons from adenovirus. *J. Mol. Biol.*, **68**, 181
122. Markham, R., Frey, S. and Hills, G. J. (1963). Methods for the enhancement of image detail and accentuation of structure in electron microscopy. *Virology*, **20**, 88

123. Laver, W. G., Wrigley, N. G., and Pereira, H. G. (1969). Removal of pentons from particles of adenovirus type 2. *Virology*, **39**, 599
124. Prage, L., Pettersson, U., Höglund, S., Lonberg-Holm, K. and Philipson, L. (1970). Structural proteins of adenovirus. IV. Sequential degradation of the adenovirus type 2 virion. *Virology*, **42** 341
125. Russell, W. C., Valentine, R. C. and Pereira, H. G. (1967). The effect of heat on the anatomy of the adenovirus. *J. Gen. Virol.*, **1**, 509
126. Neurath, A. R., Rubin, B. A. and Stasny, J. T. (1968). Cleavage by formamide of intercapsomer bonds in adenovirus types 4 and 7 virions and hemagglutinins. *J. Virol.*, **2**, 1086
127. Stasny, J. T., Neurath, A. R. and Rubin, B. A. (1968). Effect of formamide on the capsid morphology of adenovirus types 4 and 7. *J. Virol.*, **2**, 1429
128. Blomberg, J., Björck, E., Olofsson, S., Berg, G. and Lycke, E. (1976). Purification of virions and nucleocapsids of herpes simplex virus by means of metrizamide and sodium metrizoate gradients. *Arch. Virol.*, **50**, 271
129. Talbot, P. and Almeida, J. D. (1977). Human cytomegalovirus: purification of enveloped virions and dense bodies. *J. Gen. Virol.*, **36**, 345
130. Simonds, J. A., Robey, W. G., Graham, B. J., Oie, H. and Vande Woude, G. F. (1975). Purification of *Herpesvirus saimiri* and properties of the viral DNA. *Arch. Virol.*, **49**, 249
131. Barnhart, E. R. and Ash, R. J. (1975). Physical characteristics of herpesvirions: low-temperature and osmotic-shock studies. *Virology*, **66**, 563
132. Spring, S. B. and Roizman, B. (1967). Herpes simplex virus products in productive and abortive infection. I. Stabilization with formaldehyde and preliminary analyses by isopycnic centrifugation in CsCl. *J. Virol.*, **1**, 294
133. Spring, S. B. and Roizman, B. (1968). Herpes simplex virus products in productive and abortive infection. III. Differentiation of infectious virus derived from nucleus and cytoplasm with respect to stability and size. *J. Virol.*, **2**, 979
134. Spring, S. B., Roizman, B. and Schwartz, J. (1968). Herpes simplex virus products in productive and abortive infection. II. Electron microscopic and immunological evidence for failure of virus envelopment as a cause of abortive infection. *J. Virol.*, **2**, 384
135. Watson, D. H. (1968). The structure of animal viruses in relation to their biological functions. *Symp. Soc. Gen. Microbiol.*, **18**, 207
136. Watson, D. H. and Wildy, P. (1963). Some serological properties of herpes virus particles studied with the electron microscope. *Virology*, **21**, 100
137. Smith, K. O. (1963). Physical and biological observations on herpesvirus. *J. Bacteriol.*, **86**, 999
138. Abodeely, R. A., Lawson, L. A. and Randall, C. C. (1970). Morphology and entry of enveloped and de-enveloped equine abortion (herpes) virus. *J. Virol.*, **5**, 513
139. Dreesman, G. R., Suriano, J. R., Swartz, S. K. and McCombs, R. M. (1972). Characterization of the herpes virion. 1. Purification and amino acid composition of nucleocapsids. *Virology*, **50**, 528
140. Kaplan, A. S. and Ben-Porat, T. (1970). Synthesis of proteins in cells infected with herpesvirus. VI. Characterization of the proteins of the viral membrane. *Proc. Nat. Acad. Sci. USA*, **66**, 799
141. Martin, M. L., Palmer, E. L. and Kissling, R. E. (1972). Complement-fixing antigens of herpes simplex virus types 1 and 2: reactivity of capsid, envelope, and soluble antigens. *Infect. Immun.*, **5**, 248
142. Matis, J. and Golaisová, E. (1976). Influence of host cell type on the density of herpes simplex virus particles. *Acta Virol.*, **20**, 455
143. Olshevsky, U. and Becker, Y. (1970). Herpes simplex virus structural proteins. *Virology*, **40**, 948
144. Roizman, B., Spring, S. B. and Schwartz, J. (1969). The herpesvirion and its precursors made in productively and in abortively infected cells. *Fed. Proc.* **28**, 1890
145. McCombs, R. M. and Williams, G. A. (1973). Disruption of herpes virus nucleocapsids using lithium iodide, guanidine and mercaptoethanol. *J. Gen. Virol.*, **20**, 395
146. Vernon, S. K. and Rubin, B. A. (1974). Electron microscopic observations of adeno-associated satellite virus type I capsids and subunits. *Intervirology*, **2**, 114

147. Epstein, M. A. (1976). Implications of a vaccine for the prevention of Epstein-Barr virus infection: ethical and logistic considerations. *Cancer Res.*, **36**, 711
148. Epstein, M.A. (1976). Epstein-Barr virus—is it time to develop a vaccine program? *J. Nat. Cancer Inst.*, **56**, 697
149. Parks, W. P. and Rapp, F. (1975). Prospects for herpesvirus vaccination—safety and efficacy considerations. *Progr. Med. Virol.*, **21**, 188
150. Brunell, P. A., Gershon, A. A., Uduman, S. A. and Steinberg, S. (1975). Varicella-zoster immunoglobulins during varicella, latency, and zoster. *J. Infect. Dis.*, **132**, 49
151. Fiala, M., Payne, J. E., Berne, T. V., Moore, T. C., Henle, W., Montgomerie, J. Z., Chatterjee, S. N. and Guze, L. B. (1975). Epidemiology of cyto-megalovirus infection following transplantation and immunosuppresion. *J. Infect. Dis.*, **132**, 421
152. Hampar, B. and Martos, L. M. (1973). Immunological relationshîps. In A. S. Kaplan (ed.). *The Herpesviruses*, Chapter 7, pp. 221–259. (New York and London, Academic Press)
153. Carritt, B. and Goldfarb, P. (1976). A human chromosomal determinant for susceptibility to herpes simplex virus. *Nature (Lond.)*, **264**, 556

14
'Ribosomal' vaccines: A review

T. K. EISENSTEIN

INTRODUCTION

In 1965, Youmans and Youmans[1] reported that ribosomes and ribosomal RNA extracts of the avirulent strain of *Mycobacterium tuberculosis*, H37Ra, if administered to mice in incomplete Freund's adjuvant, resulted in high levels of immunity against challenge with the virulent H37Rv strain. Evidence that the active moiety was RNA was suggested by the observations that the protective activity was retained in RNA extracts of the ribosomes, and that 50% of the activity was lost after treatment with ribonuclease (RNase), but not with trypsin[2]. At the time, no explanation was apparent for why an intracellular constituent of the bacterium should confer on the host the ability to resist bacterial infection. However, the promise of a unique function of the RNA in induction of a superior immune response has led other investigators to examine the protective ability of ribosomal extracts prepared from various pathogens. Protective vaccines have been prepared from the ribosomes or ribosomal extracts of a number of micro-organisms. These include *Salmonella typhimurium*[3–5], *Pseudomonas aeruginosa*[6,7], *Staphylococcus aureus*[7,8], *Vibrio cholerae*[9,10], *Neisseria meningitidis*[11], *Streptococcus pneumoniae*[12–14], *Streptococcus pyogenes*[15], *Histoplasma capsulatum*[16], *Francisella tularensis*[17], *Haemophilus influenzae*[18] and *Pasteurella multocida*[19]. *Yersinia pestis*[5] extracts were not protective.

The observation that such diverse organisms yield protective ribosomal extracts makes it tempting to speculate that there is a single active principle in these preparations. At present, however, the evidence suggests that no generalizations can be made about the nature of the immunogen or the mechanism of action of vaccines prepared from different organisms. In the mycobacterial system, Youmans and Youmans concluded[20] that the active substance is double-stranded RNA. On the basis of studies with metabolic inhibitors, they have hypothesized that the RNA may work by forming a

DNA template in the host cell, which transcribes specific information for replication of mycobacterial RNA in a manner analogous to that of RNA tumour viruses. Alternatively, Jensen *et al.*[9], working with extracts of *Vibrio cholerae*, were able to separate, by column chromatography, the ribosomes from the immunogenic fractions. The protective fractions were complex colloidal mixtures associated with the cell wall, and composed of protein, lipid and carbohydrate. Feit and Tewari[16] studied the protection induced by ribosomes of *Histoplasma capsulatum* and concluded that the immunogen is in the ribosomal protein fraction. As will be discussed below, the investigators working on ribosomal vaccines of salmonellae have variously concluded that the active moiety is RNA[21], protein[22] or O antigens[3]. Studies on the mechanism of action of the vaccines give equally disparate results. Some investigators using the salmonella ribosomal vaccines have presented evidence that they induce a cell-mediated immune response[23] whereas the work on the pneumococcal vaccine suggests that it induces protective antibody[13]. Since the vaccines prepared from *M. tuberculosis*, *S. typhimurium* and *S. pneumoniae* have been most thoroughly investigated, they will be considered in greater detail in this review.

Mycobacterium tuberculosis

Drs Guy and Ann Youmans pioneered the study of ribosomal vaccines, using extracts of tubercle bacilli. Our current knowledge of these mycobacterial preparations comes from studies carried out in their laboratory. They prepared ribosomes from *M. tuberculosis*, H37Ra, by rupturing the bacteria in a French pressure cell, removing unbroken cells and cell walls with two low-speed centrifugations, and ultracentrifuging the supernatant to obtain a particulate or crude ribosomal fraction. This fraction was then treated with 0.5% sodium dodecyl sulphate and recentrifuged at 144 000 *g*, to yield a ribosomal pellet. To obtain RNA, the ribosomes were treated with ethanol and 2 M NaCl. Both the ribosomal and RNA fractions obtained by this procedure consist of approximately 63% RNA and 37% protein[24]. When the protective capacity of the RNA fraction in mice was compared with that of viable H37Ra cells containing a comparable amount of RNA, the RNA was found to be almost as effective as the whole cells[24]. Since killed cells were found to be inferior to live ones in inducing antituberculosis immunity, the Youmans concluded that the ribosomal preparations were unique among non-living mycobacterial vaccines in giving high levels of immunity. They suggested that the ribosomal preparation might preserve a labile intracellular substance. Further experiments with ribosomal vaccines showed that these preparations did not induce delayed hypersensitivity in mice or guinea pigs[25]. It was concluded that the ribosomal vaccine might be an excellent candidate for a non-viable vaccine against tuberculosis, because it gave high levels of immunity and did not induce tuberculin sensitivity.

Studies on the nature of the active substance in the ribosomal vaccine showed that 50% of the immunogenicity was destroyed by ribonuclease, but not by trypsin[2]. Purified ribosomal protein was not protective[26]. A high correlation was found between the immunogenic activity of a preparation of ribosomal vaccine and the percentage increase in hyperchromicity at 260 nm of a ribonuclease-treated vaccine[24]. Thermal transition point experiments and sucrose gradient analyses suggested that double-stranded RNA was necessary for highly active preparations[27,28]. No DNA or polysaccharides[24] were detected by chemical analysis. Based on this extensive analysis of the ribosomal preparations, the hypothesis favoured by the Youmans is that the active moiety in the ribosomal preparations is the double-stranded RNA[20].

Several lines of investigation were followed to elucidate how the RNA might stimulate the immune system. It was shown that the immunity was specific for *M. tuberculosis* and long-lasting, thus ruling out the possibility of a non-specific stimulation of the immune system. Since resistance to mycobacterial infection resides ultimately with the macrophage, a study was carried out to investigate the effect of immunization with ribosomal RNA on the ability of macrophages to inhibit multiplication of mycobacteria *in vitro*. Splenic lymphocytes from RNA-immunized mice were incubated with mycobacteria and shown to elaborate a filterable substance which, when applied to normal mouse peritoneal macrophages, enabled them to inhibit the intracellular growth of virulent H37Rv tubercle bacilli[29,30]. Results of studies in which metabolic inhibitors were given to mice at various times before, with, or after RNA vaccine were interpreted as being consistent with the possibility that mycobacterial RNA was behaving like the RNA of oncogenic viruses. It was suggested that the RNA might provide the macrophage with specific information to convert it to an immune cell with mycobacteriostatic capacity via formation of a DNA template[20].

Additional studies on the biological activities of the mycobacterial RNA fraction showed that it exerted adjuvant activity when mixed with bovine γ-globulin. Ribonuclease or trypsin treatment both reduced the adjuvant effect[31].

Salmonella typhimurium

Salmonella ribosomal fractions have been prepared in a number of different laboratories, with divergent conclusions emerging from each about the nature of the protective substance. Venneman and Bigley[4] used the Youmans' method to prepare ribosomes from *S. typhimurium*, strain SR-11. They found no difference in protection induced by the whole ribosomes or the 30S or 50S subunits obtained from sucrose gradients. The immunogenicity was not decreased by treatment of ribosomes with RNase, pronase, trypsin or deoxyribonuclease. Subsequently, a ribonucleic acid-rich fraction obtained by phenol extraction and ethanol precipitation of the ribosomes was found to be more immunogenic than the whole ribosomes[32].

Venneman[21] chromatographed the ribosomal RNA fractions on Biogel P-6 and Biogel P-300 columns and recovered the immunogenicity only in the RNA-containing fractions. Protein fractions were not active. He concluded that the immunogen was greater than 300 000 molecular weight and was probably RNA, although the possibility of a polysaccharide contaminant could not be ruled out.

Other investigators have concluded that the immunogen in the Salmonella vaccine is a protein. Johnson[22] immunized mice with a ribosomal protein fraction of strain SR-11 obtained by 2-chloroethanol extraction of ribosomes prepared by the method of Fogel and Sypherd. Before extraction, the ribosomes were washed seven times in Tris buffer containing 0.35 M NH_4Cl, passed through a Sephadex G-200 column, dialysed, and centrifuged again at 105 000 *g*. The protective substance was pronase–sensitive and was species–specific. From these studies it appeared that the active fraction was a ribosomal protein.

Smith and Bigley[23] used supernatants of French pressure cell lysates of strain SR-11 which were ethanol-precipitated, to yield a nucleic acid-protein fraction designated E-RNA. This E-RNA was further extracted with ammonium sulphate to yield a protein fraction, NP. Both of these fractions, which are extracts of whole cell lysates, not of ribosomal fractions, were protective, but the crude E-RNA was more active. However, combination of NP with poly A-U restored its protective capacity to levels approaching E-RNA. On the basis of these experiments, and the observation that phenol extracted E-RNA was poorly protective, it was concluded that the immunogen is protein in nature.

In 1971 Eisenstein *et al.* (*Bacteriol. Proc.*, p. 112) first suggested that the protective capacity of Salmonella ribosomes might be due to contaminating O antigens. Evidence for the presence of O antigens was obtained using genetically defined strains of Salmonella[3]. Ribosomal 'RNA' was extracted by the method of Youmans and Youmans from a mutant of *S. typhimurium*, strain TA1659, which is unable to make O antigens. Instead, this mutant makes an incomplete lipopolysaccharide (LPS) of the R_c type. A similar 'RNA' extract was also made from *S. typhimurium*, strain SL1694, which is a derivative of TA1659 whose genetic defect was corrected by acquisition of F′8-*gal*$^+$ so that it makes a complete LPS of the typhimurium serotype. Mice were challenged with virulent *S. typhimurium*, strain SL4522, and the number of bacteria in their carcasses was determined 5 days later. The extract of the rough strain, TA1659, was not protective, while the extract of the smooth strain prevented proliferation of the challenge organisms.

Other evidence for the presence of O antigens in the ribosomal vaccine was obtained using isogenic strains of Salmonella which differed only in the region of the chromosome coding for the O antigens. Because they were transductants of the same parent strain, their ribosomes were expected to be identical. If ribosomal components were the immunogens, preparations from one strain should have cross-protected against the other. Any specificity of protection would have been evidence for the presence of O antigens. Using a double-challenge technique and whole-body counts, it was shown that there was some specificity of protection as well as some cross-protection[3]. The specificity suggested O antigen contamination of the fractions. Additional evidence for O antigens as immunogens was the observation that the immunogenicity of the 'RNA' preparations was stable to boiling for 30 min, a finding which was consistent with the heat stability of LPS[3]. Furthermore, mice immunized with ribosomal preparations developed antibody to LPS as measured by passive haemagglutination[3]. Protein and RNA fractions prepared using the method of Fogel and Sypherd also showed evidence of O antigenic contamination of both the RNA and protein fractions[3].

The conclusion that the protective moiety in the Salmonella vaccines is extrinsic to the ribosomes is supported by Hoops *et al.*[33]. They reported that ribosomes washed with 1 M NH_4Cl lose their protective capacity, and the protection can be found in the wash supernatant. Washed ribosomes still retain the capacity to function in *in vitro* protein synthesis, indicating their integrity. Evidence that the contaminant might be O antigens is provided by the observation that gas-liquid chromatography of the Venneman type of RNA revealed the presence of rhamnose, galactose, and mannose; all constituents of lipopolysaccharide[34].

The studies reviewed above show that O antigens can contaminate ribosomes, RNA, and protein fractions and can contribute to the protection engendered by the vaccines. However, it is presently unclear if *all* of the protection is due to contaminants. Johnson has presented convincing evidence[5] for a protective protein antigen obtained from well-washed ribosomes. Whether it is a ribosomal structural protein or a protein contaminant remains to be determined. Eisenstein[3] reported that ribosomes prepared from *S. adelaide* protected against challenge by *S. typhimurium*, even though these organisms have no O antigens in common. Additional experiments have shown that this protection crosses genus lines, as ribosomal extracts of smooth and rough *Escherichia coli* also give heterologous protection[35]. This heterologous effect is much weaker than the homologous protection, the former giving protection against approximately 16 LD_{50} doses, and the latter against more than 1000 LD_{50} doses. The identity of the cross-protective substance is under investigation.

Immunity to Salmonella infection appears to involve two different kinds of immune responses. Cellular immunity is induced by living Salmonella or heat-killed organisms given in complete Freund's adjuvant[36,37]. The bacterial antigen against which this type of immune response is directed is unknown. The other type of immune response is induced by killed cells and lipopolysaccharide (LPS), and is assumed to be humoral. Anti-O antibody appears to be important in this type of host defence, although other undefined antigens may also play a role. Living vaccines are generally thought to provide superior protection to non-living vaccines[38–40]. In fact, in the literature the superiority of living vaccines has been so greatly emphasized that the substantial protective ability of non-living vaccines has been somewhat overlooked. The protection by non-living vaccines has been well documented in human field trials[41] and in mouse protection studies[42,43]. In the latter, levels of protection up to 1000 LD_{50} doses were found using heat-killed cells or a sodium deoxycholate cellular extract.

Living vaccines are thought to produce superior immunity because only they are presumed to result in macrophage activation, with resultant enhanced bactericidal capacity, via T-cell sensitization[44]. One of the reasons for investigating ribosomal vaccines was the hope that they would somehow mimic live cells and result in a cellular immune response. As described above, Youmans and Youmans have evidence that the ribosomal RNA of mycobacteria induces macrophage immunity, but without the concomitant appearance of delayed hypersensitivity. Thus, superior levels of immunity might be attainable without the problems associated with developing a live vaccine. Several investigators have compared the protection of Salmonella ribosomal vaccines with that of live cells, and reported that ribosomal preparations confer the same high level of protection as that produced by living, attenuated organisms[21,32]. The high protective capacity of these ribosomal vaccines has been attributed to their ability to elicit a cellular immune response in the host, as measured by passive transfer of peritoneal cells[45,46], footpad hypersensitivity[23], and cytophilic macroglobulin[47].

Although only limited comparisons with other non-living vaccines have actually been performed[32,34], several investigators have concluded that Salmonella ribosomal vaccines are superior to other non-viable Salmonella vaccines. Thus, it has been claimed that Salmonella ribosomal vaccines are unique among non-living vaccines of this organism, both in giving highest levels of protection and in inducing cellular immunity.

Studies by Angerman and Eisenstein have been carried out[48] to systematically compare the efficacy of ribosomes prepared from *S. typhimurium* with acetone-killed cells and lipopolysaccharide made from the same organism. Their results show that although the protection given by ribosomes approaches the levels of protection conferred by living organisms, acetone-killed cells administered in appropriate dosages, provide levels of protection comparable with that of ribosomes. Lipopolysaccharide was found to be significantly less protective than the other vaccines. They concluded that regardless of the mechanism of action of the Salmonella ribosomal extract, and regardless of the identity of the immunogen, the vaccine is not unique among non-living preparations in giving high levels of protection. It is noteworthy from a practical point of view that ribosomal vaccines were superior to the acetone-killed cells in the duration of protection they induced. An optimal dose of the ribosomal extract gave significantly better protection to mice challenged 6 months post-vaccination than did acetone-killed cells (C. Angerman and T. K. Eisenstein, unpublished observations).

The inferiority of the protection provided by lipopolysaccharide, as compared with that of the ribosomal vaccine or acetone-killed cells, suggests either that there are multiple antigens in the whole cells, or that the lipopolysaccharide is more immunogenic when complexed with a carrier. In this sense, the ribosomes may act as an adjuvant for the LPS[49].

Streptococcal ribosomal vaccines

Thompson and Synder[12] first reported that a crude ribosomal extract of a rough strain of type 3 *S. pneumoniae* was protective against challenge with the smooth strain. They also demonstrated two other interesting properties of the vaccine: (1) it gave cross-serotype protection against types 1, 2 and 7; and (2) the protection was abolished by RNase and markedly reduced by protease treatment. The protection did not appear to be due to capsular polysaccharide. Thompson and Eisenstein[13] confirmed the protection induced by the ribosomal vaccine using a different type 3 rough strain. They also found that the homologous protection could be passively transferred with serum, and absorbed out with both rough and smooth type 3 cells[13]. To explain these observations, it was proposed that the immunogen is a component of the rough cell wall, which contaminates the ribosomal fraction, is present on smooth cells of several serotypes, and is accessible to antibody even in the encapsulated organism[13]. The identity of the antigen has not yet been determined.

Swendsen and Johnson[14] confirmed the finding that ribosomal vaccines of *S. pneumoniae* give cross-serotype protection. They prepared their vaccine from still another rough type 3 organism, and were able to protect against subcutaneous challenge with serotypes 2, 3, 6 and 14. They confirmed that anti-ribosomal serum would passively transfer protection, and also found that smooth heterologous serotypes would absorb out the protection. Based on purification studies, they concluded that the immunogen was proteinaceous.

A cross-protective ribosomal vaccine has also been prepared by Schalla and Johnson[15] from a closely related organism, a group A *S. pyogenes*, type 14. Ribosomes from this species protected against homologous challenge as well as against challenge with *S. pyogenes* types 2, 5, 8 and 12. Whole killed cells only gave protection to challenge with the homologous strain. The homologous protective capacity was retained in the ribosomal protein subfraction, but not in the ribosomal RNA fractions. The vaccine was not protective unless given in adjuvant. To obtain effective immunization, it was necessary to give three injections of the vaccine and to use a dose of 326 μg of protein. The nature of the immunogen in this vaccine has also not been identified, although on the basis of Ouchterlony plates, it was concluded that it is not M protein or C carbohydrate.

For *S. pneumoniae* and *S. pyogenes* vaccines it has not been definitively established whether the immunogen is ribosomal or a contaminant. However, in both cases the ribosomes appear to play some role, since RNase abolishes the immunogenicity of the pneumococcal vaccine, and whole cells do not duplicate the cross-protective effects of the streptococcal subcellular vaccine. Vaccines from both these organisms also have the highly advantageous property of being cross-protective to subtypes in the species.

CONCLUSIONS

Ribosomal vaccines have been actively investigated in the past 10 years because it was hoped that they might provide a unique means of immunizing against infections for which no vaccine is presently available or for which the present vaccines are inferior. Thus, while BCG vaccine is efficacious against tuberculosis, it has not been widely used in the USA because it results in conversion to a positive tuberculin test. In the case of pneumococcal infections no vaccine was available until recently. Polyvalent polysaccharide vaccines are currently in field trials and they induce a significant antibody response[50]. They have the disadvantage, however, that they will only protect against the serotypes whose capsular polysaccharide are included in the vaccine, and thus may only protect against 75% of pneumococcal disease[51]. The present typhoid vaccine has the disadvantage that it requires multiple injections and has marked toxicity.

The ribosomal vaccines of the three organisms discussed in this chapter may each have some advantage over more conventional vaccines. Animal experiments suggest that the mycobacterial ribosomal vaccine induces immunity without tuberculin sensitivity, that the Salmonella ribosomal vaccine gives longer-lasting immunity than conventional vaccines, and that the pneumococcal ribosomal vaccine gives cross-serotype protection.

From a theoretical point of view these vaccines present a puzzle when one confronts the question of their mechanism action. If one postulates that ribosomal components function as antigens, it is difficult to see how they can be effective in the intact cell, since ribosomes are usually intracellular. To support such a hypothesis one would have to show that ribosomal components are in fact exposed to the cell surface during some phase of bacterial replication.

The studies of Eisenstein[3], Hoops[33], and Berry[34] show that non-ribosomal antigens are associated with the ribosomal fractions, and that these contaminants account for at least part of the immunogenicity observed in the Salmonella system. Thompson and Eisenstein have also concluded that the protection afforded by the pneumococcal ribosomal vaccine is due to a non-ribosomal antigen, although it is probably complexed with ribosomes, since ribonuclease and protein reduced the immunogenicity[13]. The observation that extranenous materials can fractionate with ribosomes is not new. Wicken showed that lipoteichoic acid of Group D streptococci was most easily obtained from a ribosomal fraction[52]. The question can be raised as to whether protection by ribosomal preparations from all organisms investigated to date might be due to non-ribosomal antigens that co-isolate with the ribosomes. Certainly, when ribosomes are prepared from Gram-negative bacteria, it is highly probable that lipopolysaccharide will also be present. As little as 1 μg of LPS of *S. typhimurium* extracted by phenol–water will protect 70% of injected mice against a challenge of 500 LD_{50} doses of live organisms[48]. Smaller doses of LPS may protect against smaller challenge doses. Thus, in order to say with assurance that biologically active amounts of LPS are not present in ribosomes prepared from Gram-negative organisms, very sensitive tests for LPS or endotoxin must be used.

If the ribosomes do play a role in the protection afforded by the pneumococcal and Salmonella preparations, it may be to act as an adjuvant or a carrier for a non-immunogenic or poorly immunogenic non-ribosomal antigen, in the same manner that the Youmans showed their RNA to be an adjuvant for bovine γ-globulin. There is a precedent for the idea that an antigen can be sufficiently exposed on the surface of a cell to absorb antibodies, but be immunogenic only in subcellular extracts. The Enterobacterial Common Antigen (ECA) is present on the surface of many Gram-negative organisms but is an immunogenic configuration in very few strains. However, ethanol-soluble extracts of the non-immunogenic strains do yield immunogenic preparations[53].

At present, it is not clear how the mycobacterial ribosomal preparations protect. Since tubercle bacilli have a much more intimate association with the host macrophage than Salmonella or pneumococci, and can persist intra-cellularly, it is conceivable that their nucleic acid might interact in some different way with the host cell. However, for all ribosomal preparations, the hypothesis that cell wall or membrane contaminants are the antigenic substances, and ribosomes merely the carriers, should be considered. Experiments should be designed to rigorously rule out this possibility before concluding that a ribosomal extract has a unique mechanism of action.

Acknowledgment

Dr Eisenstein was supported by Public Health Service Grant AI–11860 from the National Institute of Allergy and Infectious Diseases.

References

1. Youmans, A. S. and Youmans, G. P. (1965). Immunogenic activity of a ribosomal fraction obtained from *Mycobacterium tuberculosis*. *J. Bacteriol.*, **89**, 1291
2. Youmans, A. S. and Youmans, G. P. (1966). Effect of trypsin and ribonuclease on the

immunogenic activity of ribosomes and ribonucleic acid isolated from *Mycobacterium tuberculosis*. *J. Bacteriol.*, **91**, 2146

3. Eisenstein, T. K. (1975). Evidence for O antigens as the antigenic determinants in 'ribosomal' vaccines prepared from *Salmonella*. *Infect. Immun.*, **12**, 364
4. Venneman, M. R. and Bigley, N. J. (1969). Isolation and partial characterization of immunogenic moiety obtained from *Salmonella typhimurium*. *J. Bacteriol.*, **100**, 140
5. Johnson, W. (1972). Ribosomal vaccines. I. Immunogenicity of ribosomal fractions isolated from *Salmonella typhimurium* and *Yersinia pestis*. *Infect. Immun.*, **5**, 947
6. Smith, R. L., Wysocki, J. A., Brunn, J. N., DeCourcy, S. J. Jr., Blakemore, W. S. and Mudd, S. (1974). Efficacy of ribosomal preparations from *Pseudomonas aeruginosa* to protect against intravenous pseudomonas challenge in mice. *J. Reticuloendothelial Soc.*, **15**, 22
7. Winston, S. H. and Berry, L. J. (1970). Antibacterial immunity induced by ribosomal vaccines. *J. Reticuloendothelial Soc.*, **8**, 13
8. Winston, S. H. and Berry, L. J. (1970). Immunity induced by ribosomal extracts from *Staphylococcus aureus*. *J. Reticuloendothelial Soc.*, **8**, 66
9. Jensen, R., Gregory, B. Naylor, J. and Actor, P. (1972). Isolation of protective somatic antigen from *Vibrio cholerae* (Ogawa) ribosomal preparations. *Infect. Immun.*, **6**, 156
10. Agarwal, S. C. and Sundararaj, T. (1976). Cell-mediated immunity to *Vibrio cholerae* with ribonucleic acid-protein fractions of *V. cholerae* L-form lysates. *Infect. Immun.*, **14**, 363
11. Thomas, D. W., and Weiss, E. (1972). Response of mice to injection of ribosomal fractions from group B *Neisseria meningitidis*. *Infect. Immun.*, **6**, 355
12. Thompson, H. C. W. and Snyder, I. S. (1971). Protection against pneumococcal infection by a ribosomal preparation. *Infect. Immun.*, **3**, 16
13. Thompson, H. C. W. and Eisenstein, T. K. (1975). Biological properties of an immunogenic pneumococcal subcellular preparation. *Infect. Immun.*, **13**, 750
14. Swendsen, C. L. and Johnson, W. (1976). Humoral immunity to *Streptococcus pneumoniae* induced by a pneumococcal ribosomal protein fraction. *Infect. Immun.*, **14**, 345
15. Schalla, W. O. and Johnson, W. (1975). Immunogenicity of ribosomal vaccines isolated from group A, type 14 *Streptococcus pyogenes*. *Infect. Immun.* **11**, 1195
16. Feit, C. and Tewari, R. P. (1974). Immunogenicity of ribosomal preparations from yeast cells of *Histoplasma capsulatum*. *Infect. Immun.*, **10**, 1091
17. Andron, L. A. and Eigelsbach, H. T. (1975). Biochemical and immunological properties of ribonucleic acid-rich extracts from *Francisella tularensis*. *Infect. Immun.*, **12**, 137
18. Lynn, M., Tewari, R. P. and Solotorovsky, M. (1977). Immunoprotective activity of ribosomes of *Haemophilus influenzae*. *Infect. Immun.*, **15**, 453
19. Baba, T. (1977). Immunogenic activity of a ribosomal fraction obtained from *Pasteurella multocida*. *Infect. Immun.*, **15**, 1
20. Youmans, A. S. and Youmans, G. P. (1974). The effect of metabolic inhibitors and hydroxylamine on the immune response in mice to mycobacterial ribonucleic acid vaccines. *J. Immunol.*, **112**, 271
21. Venneman, M. R. (1972). Purification of immunogenically active ribonucleic acid preparations of *Salmonella typhimurium*: molecular-sieve and anion-exchange chromatography. *Infect. Immun.*, **5**, 269
22. Johnson, W. (1973). Ribosomal vaccines. II. Specificity of the immune response to ribosomal ribonucleic acid and protein isolated from *Salmonella typhimurium*. *Infect. Immun.*, **8**, 395
23. Smith, R. A., and Bigley, N. J. (1972). Detection of delayed hypersensitivity in mice injected with ribonucleic acid-protein fractions of *Salmonella typhimurium*. *Infect. Immun.*, **6**, 384
24. Youmans, A. S. and Youmans, G. P. (1969). Factors affecting immunogenic activity of mycobacterial ribosomal and ribonucleic acid preparations. *J. Bacteriol.*, **99**, 42
25. Youmans, G. P. and Youmans, A. S. (1969). Allergenicity of mycobacterial ribosomal and ribonucleic acid preparations in mice and guinea pigs. *J. Bacteriol.*, **97**, 134
26. Youmans, A. S. and Youmans, G. P. (1971). Failure of synthetic polynucleotides to affect the immunogenicity of mycobacterial ribonucleic acid and ribosomal protein preparations. *Infect. Immun.*, **3**, 149

27. Youmans, A. S. and Youmans G. P. (1973). The relationship between sedimentation value and immunogenic activity of mycobacterial ribonucleic acid. *J. Immunol.*, **110**, 581
28. Youmans, A. S., and Youmans, G. P. (1970) Immunogenic mycobacterial ribosomal and ribonucleic acid preparations: chemical and physical characteristics. *Infect. Immun.*, **2**, 659
29. Patterson, R. J. and Youmans, G. P. (1970). Demonstration in tissue culture of lymphocyte-mediated immunity ɉo tuberculosis. *Infect. Immun.*, **1**, 600
30. Klun, C. L. and Youmans, G. P. (1973). The effect of lymphocyte supernatant fluids on the intracellular growth of virulent tubercle bacilli. *J. Reticuloendothelial Soc.*, **13**, 263
31. Youmans, G. P. and Youmans, A. S. (1972). The effect of mycobacterial RNA on the primary antibody response of mice to bovine γ globulin. *J. Immunol.*, **109**, 217
32. Venneman, M. R., Bigley, N. J. and Berry, L. J. (1970). Immunogenicity of ribonucleic acid preparations obtained from *Salmonella typhimurium. Infect. Immun.*, **1**, 574
33. Hoops, P., Prather, N. E., Berry, L. J. and Ravel, J. M. (1976). Evidence for an extrinsic immunogen in effective ribosomal vaccines from *Salmonella typhimurium. Infect. Immun.*, **13**, 1184
34. Berry, L. J., Douglas, G. N. Hoops, P. and Prather, N. E. (1975). The background of immunization against Salmonellosis. In E. Neter and F. Milgrom (eds.) *4th International Convocation of Immunology*, pp. 388–398
35. Eisenstein, T. K. and O'Donnell, S. (1978). Intergenus cross-protection afforded by RNA-rich subcellular fractions prepared from *Salmonellae* and *Escherichia coli*. Manuscript
36. Mackaness, G. B., Blanden, R. V. and Collins, F. M. (1966). Host–parasite relations in mouse typhoid. *J. Exp. Med.*, **124**, 573
37. Collins, F. M. (1972). Effect of adjuvant on immunogenicity of a heat-killed Salmonella vaccine. *J. Infect. Dis.*, **126**, 69
38. Blanden, R. V., Mackaness, G. B. and Collins, F. M. (1966). Mechanisms of acquired resistance in mouse typhoid. *J. Exp. Med.*, **124**, 585
39. Rowley, D., Auzins, I. and Jenkin, C. R. (1968). Further studies regarding the questions of cellular immunity in mouse typhoid. *Aust. J. Exp. Biol. Med. Sci.*, **46**, 447
40. Ushiba, D., Saito, K., Akiyama, T., Nakano, M., Sugiyama, T. and Shirono, S. (1959). Studies on experimental typhoid: bacterial multiplication and host cell response after infection with *Salmonella enteriditis* in mice immunized with live and killed vaccines. *Japan. J. Microbiol.*, **3**, 231
41. Joō, I. (1971). Present status and perspectives of vaccination against typhoid fever. In *International Conference on the Application of Vaccines Against Viral, Rickettsial, and Bacterial Diseases of Man*, pp. 329–341 (Washington DC: Pan American Health Organization)
42. Ornellas, E. P., Roantree, R. J. and Steward, J. P. (1970). The specificity and importance of humoral antibody in the protection of mice against intraperitoneal challenge with complement-sensitive and complement-resistant Salmonella. *J. Infect. Dis.*, **112**, 113
43. Herzberg, M., Nash, P. and Hino, S. (1972). Degree of immunity induced by killed vaccines to experimental salmonellosis in mice. *Infect. Immun.*, **5**, 83
44. Mackaness, G. B. (1971). Resistance to intracellular infection. *J. Infect. Dis.*, **123**, 439
45. Venneman, M. R. and Berry, L. J. (1971). Cell-mediated resistance induced with immunogenic preparations of *Salmonella typhimurium. Infect. Immun.* **4**, 381
46. Venneman, M. R. and Berry, L. J. (1971) Experimental samonellosis: differential passive transfer of immunity with serum and cells obtained from ribosomal and RNA immunized mice. *J. Reticuloendothelial Soc.*, **9**, 491
47. Margolis, J. M. and Bigley, N. J. (1972). Cytophilic macroglobulin reactive with bacterial protein in mice immunized with ribonucleic acid-protein fractions of virulent *Salmonella typhimurium. Infect. Immun.*, **6**, 390
48. Angerman, C. R. and Eisenstein, T. K. (1977). Comparative efficacy and toxicity of a 'ribosomal' vaccine, acetone-killed cells, lipopolysaccharide, and a live cell vaccine prepared from *Salmonella typhimurium. Infect. Immun.* (in press)
49. Eisenstein, T. K., Angerman, C. Thompson, H. C. W. and Wolde-Mariam, W. (1976). Ribosomal vaccines, In W. H. Bowen *et al.* (eds.). *Immunologic Aspects of Dental Caries.*

(Proceedings of a Workshop on Selection of Immunogens for a Caries Vaccine), Suppl. to *Immunology Abstracts*, pp. 149–157

50. Austrian, R. (1976). Pneumococcal vaccines. In W. H. Bowen *et al.* (eds.). *Immunologic Aspects of Dental Caries*. (Proceedings of a Workshop on Selection of Immunogens for a Caries Vaccine), Suppl. to *Immunology Abstracts*, pp. 125–130
51. Austrian, R. 1971. The current status of pneumococcal disease and the potential utility of a polyvalent pneumococcal vaccine, In *International Conference on the Application of Vaccines against Viral, Rickettsial, and Bacterial Diseases of Man*, pp. 359–363. (Washington, DC; Pan American Health Organization, publ. 226)
52. Wicken, A. J. and Baddiley, J. (1963). Structure of intracellular teichoic acid from group D streptococci. *Biochem. J.*, **87**, 54
53. Suzuki, T., Gorzynski, E. A. and Neter, E. (1964). Separation by ethanol of common and somatic antigens of *Enterobacteriaceae*. *J. Bacteriol*, **88**, 1240

15
Cholera vaccines

H. FRIEDMAN

INTRODUCTION

Bacterial vaccines have generally been the first line of defence in many areas of the world in protecting individuals against lethal infection by pathogenic micro-organisms. Although the introduction of sanitation, and generally improved hygiene during the last century or so has resulted in the elimination of many microbial epidemics, there is still widespread potential for uncontrolled infections in many populations throughout the world. This is especially true for those individuals living in underdeveloped countries and in crowded and substandard socio-economic conditions. In recent years there has been a re-emergence of interest concerning microbial vaccines, including vaccines to protect individuals against both bacterial and viral infections.

Cholera, the disease caused by vibrios spread by contaminated water and food, is one of the most feared infectious diseases of man, and indeed pandemics of cholera have raged throughout the world even in recent decades. Although it is conceivable that cholera could be eliminated as an important contagious disease by improved sanitary conditions and public health measures, it is widely recognized that such measures are impractical in many highly populated but underdeveloped countries. The disease is spread by direct contact among individuals, or by food and water contaminated with human faeces. Protective vaccination of individuals in endemic areas is a major goal for public health officials, including those associated with world health organizations[1–4]. The recent discovery that an exo-enterotoxin produced by *Vibrio cholerae* is responsible for the massive fluid loss from the small bowel (a characteristic of this disease) has led to attempts to develop effective vaccines[2,6].

Cholera is endemic in the Indian subcontinent and Southeast Asia, but has also spread within the last decade not only to Africa and the Middle East, but also to portions of Europe. Thus, public health officials responsible for the prevention of disease in the Western hemisphere and the industrialized nations of Europe and North America are concerned that cholera may spread rapidly, especially by airborne travellers and by tourists. Consequently, much effort has been given to developing an effective vaccine derived from inactivated vibrios or their products. Initial tests utilizing formalinized enterotoxin devised from vibrios in man have been complicated by a variety of factors, including the observation, in a number of studies, that protection against the symptoms of infection may be quite weak or actually absent. Although detoxified toxoids from vibrios have been found effective in some animal studies, there is still much to be done concerning development of a suitable toxoid for protection of man against this disease.

Cholera vaccines prepared from phenol-inactivated suspensions of the classic strains of cholera bacteria grown on agar or in broth have been widely utilized in endemic areas. However, most public health officials now recognize that inactivated whole-cell vaccines are minimally effective, if at all, and do not prevent disease transmission. For such reasons the US Public Health Service recently removed the requirement that immigrants or visitors to the USA from infected areas be vaccinated with such cholera preparations. Surveillance and treatment of the disease are considered sufficient to contain cholera if introduced into the USA, since the vaccine *per se* is considered very limited in effectiveness.

It is apparent that much still must be done concerning development of safe and effective vaccines to prevent cholera infection in man, as has been so successfully done with a number of other bacterial and viral diseases. It is also apparent that development of successful vaccines for cholera depends not only on an understanding of immune responses *per se*, but also on an understanding of how cholera bacillus causes disease. In this regard, much information has recently been discovered concerning the biochemical aspects of the diarrhoea in patients with cholera, and pharmacological aspects of the fluid loss. Furthermore, animal experiments have shown that the immune response to the cholera vibrios may be significantly different from the typical 'immune response' to antigens such as serum proteins or xenogenic erythrocytes, the favourite antigens used by experimental immunologists in studying the immune response mechanism[2,6–11].

It is the purpose of this review to describe in general terms the pathogenesis of the disease caused by these micro-organisms. A brief description of the whole-cell vaccines currently used both in experimental work and for immunization of man in other countries will be described. Newer studies concerning the development of inactivated toxoids derived from the cholera exo-enterotoxin will then be described. The shortcoming of these two distinct types of vaccines for protection against cholera will be briefly mentioned. The development of immunity to cholera, as determined mostly in experimental animals, as well as some serologic studies in man, will then be discussed and related to current concepts of how anticholera immunity may be elicited to prevent both disease symptoms and transmission of the disease.

PATHOGENESIS OF CHOLERA

There is still much to be learned concerning the mechanism(s) whereby cholera vibrios infect, establish residence in the small bowel, multiply, cause symptoms of cholera and then, in patients who recover, become cleared. However, some of the details of these steps are beginning to emerge from studies in human volunteers, infected patients and experimental animals. Vibrios gain entry into the human host by the oral route through ingestion of contaminated water or food, but must then overcome several levels of effective resistance in order to cause cholera. Gastric acidity, various enzymes in the digestive tract, as well as 'normal' microbial flora are involved in maintaining a non-immunologic defence against cholera. It is now recognized, however, that once the cholera bacillus gains a foothold in the intestinal tract, marked physiological changes occur, probably because of the release of exo-enterotoxin by the vibrios. This results in an increase of intestinal capillary permeability, as evidenced by the high albumin content of fluid and leakage of intravenously administered Evans blue dye. Studies with experimental animals as well as man showed that the diarrhoea may be due to a factor actively secreted by the bacteria. A toxin purified from culture supernatants of vibrios grown *in vitro* similarly stimulates marked physiological changes in the intestine. Purification of this material (i.e. the cholera toxin) has permitted a wide variety of experimental studies, culminating in the finding that the sodium transport mechanism of the intestine is affected by the toxin.

The effect of the toxin is thought to occur as follows: enterotoxin introduced into the lumen of the small intestine is rapidly and irreversibly bound to the epithelium. After a lag period of about 30 min, fluid outpouring occurs, reaching a peak in 3–4 h. Secretion of fluid and water into the lumen of the intestine is not accompanied by any histopathological change in the tissues. Much evidence rules out changes in capillary permeability. It appears that the enterotoxin stimulates adenyl cyclase activity in the intestinal epithelial cells, thereby increasing cyclic adenosine monophosphate (AMP) levels which, in turn leads to increased electrolyte secretion. Immunization of experimental animals with toxoid (see below) prevents not only the symptoms of cholera *per se*, but also the increase in cyclase activity in gut epithelial cells, as well as in other cells which would normally respond to small amounts of the toxin.

ANTIGENS OF CHOLERA BACILLI

The cholera vibrios are classified serologically by use of typing sera which detect a common group-specific antigen present in all serotypes of these bacilli, as well as type-specific antigens, one of which is distinctive for the Inaba serotype and the other for the Ogawa serotype. The most recent cholera pandemic, however, was caused by the El tor cholera bacillus which was initially differentiated from classical vibrios because of the distinct geographical location of the disease. However, classical *Vibrio cholerae* as well as the more recent El tor biotype are immunologically similar. Nevertheless, there are non-cholera vibrios, as well as vibrios which are not agglutinated by the usual antisera used to detect cholera serotypes and the El tor vibrios[2].

The strains which are considered the cause of cholera as a disease are agglutinated characteristically by O group 1 antiserum, which has been standardized by WHO reference laboratories. Somatic O antigens differentiate the classical and El tor vibrios into the Inaba and Ogawa strains, as determined by agglutination and agglutination-absorption tests based on the presence of three antigens designated A, B, and C. Antigen A is the common group-reactive antigen possessed by all members of O group 1 cholera bacilli, whereas antigen B is the type-specific antigen for the Ogawa serotype, and antigen C is the type-specific antigen for the Inaba serotype. Other intermediate serotypes, however, have been suggested. There are also other types of variations, including variations due to transformation of antigens on the vibrio surface so as to cause smooth to rough transformation, this in turn causing the loss of reactivity of the vibrios to type-specific antisera. The vibrios also have flagellar antigens (H antigens), which are also shared by non-cholera vibrios.

Isolated somatic antigen preparations have been prepared, usually resulting in lipopolysaccharide-rich materials which are obtained either from whole cells by appropriate means or from culture supernatants. Most antisera are defined immunologically by their ability to inhibit or neutralize the vibriocidal activity of known antisera against intact bacteria. During cell death, both *in vivo* and *in vitro*, excessive amounts of somatic antigens are often released. However, the presence of antigen in culture fluids does not always depend upon cell lysis or death. Extensive biochemical, as well as immunochemical, studies have been performed to analyze the somatic antigens of vibrios, with a great deal of information now available about the ubiquitous sialidase-resistant monosialosyl ganglioside, Gm, moiety of vibrios. The interaction with ganglioside receptor on the surface of intestinal epithelium, after a characteristic latent period, activates adenylcyclase, which in turn catalyses conversion of ATP to cAMP, causing the characteristic changes in cell fluid reactivity. The toxin can be measured by its effects on a variety of cell systems both *in vivo* and *in vitro*. In animal models, including ligated rabbit ileal loop system, the development of fluid after injection of extremely small amounts of toxin is quite characteristic. Furthermore, the cholera enterotoxin induces other characteristic reactivities. Various *in vitro* biochemical assays have been developed for detecting and quantitating the toxin, including lipolysis of fat cells, induction of cAMP, stimulation of stereogenesis, as well as morphological alteration of target cells in culture.

SEROLOGIC RESPONSES IN CHOLERA

Although cholera is a disease in which vibrios and their enterotoxin are confined to the lumen and cell surfaces of the small bowel, cholera patients and even individuals with inapparent disease (i.e. asymptomatically infected individuals) develop vigorous serologic responses to the bacilli and the toxin. Antibody to the vibrios can readily be detected by agglutination tests *in vitro*, as well as by using the sensitive vibriolytic antibody procedure based upon the Pfeiffer phenomenon in which target vibrios are lysed by antibody and complement[12]. Indirect haemagglutination assays have also been developed whereby vibrio extracts, as well as enterotoxin, can be coated onto indicator red blood cells or other particular substances such as latex or charcoal particles and antibody to the appropriate antigen detected by the indirect agglutination of the erythrocyte or carrier particle[13]. Fluorescent antibody techniques have also been developed whereby specific antibody to cholera antigens can be tagged with a fluorochrome and used to monitor the interaction of antibody with the appropriate bacterial surface antigens.

More recently a cellular assay has been developed whereby individual antibody plaque-forming cells releasing specific vibriocidal antibody to the somatic group and type-specific antigens of the cholera bacillus can be measured quite accurately *in vitro*. For this procedure lymphoid cell suspensions containing immunocytes reactive to vibrios are added to melted agar gel to which is added a washed suspension of the appropriate strain of living vibrios. After incubation in agar plates for an hour, the plates are treated with guinea pig complement for an additional hour, washed and then incubated further for 3–6 h until a 'lawn' of vibrios grows on the surface of the agar plate except in those areas where vibriocidal antibody secreted by the immunocytes results in lysis of the bacteria, preventing growth. Larger numbers of antibody-producing cells can thus be enumerated very readily by the direct vibriocidal plaque assay[14,15]. Detection of lymphocytes reactive to vibrios by a rosette assay is also available whereby heat-killed vibrios, or carrier erythrocytes sensitized with the appropriate antigens derived from vibrios, are mixed with suspensions of lymphoid cells for short periods of time and then examined by high-power microscopy for enumeration of those immunocytes which bind bacteria to their surface.

IMMUNITY IN CHOLERA

The problem of inducing effective immunity against cholera, an infection strictly localized in the gut, is a difficult one, especially since the bacteria are essentially restricted to the surface and lumen of the small bowel where it appears difficult for the immune mechanism of the host to be effective. The production of antibodies or other immune factors to vibrios or their enterotoxin has little or no bearing on the disease unless causally related to or correlated with events happening at the site of infection. Thus, local immune mechanisms must play a dominant role in protection. Nevertheless, much effort has been directed at inducing effective systemic immunity against cholera. Individuals convalescing after cholera infection are refractory to reinfection for several months. This observation argues against the conclusion by some investigators that the risk of reinfection with cholera is probably only slightly less than the risk of initial infection. It now seems clear that cholera vaccines, composed of killed vibrios or isolated somatic antigen preparations, administered parenterally, do stimulate significant, although limited, immunity in some human population groups. However, it is felt that such vaccine preparations do not elicit antitoxic immunity *per se*, merely antibacterial immunity.

Immune protection against cholera is based on several distinct events. Firstly, it is felt that vibrios have an adhesive factor for the surface of the intestinal mucosa and prevention of implantation of vibrios onto the surface of intestinal cells is an important event for prevention from disease. Thus local immune factors which prevent implantation of bacteria should certainly be protective. Inhibiting effects of antibody against the somatic antigens on vibrio motility and attachment to intestinal cell lining have been observed. Antivibrio antibody in the lumen of the gut, while not significantly affecting viable vibrio populations, apparently may reduce the proportion of vibrios which are adherent to the mucosa. Coproantibody against vibrios in the gut of cholera patients, usually of the IgA class (although IgG and IgM antibody have also been detected), may prevent multiplication of the bacteria. However, vibriocidal activity *per se* may not be essential for protection if the vibrios can be prevented from attaching to surface cells in the small bowel.

Antitoxin immunity is thought by some investigators to be the most effective means of protecting individuals against the pathogenesis of the disease[2,8–10]. Even if the vibrios manage to become implanted and colonize the intestinal mucosa, intervention of antibody against the cholera enterotoxin may prevent disease symptoms. Many studies in recent years have been performed which show that a toxoid prepared from the enterotoxin may protect both patients and animals against live vibrio challenge, as well as against intestinal challenge with toxin (mainly animal studies). It is felt that the toxins from various strains of vibrios are similar and that an antibody against toxin from one strain will protect against the toxin from another serotype. However, the physical state of the immunizing toxin is important and it has been reported that toxin given together with adjuvants will stimulate a higher antibody titre, and possibly induces a greater degree of resistance against experimental cholera as compared to toxin alone. Booster injections are even more effective in experimental animals.

It is important to note that cholera is often a self-limiting disease and that once the patient recovers biochemically from the physiological insult to the gut lumen, the bacteria disappear. Since spontaneous disappearance of vibrios may be a result of the host's own antibacterial response, it has been suggested that effective prophylaxis with a vaccine or antitoxin will contribute to natural recovery. A number of large field studies have been undertaken, both with whole-cell vaccines and toxoids, with a variety of results. Results of field tests with killed cellular vaccines suggest that some protection against cholera may be achieved by protective vaccination. However, in almost every instance such trials have been performed without significant controls, including double-blind procedures with placebo, groups at equal risk, etc. Thus, although cholera vaccines have been in use since the introduction of living bacterial cell vaccines during the last century, and despite availability of both live attenuated and killed vaccines, it was not until studies during the last decade with well-matched and untreated control groups that conclusive and quantitative evidence of partial efficacy of cholera vaccine was developed. Nevertheless, it is evident that conventional killed vibrio vaccines do not provide a effective barrier for the spread of cholera and, moreover, are economically unsound.

WHOLE-CELL VERSUS TOXOID VACCINES

Despite the extensive work over quite a few decades concerning vaccines for cholera, there is at present no adequate immunizing agent to prevent *both* the disease *per se* and the spread of infection in human populations. Vaccines are prepared usually by chemical or heat inactivation of living vibrios grown in a variety of media *in vitro*. Various strains of vibrios have been used. In many cases several serotypes are combined. In some instances only one serotype is used, since all of the common disease cholera organisms share a common cross-reacting antigen. For example, immunization of man or animals with a heat-killed vaccine, regardless of serotype, usually results in appearance of agglutinating and/or vibriocidal antibody equally reactive both to homologous and heterologous vibrio serotypes. However, recent studies in this laboratory have indicated that mice, which show no pre-existing antibody to vibrios and which respond to these organisms in a true primary response (i.e. they apparently have never been sensitized to vibrio antigens in nature), initially recognize the type-specific antigen of the homologous vibrios, since over 90% of the antibody-forming cells appearing during the 2–3 weeks after immunization with heat-killed organisms are specific for the homologous vibrios (type-specific antigens) with less than 10% of the antibody-forming cells reactive to the common group antigen[12,14,15].

Many attempts have been made to isolate specific vibrio somatic antigens (A, B and C), but generally with very poor results. For example, experiments in this and other laboratories have shown that whole-cell vaccines, either

Table 1 Vaccines

A.	*Type*
1.	Cellular – heat- or chemical-killed whole-cell vaccines (with Ogawa, Inaba or both)
2.	Cell-derived: LPS, somatic extract, etc.
3.	Toxin – exo-enterotoxin – heat- or chemical-inactivated
4.	Mixture – cells plus toxoid
B.	*Experimentation*
1.	Vaccines (bacterial cells or toxin) normally poorly effective as judged by protection, though effective immunogen by *in vitro* serologic or neutralization assays
2.	Animal models may not reflect human experience
C.	*Properties*
1.	Vaccines induce serum antibody: Measured serologically by agglutination passive haemagglutination (LPS–RBC)
2.	Toxoid – induces antitoxin: Measured serologically by precipitation, passive haemagglutination (Tx-RBC) or neutralization of foot pad reaction, cyclase induction (fat cells, etc.)
3.	Protection assays – protection from challenge with bacteria or toxin, *in vivo* versus *in vitro*

from the Inaba or Ogawa strains, can be subjected to differential fractionation or extraction procedures and the resulting materials concentrated by lyophilization and then used as an immunogen. Fractions have been prepared which are much more efficient in stimulating type-specific responses as compared to the common antigen. For example, unfractionated whole-cell vaccines, as indicated before, induce a significant number of antibody-forming cells to the common antigen present in both the homologous and heterologous strains. However, a fraction was prepared by ammonium sulphate precipitation procedures which stimulated, almost exclusively, antibody-producing cells to the type-specific antigen; fewer than 1% of the antibody-forming cells reacted with the common class-specific antigen[16].

Similar approaches have been used in a number of laboratories with acellular vaccines derived from vibrios. However, there is no information at present as to whether such purified type-specific antigens are protective in man. There is the likelihood, however, that such fractionated and purified antigens may be less likely to cause untoward reactions, such as pyrogenicity or swelling at the site of inoculation. Such reactions are often due to pre-existing immunity, both humoral and cellular, to vibrio antigens, even though such immunity may be systemic and not protective in the sense that there is little or no local resistance to implantation and replication of the bacteria in the intestine. However, in the presence of such pre-existing immunity a subsequent parenteral injection of killed vibrios or subcellular somatic antigen fractions may elicit a secondary type-allergic reaction which, although not protective, may cause discomfort and/or various side-reactions.

The purified enterotoxin has been shown to stimulate antitoxin immunity both in animals and man. However, experimental trials with animals, including dogs, as well as field studies with man, have shown that toxoid,

Table 2 Biologic properties of cholera toxin versus toxoid

Assay	*Toxin*	*Toxoid*
Rabbit		
Cholerogenesis (infant)	0.25 μg	>100
Ileal loop reaction	0.20 μg	>100
Skin reaction (adult)	0.0001 μg	>0.1
Mouse		
Cholerogenesis (adult)	4.0 μg	>100
Food oedema	0.4 μg	>100
Immunizing dose	0.1	0.1
Lf dose	0.9 μg	0.6 μg

regardless of its method of preparation, is not very effective in preventing either the disease or the symptoms of cholera. Moreover, some of the commercial preparations of toxoid have been shown to contain some lipopolysaccharides (endotoxins) from the whole bacterial cells. This material is pyrogenic and causes untoward reactions in vaccinated individuals. However, some of the efficacy of toxoid preparations, especially in experimental animals, has been attributed to contamination with lipopolysaccharides which serve as an adjuvant or nonspecific stimulator of immunity. Nevertheless, as indicated before, there is no definitive evidence that parenteral immunization, either with toxoid or whole-cell vaccines, effectively stimulates local immunity in the intestinal tract.

PROSPECTS FOR FUTURE DEVELOPMENTS

The official action of US Government Agencies implies that there are essentially no efficacious vaccines at present for definitive prevention of cholera. Thus mandatory vaccination against cholera has been discontinued for US travellers. Nevertheless, pandemics caused by cholera vibrios are potentially ever-present throughout many parts of the world, and in the absence of adequate public health and sanitation capabilities preventive vaccination seems to be the ideal goal for controlling this highly contagious disease. Field trials with currently available vaccines, either whole bacteria or toxoid derivatives, apparently leave much to be desired since resistance of vaccinated individuals either to primary infection or reinfection with cholera vibrios is not satisfactory. Therefore, the potential usefulness of an efficacious vaccine is essentially unlimited.

One approach suggested by some investigators is the development of a combined vaccine, i.e. containing heat or chemically inactivated whole-cell vaccine together with a toxoid administered parenterally with an adjuvant. Other approaches are to 'immunize' persons at risk by the oral route with an attenuated vibrio. It is presumed that such an organism would not release toxin (thus it would not be a disease producer), precluding immunization against the soluble products of the vibrios. Alternatively, oral immunization might be possible using an attenuated vibrio *plus* multiple oral administration of a toxoid. Extensive laboratory studies would be necessary to establish both the efficacy of such immunogens and optimum means of achieving satisfactory results.

A non-immunologic approach, considered by some, is to develop substances which could counteract the cyclase-inducing activity of cholera toxin, thus achieving protection from disease by pharmacological intervention of the biochemical events which are associated with vibrio infection. Such an approach would be more in the nature of treatment rather than prophylaxis. At present individuals who are actively infected with vibrios and show severe symptoms of diarrhoea can be medically treated by supportive measures, rather than antimicrobial therapy. Thus a pharmacological approach would have little impact on preventing the widespread dissemination of the disease organism and the rapid development of an epidemic in a susceptible population. The goal, therefore, in achieving a successful vaccine for prevention of cholera is certainly important, but the means of achieving this goal is not certain at present.

ECONOMIC CONSIDERATIONS

Cholera is a major contributor to the economic problems of many underdeveloped countries. Pandemics of this disease decimate populations, disrupt the ability of individuals at a marginal subsistence level from achieving economic stability, and certainly, in terms of public health and medical costs, are a major drain of resources of various areas of the globe as well as of international agencies, supported mainly by financial aid from the developed and industrialized nations. It is estimated that an effective vaccine which would prevent the spread of cholera would reduce world expenditure for medical purposes by billions of dollars. The cost of developing and administering a prophylactic vaccine for cholera would probably be less than one year's cost for present worldwide cholera control. It is widely accepted that successful vaccine programmes, such as the one which essentially eliminated polio in the USA, resulted in a ratio of $100.00 saving of public tax money per year for *every* dollar of expense for developing the vaccine (i.e., based on the estimated cost of hospitalization and institutional care for persons who would otherwise have developed polio in the absence of the vaccine *and* the tax revenue obtained from individuals who reach maturity, had gainful employment and thus become a taxpayer rather than recipient). A probably greater financial return would occur with the availability of a satisfactory vaccine. In terms of actual worldwide value, it is estimated that hundreds of millions of doses of cholera vaccine would be utilized throughout the world. Even at a minimal one-dose schedule per individual at risk, this would represent a market value of several hundred million dollars per year.

The preparation of a cholera vaccine derived either from whole bacteria or from detoxified entero-exotoxin would certainly cost much less than developing and manufacturing virus vaccines which depend upon the cumbersome technique of propagating viruses in either expensive eggs or tissue cultures and then processing the virus-containing fluid to obtain a concentrated and inactivated virus preparation. Even the most complex cholera vaccine envisioned at present, i.e. a whole-cell killed vaccine *plus* a toxoid, could be prepared in readily available bacteriologic medium using large-scale fermenting apparatuses already available in the microbiologic/pharmaceutical industry.

The procedure for separating bacteria from the culture broth has been standardized over the last few decades in bacteriology and methods for inactivating bacteria and preparing toxoids are quite straightforward. Thus, the cost of preparing a bacteria plus toxoid vaccine would be very minimal, as compared with the cost of preparing viral vaccines. As indicated above, however, such vaccines are not useful unless proven efficacious in *preventing* disease. As a result the extremely large potential market for such a vaccine will never be achieved until a more successful preparation becomes available.

SUMMARY

Cholera is still one of the most feared and widespread bacterial diseases of man. Although vaccines to prevent cholera have been developed and utilized for over six decades, it is now quite apparent that protective immunization against this disease, caused by a localized infection in the intestinal tract of man, is quite difficult to achieve. Vaccines prepared by either attenuating or killing intact bacteria or, alternatively, by detoxifying the exo-enterotoxin which is the major cause of the symptoms of the disease, i.e. rapid dehydration because of fluid loss in the intestine, also are not satisfactory.

The mechanism of immunity to cholera is poorly understood, but it appears that only local immunity in the intestinal tract and not systemic immunity is important in either natural or induced resistance to infection, which is generally quite short-lived. It is now widely accepted that the symptoms of cholera are caused by the toxin elaborated by this organism growing on the surface of the intestinal lumen. The toxin stimulates the cyclase enzyme system which results in enhanced levels of cyclic AMP which, in turn, causes a major shift in the sodium–potassium 'pump' of the intestinal cells and the outpouring of fluid. Successful clinical treatment of the symptoms of cholera is based on restoring the salt/water balance of a patient and, in most cases, the patient recovers from the disease and eliminates the bacteria from the intestine.

Protective immunity by vaccination is essentially ineffectual. Vaccines prepared from whole cells or from toxoids must still be improved and shown to be efficacious. However, there is potentially a huge market for an effective vaccine among the underdeveloped and overpopulated countries of the globe. There is also a significant market for an efficacious vaccine for travellers from developed, industrialized countries for business or pleasure to areas such as the Indian sub-continent, Asia, North Africa and the Middle East. This potential market cannot be utilized until a satisfactory vaccine is developed.

References

1. Mosley, W. H. (1969). The role of immunity in cholera, A review of epidemiologic and serologic studies. *Tex. Rep. Biol. Med.*, **27**, 227
2. Finkelstein, R. (1973). Cholera. *CRC Crit. Rev. Microbiol.*, **2**, 553
   Sharp, G. W. G. and Hynie, S. (1971). Stimulation of intestinal adenyl-cyclase by cholera toxin, *Nature*, **229**, 266
3. Cash, R., Music, S., Libonati, J., Snyder, M., Wenzel, R., and Hornick, B. (1974). Response of man to infection with V. cholerae, *J. Infect. Dis.*, **129**, 45
4. Holmgren, J. and Svennerholm, A. (1977). Mechanisms of disease and immunity in cholera: A review, *J. Infect. Dis.*, **136**, 5105
5. Field, M. (1971). Intestinal secretion of cyclin AMP and its role in cholera, *N. Engl. J. Med.*, **284**, 1137
6. Pierce, N. F., Kaniecki, L. A., and Northrup, R. S. (1972). Antitoxin protection against experimental cholera. *J. Infect. Dis.*, **126**, 606
7. Nesh, S. H. and Rowley, D. (1970). The antigens of *Vibrio cholersae* involved in the vibriocidal action of antibody and complement. *J. Infect. Dis.*, **121**, 505
8. Carlin, G., Craig, J. P., Sulong, P. and Carpenter, C. C. (1970). Antitoxic immunity in experimental cholera. *J. Infect. Dis.*, **121**, 463
9. Svennerholm, A. M. (1975). Experimental studies in cholera immunocytes. *Int. Arch. Allerg. Appl. Immunol.*, **49**, 434
10. Svennerholm, A. M. and Holmgren, J. (1976). Synergistic protective effect on rabbits of immunocytes with *Vibrio cholerae* lipopolysaccharide and toxin/toxoid. *Infect. Immun.*, **13**, 735
11. Pierce, N. F. and Sack, R. B. (1977). Immune response of the intestinal mucosa to cholera toxoid, *J. Infect. Dis.*, **136**, 5113

12. McAlack, R. F., Cerny, J., Allen, J. L., and Friedman, H. (1970). Vibriolytic antibody forming cells: A new application of the Pfeiffer phenomenon, *Science*, **168**, 141
13. Kateley, J. R. and Friedman, H. (1975). The use of erythrocytes sensitized with purified enterotoxin from cholera vibrios for the assay of antibody and antibody forming cells, *J. Infect. Dis.*, **131**, 144
14. McAlack, R. F., Cerny, J. and Friedman, H. (1971). Cellular formation of vibriolytic antibody by mouse immunocytes: Cytokinetics and specificity of the response, *J. Immunol.*, **107**, 1752.
15. Cerny, J., McAlack, R. F., Sajid, M. A., Fronton, J. and Friedman, H. (1971). Early accumulation of antibody plaque forming cells in mouse spleens lacking a pre-existing immune background. *J. Immunol.*, **106**, 1331
16. Sajid, M. A., McAlack, R. F., Cerny, J. and Friedman, H. (1971). Antibody plaque responses of mice given *Vibrio cholerae* antigensin neonates. *J. Immunol.*, **106**, 1301

16
A vaccine for the prevention of pneumococcal infections

G. SCHIFFMAN

A vaccine against pneumococcal infections is needed for many reasons. First, despite extensive use of antibiotics deaths due to pneumonia were 35 per 100 000 in 1968 or approximately 70 000 people, enough to rank fifth among the leading causes of death in the USA. Second, the cost of hospitalization has been estimated to be several billions of dollars. Third, a number of illnesses other than pneumonia exist in which infection with pneumococcal organisms represent a major or contributing cause to morbidity or death; e.g. otitis media, lipoid nephrosis, sickle-cell disease, Hodgkin's disease, immunodeficiency syndromes, etc. Numerous attempts to prevent pneumonia by vaccines have been reported[1–6]. MacLeod, Hodges, Heidelberger and Bernhard[2] concluded that 30–60 μg of capsular polysaccharide of types 1, 2, 5 and 7, given in a single subcutaneous injection, was effective in preventing pneumonia caused by these types but not heterologous types. The immunees were recruits in an Army Air Force Technical School.

In this landmark study the authors used a vaccine of purified capsular polysaccharide prepared as a 'water-clear' solution of known composition, rather than whole bacteria which frequently caused local abscesses. The purified polysaccharide preparation allowed the dose to be standardized on a weight basis. Type-specific immunity was shown to be relatively long-lasting; a minimum of 6 months.

Subsequent studies expanded the number of polysaccharides in the vaccine to six[3] and evaluated the persistence of antibodies in humans injected with pneumococcal polysaccharide[7]. After 3 years most subjects showed one-fifth to one-half of maximal values, a surprisingly small decrease in titre for such a long time-span. The Air Force field trials were conducted on young men. The question whether pneumonia in the aged could be prevented by a vaccine of soluble capsular polysaccharide was answered by a 6-year study reported by Kaufman[4]. The administration of 1 mg of each of types 1, 2 and 3 significantly reduced the incident rate of pneumonia in the aged population studied.

Studies recently conducted by Austrian and collaborators as well as others[5] addressed the problem of antigenic competition: *viz.*, how many polysaccharides, at 50 μg each, can be combined to give a single vaccine capable of inducing antibody to each type in sufficient amounts to protect against disease for a reasonable length of time. In 1964 and 1974 Austrian and Gold reported on a 10-year study of pneumococcal bacteraemia[18,19]. They found that nearly three-fifths of all deaths from pneumococcal pneumonia and bacteraemia in the absence of an extrapulmonary focus of infection resulted from infection with one of six capsular types in persons 50 years of age or older, or with complicating systemic disease, or both. Continued surveillence reported later[5] indicated that bacteraemia caused by pneumococci in 3644 infections occurred in the following order of decreasing frequency: types 8, 4, 1, 14, 3, 7, 12, 6, 18, 9, 19, 23, 5, 20, 22, 11, 16, 15, 17, 13, 10, 2, 21. These twenty-three types accounted for 90% of all bacteraemias. A duodecavalent vaccine consisting of the twelve most common types would be expected to protect against about 80% of infections caused by pneumococcus. To test this hypothesis a series of multivalent vaccines were produced culminating in a 14-valent vaccine consisting of types 1, 2, 3, 4, 6, 7, 8, 9, 12, 14, 18, 19, 23 and 25. These vaccines were tested for safety, immunogenicity and efficacy.

The majority of recipients experience no untoward reactions. Of those that did show reactions to the vaccine the majority consisted of pain and or local erythema.

The immunogenicity was tested by measurement of antibody production by a radioimmunoassay procedure employing [^{14}C]-labelled capsular polysaccharides[8].

The technique is specific for each type of capsular polysaccharide[9]. By inhibiting the precipitation of [^{14}C]-labelled antigen–antibody complexes with unlabelled polysaccharide the method can be used: (1) to measure antigen in the sera of patients with pneumococcal infections[10]; (2) to assay purity as an aid in preparation and in final vaccine prepared for human use even in a mixture of eleven other polysaccharides; (3) for typing of pneumococci by RIA[11]; (4) to measure the amount of antigen in antigen–antibody complexes[12].

The results of a dose–response study, utilizing 12.5–1000 μg of each pneumococcal polysaccharide, showed a broad plateau at 25–100 μg, confirming previous work.

Fifty μg of each polysaccharide was then combined to give a multivalent vaccine. Results using several vaccines prepared by different pharmaceutical firms and many other tests showed that antibody levels can be raised two to ten times, or more, above pre-immunization levels by each component in a multivalent vaccine. The question remains, however, how much antibody is required to protect against disease. A report on the efficacy of the pneumococcal vaccine has been referred to previously, and indicates that the vaccine is at least 78.5% effective in providing protection against type-specific putitive pneumococcal pneumonia, and 82.3% effective in prevention of bacterial infections with homologous organism.

As hopeful as these results are, modification of the vaccine composition could improve the efficacy. At present the vaccine contains, among other types, 6A, 7(51), 18C and 19F. These correspond to American types 6, 51, 56 and 19. The relationship between American and Danish nomenclature is seen in Table 1.

Table 1 Correlation of American and Danish pneumococcal capsular polysaccharide type designations

USA	*Denmark*	*USA*	*Denmark*	*USA*	*Denmark*
1	1	29	29	57	19A
2	2	30	15A	58	19B
3	3	31	31	59	19C
4	4	32	32F	60	24B?
5	5	33	9A	61	35C
6	6A	34	10A	62	35A
7	7A	35	35F	63	22A
8	8	36	36	64	23B
9	9N	37	37	65	24A
10	10F	38	41F	66	35B
11	11F	39	33C	67	32A
12	12F	40	33A	68	9V
13	13	41	34	69	39
14	14	42	33B	70	33F
15	15F	43	11A	71	38
16	16	44	18A	72	45
17	17	45	40	73	46
18	18F	46	23A	74	41A
19	19F	47	35A	75	43
20	20	48	7B	76	11B
21	21	49	9L	77	15C
22	22F	50	7C	78	17A
23	23F	51	7F	79	28A
24	24F	52	47F	80	42
25	25	53	11C	81	44
26	6B	54	15B	82	48
27	27	55	18B	83	12A
28	28	56	18C	84	47A

Data taken from Reference 13

The American system has the advantage of assigning one number for each type, avoiding the ambiguity which now exists; e.g., if an aetiological agent is reported as type 19 it could be 19, 19A(57), 19B(58), or 19C(59) since the only commercially available typing sera contain pools of related types.

Monospecific sera for sub-typing are extremely rare. A method for sub-typing, independent of monospecific sera, has been reported[11]. E. Lund[14] showed that of the number of isolates from diseases caused by pneumococcus type 19, twenty-four out of thirty-nine were caused by types 19(19) and fifteen out of thirty-nine were caused by type 19A(57). Serological data can be extrapolated to infer that antibody raised to type 19(19) in the vaccine need not protect[11] against type 19A(57) infection. On the other hand, it is possible to predict that antibody to 19A(57) would protect completely against an infection of pneumococcus type 19(19). It remains to be seen if humans will respond favourably to a preparation of pneumococcal capsular type 19A(57) to offer protection against both types.

Additional studies will be required to determine the best formulation of the vaccine to obtain maximally beneficial results.

In addition to prevention of pneumococcal pneumonia, a vaccine of pneumococcal capsular polysaccharides can be used to prevent pneumococcal infections in a wide variety of other cases. Otitis media is a disease caused by an infection of the middle ear occurring principally in infants. The major aetiological agents are the pneumococcus and *Haemophilus influenzae*. Attempts to evaluate the use of the vaccine in the prevention of otitis media are now underway.

Similarly children with sickle-cell anemia run 200 times the risk of pneumococcal infection than disease-free children. A report on the efficacy of the vaccine in a 2-year study has just been released[15]. This report shows complete protection of the children vaccinated against pneumococcus as compared to the non-vaccinated controls. Other pneumococcus diseases will undoubtedly be attacked by the vaccine.

The vaccine has been applied to patients with chronic nephrotic syndrome or lipoid nephrosis (LN). Shalhoub[16] proposed that LN is produced by a systemic abnormality of T-cell function—suppressor T cells—resulting in reduced immunoglobulin synthesis by B-cells and in secretion of chemical mediators toxic to glomerular basement membranes.

One of the features of LN is the susceptibility of the patients to bacterial, particularly pneumococcal, infections[16]. Even though antibody production to pneumococcal capsular polysaccharides in the mouse is T-cell-independent, Baker[17] has shown that suppressor and helper T-cells modulate the response. Thus, in LN a T-cell abnormality culminating in the production of excessive amounts of suppressor T-cells will result in inadequate response against pneumococcal capsular antigens, low host defence and increased susceptibility to pneumococcal disease.

A direct test of this hypothesis was undertaken by immunization of age- and sex-matched control and nephrotic children with polyvalent pneumococcal vaccines, and by measuring and comparing their antibody responses to the capsular antigens. If increased suppressor T-cell activity plays a role in the pathogenesis of LN, then patients with this disease will be expected to

Table 2 *Rise in antibody levels at 4 and 6 weeks*

Vaccine Dose		Time	1A	3	4	6A	7	8	9	12	14	18C	19	23
25 μg	Control	At 4 Wks	5.49	6.30	4.89	5.51	3.16	11.46	10.72	3.51	2.34	6.92	1.11	3.98
25 μg	Non-L.N.	At 4 Wks	1.69	8.12	7.76	3.98	1.81	25.70	6.75	2.88	3.46	8.50	1.07	8.32
25 μg	L.N.	At 4 Wks	—	—	—	—	—	—	—	—	—	—	—	—
50 μg	Control	At 4 Wks	5.52	6.46	5.24	2.38	2.19	15.10	11.50	3.55	2.75	8.53	1.14	3.03
50 μg	Non-L.N.	At 4 Wks	3.16	4.68	6.45	6.41	4.70	18.20	10.50	7.46	2.95	7.06	1.00	3.89
50 μg	L.N.	At 4 Wks	9.26	23.25	10.90	7.15	2.63	14.10	18.20	11.60	5.50	15.90	1.63	2.63
25 μg	Control	At 6 Wks	5.01	5.48	2.69	5.15	3.24	10.21	10.47	4.13	2.34	7.42	1.57	3.89
25 μg	Non-L.N.	At 6 Wks	1.62	7.58	8.57	3.90	1.86	26.30	6.75	2.88	3.63	7.94	0.97	8.13
25 μg	L.N.	At 6 Wks	5.62	13.10	6.91	2.57	4.58	21.50	4.07	3.02	2.34	2.13	1.26	3.88
50 μg	Control	At 6 Wks	4.91	6.17	5.36	2.33	2.24	15.10	12.08	3.24	2.75	9.58	1.09	3.03
50 μg	Non-L.N.	At 6 Wks	2.82	4.47	5.88	5.86	4.58	16.60	8.34	5.67	2.88	6.16	0.97	3.06
50 μg	L.N.	At 6 Wks	7.52	14.60	10.90	9.00	12.80	12.60	15.80	8.25	5.91	10.5	1.61	2.75

* Pneumococcal polysaccharide type
† Expressed as multiples of pre-immunization levels

have a poor antibody response to each and all of the individual components of the vaccine. Furthermore, since antibody suppression may be specific as well as non-specific, the pattern of response to the twelve seriologically non-cross-reacting antigens would be informative as to the nature of the immunological lesion. Therefore, twenty-seven normal subjects with no evidence of renal disease, as well as twenty-one patients with nephrotic syndrome, were studied[18].

The vaccine was kindly provided by Lederle Laboratories of Pearl River, New York (Lot Nos. 7–1348–155 and 7–1347–180). It contained purified pneumococcal capsular polysaccharides to types 1, 3, 4, 6A(6), 6B(26), 7(51), 8, 9, 12, 14, 18C(56), 19 (known to be non-immunogenic in this lot) and 23 (Danish nomenclature, with USA counterparts in parentheses) and was supplied in vials of 25 μg or 50 μg.

The geometric means of pre-immunization titres for the 12 types of polysaccharides from the control subjects were higher than the titres of the nephrotic patients. The lower titres can be due to the loss of protein in the urine or increased catabolism. However, the nephrotic (LN as well as other types of nephrosis) subjects responded promptly to all of the twelve types of capsular polysaccharides, and the rise in the antibody titre expressed as multiples of the pre-immunization titre was well sustained at the end of the 4th and 6th weeks. These values compared favourably with the results obtained from the control subjects immunized with similar doses of the vaccine. These results are summarized in Table 2.

The response of the nephrotic patients to the vaccine was equal to that of the control subjects. These findings indicate that the nephrotics, in spite of the hypogamma-blobulinemia, can mount an adequate response to pneumococcal capsular polysaccharides, and that there is no evidence for suppressor T-cells or dysfunctioning B-cells.

Acknowledgment

This study was supported in part by USPHS Grant AI 42521.

References

1. White, B. (1938). *The Biology of Pneumococcus.* (New York: The Commonwealth Fund)
2. MacLeod, C. M., Hodges, R. G., Heidelberger, M. and Bernhard, W. G. (1945). Prevention of pneumococcal pneumonia by immunization with specific capsular polysaccharides. *J. Exp. Med.*, **82**, 445
3. Heidelberger, M., MacLeod, C. M. and DiLapi, M. M. (1948). The human antibody response to simultaneous injection of six specific polysaccharides of pneumococcus. *J. Exp. Med.*, **88**, 369
4. Kaufman, P. (1947). Pneumonia in old age. Active immunization against pneumonia with pneumococcus polysaccharide; results of a six year study. *Arch. Intern. Med.*, **79**, 518

5. Austrian, R., Douglas, R. M., Schiffman, G., Coetzee, A. M., Koornhof, H. J., Hayden-Smith, S. and Reid, R. D. W. (1976). Prevention of pneumococcal pneumonia by vaccination. *Trans. Assoc. Amr. Physicians*, **lxxxix**, 184
6. Weibel, R. E., Vella, P. P., McLean, A. A., Woodhour, A. F., Davidson, W. L. and Hilleman, M. R. (1977). Studies in human subjects of polyvalent pneumococcal vaccines (39894). *Proc. Soc. Exp. Biol. Med.*, **156**, 144
7. Heidelberger, M., DiLapi, M. M., Siegel, M. and Walter, A. W. (1950). Persistence of antibodies in human subjects injected with pneumococcal polysaccharides. *J. Immunol.* **65**, 535
8. Schiffman, G. and Austrian, R. (1971). A radioimmunoassay for the measurement of pneumococcal capsular antigen and of antibodies thereto. *Fed. Proc.*, **30**, 658
9. Schiffman, G., Summerville, J. E. and Castagna, R. (1973). *Immunologic specificity in the pneumococcal radioimmunoassay system*; presented at 'New Approaches for Inducing Natural Immunity to Pyogenic Organisms' which was held on March 21–23, 1973 in Winter Park, Florida. DHEW Publication No. (NIH) 74–553.
10. Dee, T. H., Schiffman, G., Sottile, M. I. and Rytel, M. W. (1977). Immunologic studies in pneumococcal disease. *J. Lab. Clin. Med.*, **89**, 1198
11. Schiffman, G., Castagna, R., and Boudreault, J. (1975). Typing of pneumococci by radioimmunoassay: identification of sub-types isolated from middle ear fluids of patients with otitis media. Annual Meeting of the American Society of Microbiology, Washington, DC, September, 1975 (abs.)
12. Schiffman, G., Summerville, J. E., Castagna, R., Douglas, R., Bonner, M. J. and Austrian, R. (1974). Quantitation of antibody, antigen, and antigen–antibody complexes in sera of patients with pneumococcal pneumonia. *Fed. Proc.*, **33**, 758
13. Kauffman, F., Lund, E. and Eddy, B. (1970). *International Bulletin of Bacterial Nomenclature and Taxonomy*, **10**, 31
14. Lund, E. (1971). Distribution of pneumococcus types at different times and different areas. In Bayer Symposium III. *Bacterial Infections. Changes in their Causative Agents–Trends* and *Possible Basis.* M. Finalnd, W. Marget and K. Bartman (eds.) pp. 49–59 (Berlin: Springer-Verlag)
15. Ammann, A. J., Addiego, J., Wara, D. W., Lubin, B., Smith, W. B. and Mentzer, W. G. (1977). Polyvalent pneumococcal polysaccharide immunization of patients with sickle-cell anemia and patients with splenectomy. *New Eng. J. Med.*, **297**, 897
16. Shalhoub, R. J. (1974). Pathogenesis of lipoid nephrosis: A disorder of T-cell function. *Lancet*, **2**, 556
17. Baker, P. J., Stashak, P. W., Amsbaugh, D. F., Prescott, B., and Barth, R. F. (1970). Evidence for the existence of two functionally distinct types of cells which regulate the antibody response to type III pneumococcal polysaccharide. *J. Immunol.*, **105**, 1581
18. Fikrig, S. M., Schiffman, G., Phillipp, J. C. and Moel, D. I. (1978). Nephrotic syndrome and pneumococcal vaccine (submitted for publication)

17
Meningococcal vaccines

W. A. HANKINS

The bacterium *Neisseria meningitidis*, while not exclusively a pathogen of infants and children, has a predilection for the very young. In addition, young adults (18–20 years of age) that congregate in certain environmental circumstances, such as barracks, have an increased susceptibility to meningococcal disease. Problems also arise concerning the prophylaxis of close contacts with individuals having confirmed meningococcal disease. Meningococcal disease[1] and chemoprophylaxis of meningococcal disease have been reviewed elsewhere[2,3].

Neisseria meningitidis has been subdivided into several serogroups, i.e., A, B, C, D, X, Y, Z, W-135 and 29E. Meningococcal isolates not identifiable in this system are categorized as 'non-typable', and each serogroup can be characterized by its capsular polysaccharide. Precise biochemical analyses of several serogroup polysaccharides have been completed. The structure of the group A polysaccharide is one of repeating units of 2-acetamido-2-deoxy-D-mannopyranosylphosphate with O-acetyl groups present[4]. The group B polysaccharide is composed of N-acetyl neuraminic acid[5]. The structure of the group C polysaccharide has also been defined[5,6] and is a polymer of N-acetyl neuraminic acid, with some O-acetyl substitutions. The group X polysaccharide has been identified as a polymer of 2-acetamido-2-deoxy-D-glucopyranosylphosphate[7]. The group Y polysaccharide consists of repeating units of 4–O-alpha-D-glucopyranosyl-N-acetylneuraminic acid[8]. The W-135 strain polysaccharide is very similar to the group Y polysaccharide; the difference being the presence of galactose rather than glucose[8]. Work in our laboratory suggests that the degree of O-acetylation of these two polysaccharides, along with the group C polysaccharide, may vary with different culture conditions such as pH of media and substrate (glucose or glycerol phosphoric acid), and the method of extraction. Jennings and his co-workers[9] have been instrumental in defining the structure of meningococcal polysaccharides.

Groups A, B, and C meningococci are considered to be of major medical significance and, historically, the greatest number of cases of meningococcal disease have been associated with one of these three groups. The prominence of any one of these serogroups has varied with a particular period of history and/or geographical area, typifying one of the many still unsolved mysteries of the meningococcus. The designation of this micro-organism as 'an enigma coated with sugar', is quite apropos. Instances of disease are rarely associated with the other serogroups[10–14]; they are identified more often in surveillance studies to identify carriers of *Neisseria* species[15,16].

Group A meningococcal disease has occurred sporadically in North America in the 1970s. Cases have been documented in the Pacific Northwest, Alaska, and Manitoba (G. W. Counts and K. K. Holmes, University of Washington; A. Ronald, University of Manitoba). Group A meningococcal disease has occurred in recruit gold miners in South Africa, also in the 'meningitis belt' of Africa[17] and in Finland[18]. Groups A and C meningococcal epidemics have occurred in Brazil[19–21]. The group B meningococcus continues to be a substantial hurdle in the control of meningococcal disease in the USA[15, 16]. Group B disease has been recognized in Belgium[22, 23], and Norway[24].

The problem of group C meningococcal disease in American military personnel served as a catalyst for investigators at the Walter Reed Army Institute of Research, to focus their resources, in the late 1960s, on conducting fundamental studies that led to effective vaccines against group A and group C meningococcal disease. In a series of five papers[25–29], Artenstein and his co-workers established the relationship of anti-capsular antibody and protection, and set criteria of composition and purity of capsular polysaccharide that could effectively induce protective antibody. Of particular significance was the observation that the molecular size of the polysaccharide is critical; i.e., molecular size of 100 000 daltons or more was essential for an effective vaccine. Technology available in the late 1960s and 1970s permitted the preparation of sufficient quantities of highly purified polysaccharides, and allowed critical evaluation of their biochemical and biological properties. Berman *et al.*[30] established methods for the pilot production of purified polysaccharides, while the method developed by Gotschlich[31] has been found very satisfactory for the purification of large quantities of high molecular weight polysaccharide (10^6 daltons). A third purification method has also been reported[32].

The current American licensed vaccines, group A, group C, and combined groups A and C, must meet rigid standards and control testing established by the Bureau of Biologics, Food and Drug Administration[33]. Specifications have also been established by the World Health Organization[34]. The standards essentially can be divided into two general areas. The first relates to the potency of the vaccine, with molecular weight being the key factor since immunogenicity in man is related to molecular size of the polysaccharide[29, 31, 33]. The second general area governed by the standards relates to purity. Criteria of, and methods to determine levels of, non-polysaccharide contaminants (proteins and nucleic acid, both less than 1 %), are described. In addition, levels of lipopolysaccharide endotoxin (LPS) are determined by standard pyrogenicity tests using rabbits. A cause-and-effect relationship with levels of pyrogenicity, Limulus activity, and the clinical response of individuals receiving the vaccine, has been postulated. Methods of purification, levels of LPS and response to immunization, are areas of investigation that require continued study.

The vaccine is a lyophilized preparation requiring rehydration with diluent prior to use. The vaccine is packaged in two sizes, i.e., a 10-dose vial and a 50-dose vial; the latter is intended for jet gun administration. The recommended dosage is 50 μg of each polysaccharide, administered subcutaneously. Thiomersal is used as a preservative for multi-dose containers and has no effect on the polysaccharide[35]. Proper storage of the lyophilized vaccine is important, particularly the group A polysaccharide which is somewhat labile. Some field trials in the 'meningitis belt' of Africa with improperly stored group A vaccine emphasized this fact[31]. Current studies are directed towards improving the shelf-life of the vaccines by incorporating suitable bulking agents in the lyophilization process[36].

The Bureau of Biologics has the prerogative to require the periodic testing of vaccine lots in humans (minimum of twenty-five individuals). No suitable animal model exists to evaluate potency of meningococcal vaccines. The formation of bactericidal antibodies in at least 90 % of the individuals is required. The correlation between resistance to disease and the formation of bactericidal antibody has been established[25]. Other serological tests that have been investigated include indirect hemagglutination, complement-fixation, precipitin reactions, and immunofluorescence[37, 38]. The bactericidal test remains the assay of choice for predicting resistance to meningococcal disease. Results of radioimmune assays (RIA) of clinical sera, by McVerry and Herrmann of our laboratory using the method of Gotschlich[39], have correlated very well with bactericidal testing, and offer more precision and sensitivity in measuring the response to vaccines. Further comparison of serological testing and standardization of methods between laboratories will serve to elucidate the role of humoral immunity to the meningococcus.

The clinical evaluation and efficacy studies of groups A and C meningococcal polysaccharide vaccines have been worldwide. With respect to adults, the evaluation of the group C vaccine has been made in American military personnel[40–43]. The routine use of this vaccine in recruits, since 1972, has virtually eliminated group C meningococcal disease in American personnel (efficacy near 100 %). In 1977, the Armed Forces Epidemiological Board recommended the routine use of a group A and group C combined vaccine in recruits. The group A polysaccharide has been shown to be efficacious in South African gold miners of the same age group. Group A vaccine has been used in Army recruits in Finland[44].

Duration of antibody to group C meningococcus has been estimated to be at least 5 years[45]. Studies in our laboratory (unpublished) confirm that group A and group C antibody, as determined by radioimmune assay, persists for at least 3 years and, in addition, an immunization with a combined group A, group C, and group Y vaccine resulted in elevation in group A and C antibodies, as determined by bactericidal and/or radioimmune assay.

With regard to the immunization of infants and young children, the group most in need of protection, the situation is slowly being clarified. This is an area of ongoing research. The Advisory Committee of Immunization Practices, and the Center for Disease Control recommend, for special and epidemic situations, that the group A vaccine be used in children above the age of 2 years, and that the group C vaccine be used in children above the age of 6 years. A dose of 50 μg of each polysaccharide is recommended.

Studies to determine the suitability of meningococcal vaccines for infants and children have been done worldwide. Studies in Connecticut by Gold, Lepow, Goldschneider and their associates, established the relative safety and immunogenicity of group A and group C vaccines in infants and children [44–49]. Infants as young as 3 months of age were given the vaccines. Serological responses to the group A vaccine improved with age of the recipient and the antibody levels could be increased by a booster immunization. With the group C vaccine, the primary serological response was better with increased age of the recipients, i.e., 7 and 12 months, rather than 3 months of age. A booster response was not seen, as secondary responses were lower than after the primary immunization[49].

Field trials in Egypt and Sudan[50,51] in 1971–1972, have shown that the group A vaccine is efficacious in children above the age of 6 years. Recently[52] the report of field trials in Finland has shown efficacy using group A meningococcal vaccine in children 3 months to 5 years of age.

An effective vaccine against the group B meningococcus has eluded discovery. A polysaccharide preparation tested in 1972 was found to be non-immunogenic in man[53]. Group B meningococcal polysaccharide preparations, using techniques developed in our laboratory for other group-specific polymers, are currently being studied as potential vaccines. Polysaccharide antigens from *Escherichia coli*, which are biochemically and immunologically similar to the group B meningococcal capsular antigen, have also been studied as possible vaccine candidates[54,55].

Other group B meningococcal antigens have been studied as possible vaccine components. Most interestingly, a protein antigen, or antigens located at the cell surface, appear to have promise as effect immunogens. Serogroups C[56, 57] and B meningococci have been subdivided into serotypes based on protein surface antigens[58]. The experiments of Frasch and co-workers[59–62], and Zollinger[63,64], have referred to the possibility of using purified serotyping antigens of meningococci as vaccines. These antigens stimulate the formation of bactericidal antibodies in several laboratory animals (rabbits, mice, guinea-pigs and monkeys). Under development now are methods to define and eliminate possible toxic components such as LPS. Complete evaluation of the immunogenicity of these protein antigens in man is still in the future. Since common serotype antigens occur in both group B and group C, and possibly group Y meningococci, a vaccine with a wider coverage is possible[65]. Serogroup A meningococci appears to have distinctly different serotype antigens as compared to groups B and C[66].

Another independent meningococcal antigen under current investigation is the lipopolysaccharide antigen[67]. Zollinger has established at least eight different LPS antigens among several serogroups of meningococci. More than one LPS antigen can be present with one serotype protein, and thus appears to be independent of serotype and serogroup.

In attempts to develop a vaccine that will have the broadest coverage against meningococcal disease, a group Y polysaccharide vaccine has been developed in our laboratory[68]. The apparent molecular size is 10^7 daltons, which is several times larger than the group A or group C polysaccharides. Group Y meningococcal disease occurs sporadically in military personnel[12]. A vaccine developed in our laboratory containing the three group-specific capsular polysaccharides (A, C, and Y), has been evaluated in young adults[69]. One dose administered subcutaneously contained 50 μg of each component; over 90% of the individuals developed bactericidal antibodies and antibodies detected by the radioimmune assay. Each component appeared to act independently. Further clinical trials are planned to evaluate the dose–response of the group Y polysaccharide and to study the immunologic response of younger age groups.

The development of meningococcal vaccines has served as a good example of collaborative research between many public and private laboratories. Credit is due to many investigators over the last 10 years. Not only have specific vaccines become available for meningococcal disease, but precedents have been set for further studies on other bacterial vaccines including pneumococcal, *Haemophilus influenzae* type b and perhaps even the gonococcus. Since meningococcal vaccines have been made that are biochemically well defined and technically feasible to produce on a manufacturing scale, then serious efforts to refine other bacterial vaccines should be made to maximize potency and minimize untoward reactions.

References

1. Bell, W. E. and Silber, D. L. (1971). Meningococcal meningitis: past and present concepts. *Mil. Med.* **136,** 601
2. Meningococcal Disease Surveillance Group. (1976). Meningococcal disease secondary attack rate and chemoprophylaxis in the United States, 1974. *J. Am. Med. Assoc.*, **235,** 261

3. Kagan, B. M. and Hendeles, L. (1977). Meningococcal prophylaxis in 1977. *Infect. Dis.*, **7**(8), 4, 14
4. Liu, T. Y., Gotschlich, E. C. Jonssen, E. K. and Wysocki, J. R. (1971). Studies on the meningococcal polysaccharides. I. Composition and chemical properties of the group A polysaccharide. *J. Biol. Chem.*, **246**(9), 2849
5. Bhattacharjee, A. K., Jennings, H. J., Kenny, C. P., Martin, A. and Smith, I. C. P. (1975). Structural determination of the sialic acid polysaccharide antigens of *Neisseria meningitidis* serogroups B and C with Carbon 13 nuclear magnetic resonance. *J. Biol. Chem.*, **250**(5), 1926
6. Bhattacharjee, A. K. and Jennings, H. J. (1976). Determination of the linkages in some methylated, sialic acid-containing, meningococcal polysaccharides by mass spectrometry. *Carbohydr. Res.*, **51**, 253
7. Bundle, D. R., Jennings, H. J. and Kenny, C. P. (1974). Studies on the group specific polysaccharide of *Neisseria meningitidis* serogroup X and an improved procedure for its isolation. *J. Biol. Chem.*, **249**(15), 4797
8. Bhattacharjee, A. K., Jennings, H. J., Kenny, C. P., Martin, A., and Smith, I. C. P., (1976). Structural determination of the polysaccharide antigens of *Neisseria meningitidis* serogroups Y, W-135, and BO[1]. *Can. J. Biochem.*, **54**(1), 1
9. Jennings, H. J., Bhattacharjee, A. K., Bundle, D. R., Kenny, C. P., Martin, A. and Smith, I. C. P., (1977). Structures of the capsular polysaccharides of *Neisseria meningitidis* as determined by ^{13}C-nuclear magnetic resonance spectroscopy. *J. Infect. Dis.*, **136**, S78
10. Risko, J. A. and Hodges, G. R. (1974). *Neisseria meningitidis* serogroup Y: incidence and description of clinical illness. *Am. J. Med. Sci.*, **267**(6), 345
11. Sorensen, K., Girgis, N. I. and Sanborn, W. R. (1974). Meningococcemia due to *Neisseria meningitidis* serogroup D. *Scand. J. Infect. Dis.*, **6**, 365
12. Smilack, J. D. (1974). Group-Y meningococcal disease: twelve cases at an Army training center. *Ann. Intern. Med.*, **81**, 740
13. Fallon, R. J. and Brown, W. (1974). Group-Z meningococci. *Lancet*, Aug. 24, 460
14. Fallon, R. J. (1976). The relationship between *Neisseria meningitidis* of serogroups Z[1] and 29E. *J. Med. Microbiol.*, **9**, 239
15. Greenfield, S., Sheehe, P. R. and Feldman, H. A. (1971). Meningococcal carriage in a population of 'normal' families. *J. Infect. Dis.*, **123**(1), 67
16. Meningococcal Disease Surveillance Group. (1976). Analysis of endemic meningococcal disease by serogroup and evaluation of chemoprophylaxis. *J. Infect. Dis.*, **134**(2), 201
17. WHO Seminar. (1973). Epidemiological surveillance and control of cerebrospinal meningitis in Africa. *WHO Chronicle*, **27**, 347
18. Mäkelä, P. H., Peltola, H. Käyhty, H., Jousimies, H., Pettay, O., Ruoslahti, E., Sivonen, A. and Renkonen, O. V. (1977). Polysaccharide vaccines of Group A *Neisseria meningitidis* and *Haemophilus influenzae* type b: a field trial in Finland. *J. Infect. Dis.*, **136**, S43
19. Jacobson, J. A., Camargos, P. A. M., Ferreira, J. T. and McCormick, J. B. (1976). The risk of meningitis among classroom contacts during an epidemic of meningococcal disease. *Am. J. Epidemiol.*, **104**, 552
20. DeMorais, J. S., Munford, R. S., Risi, J. B., Antezanna, E., and Feldman, R. A. (1974). Epidemic disease due to serogroup C *Neisseria meningitidis* in Saõ Paulo, Brazil. *J. Infect. Dis.*, **129**(5), 568
21. Munford, R. S., DeVasconcelos, Z. J. S., Phillips, C. J., Gelli, D. S., Gorman, G. W., Risi, J. B. and Feldman, R. A. (1974). Eradication of carriage of *Neisseria meningitidis* in families: a study in Brazil. *J. Infect. Dis.*, **129**(6), 644
22. Gilguin, C. C. (1972). Studies on the strains of *N. meningitidis* isolated in Belgium from 1969–1973. *Acta Clin. Belg.*, **27**, 548
23. WHO. (1976). Meningococcal meningitis. *Wkly Epidem. Rec.*, **51**, 333
24. Bøvre, K., Holten, E., Vik-Mo, H., Brøndo, A., Bratlid, D., Bjark, P., and Moe, P. J. (1977). *Neisseria meningitidis* infections in northern Norway: an epidemic in 1974–1975 due mainly to group B organisms. *J. Infect. Dis.*, **135**(4), 669
25. Goldschneider, I., Gotschlich, E. C., and Artenstein, M. S. (1969). Human immunity to the meningococcus. I. The role of humoral antibodies. *J. Exp. Med.*, **129**, 1307

26. Goldschneider, I., Gotschlich, E. C. and Artenstein, M. S. (1969). Human immunity to the meningococcus. II. Development of natural immunity. *J. Exp. Med.*, **129**, 1327
27. Gotschlich, E. C., Liu, T. Y. and Artenstein, M. S. (1969). Human immunity to the meningococcus. III. Preparation and immunochemical properties of the group A, group B, and group C meningococcal polysaccharides. *J. Exp. Med.*, **129**, 1349
28. Gotschlich, E. C., Goldschneider, I. and Artenstein, M. S. (1969). Human immunity to the meningococcus. IV. Immunogenicity of group A and group C meningococcal polysaccharides in human volunteers. *J. Exp. Med.*, **129**, 1367
29. Gotschlich, E. C., Goldschneider, I. and Artenstein, M. S. (1969). Human immunity to the meningococcus. V. The effect of immunization with meningococcal group C polysaccharide on the carrier state. *J. Exp. Med.*, **129**, 1385
30. Berman, S., Altieri, P. L., Groffinger, A. and Lowenthal, J. P. (1970). Pilot-scale production of group A and group C meningococcal polysaccharide immunogens. *Infect. Immun.*, **2**(5), 640
31. Gotschlich, E. C., Rey, M., Etienne, J., Sanborn, W. R., Triau, R. and Cvjetanović, B. (1972). The immunological responses observed in field studies in Africa with group A meningococcal vaccines. *Progr. Immunobiol. Stand.*, **5**, 485
32. Triau, R. (1974). New meningococcal vaccines. *Nouv. Presse Med.*, **3**(36), 2325
33. Wong, K. H., Barrera, O., Sutton, A., May, J., Hochstein, D. H., Robbins, J. D., Robbins, J. B., Parkman, P. D. and Seligmann, E. B., Jr. (1977). Standardization and control of meningococcal vaccines, group A and group C polysaccharides. *J. Biol. Stand.*, **5**, 197
34. WHO Expert Committee on Biological Standardization. (1976). Requirements for meningococcal polysaccharide vaccine. *Wld Hlth Org. Tech. Report Series* **594**, 19
35. Sorrentino, J. V. and Hankins, W. A. (1974). Effect of thimerosal on purified meningococcal polysaccharide vaccines. *Develop. Biol. Stand.*, **24**, 107
36. Tiesjema, R. H., Beuvery, E. C. and TePas, B. J. (1977). Enhanced stability of meningococcal polysaccharide vaccines by using lactose as a menstruum for lyophilization. *Bull Wld Hlth Org.*, **55**, 43
37. Artenstein, M. S., Brandt, B. L., Tramont, E. C., Branche, W. C., Jr., Fleet, H. D. and Cohen, R. L. (1971). Serologic studies of meningococcal infection and polysaccharide vaccination. *J. Infect. Dis.*, **124**(3), 277
38. Brandt, B. L., Artenstein, M. S. and Smith, C. D. (1973). Antibody responses to meningococcal polysaccharide vaccines. *Infect. Immun.*, **8**, 590
39. Gotschlich, E. C., Rey, M., Triau, R. and Sparks, K. J. (1972). Quantitative determination of the human immune response to immunization with meningococcal vaccines. *J. Clin. Invest.*, **51**, 89
40. Artenstein, M. S., Gold, R., Zimmerly, J. G., Wyle, F. A., Schneider, H. and Harkins, C. (1970). Prevention of meningococcal disease by group C polysaccharide vaccine. *N. Engl. J. Med.*, **282**,(8), 417
41. Artenstein, M. S., Gold, R., Zimmerly, J. G., Wyle, F. A., Branche, W. C., Jr. and Harkins, C. (1970). Cutaneous reactions and antibody response to meningococcal group C polysaccharide vaccines in man. *J. Infect. Dis.*, **121**,(4), 372
42. Artenstein, M. S., Winter, P. E., Gold, R. and Smith, C. D. (1974). Immunoprophylaxis of meningococcal infection. *Mil. Med.*, **139**(2), 91
43. Artenstein, M. S. (1975). Control of meningococcal meningitis with meningococcal vaccines. *Yale J. Biol. Med.*, **48**(3), 197
44. Mäkelä, P. H.,, Käyhty, H. Weckström, P. Sivonen, A. and Renkonen, O. V. (1975). Effect of group-A meningococcal vaccine in Army recruits in Finland. *Lancet*, Nov. 8, 883
45. Brandt, B. L., and Artenstein, M. S. (1975). Duration of antibody responses after vaccination with group C *Neisseria meningitidis* polysaccharide. *J. Infect. Dis.*, **121**, S69
46. Goldschneider, I., Lepow, M. L. and Gotschlich, E. C. (1972). Immunogenicity of the group A and group C meningococcal polysaccharides in children. *J. Infect. Dis.*, **125** (5), 509
47. Goldschneider, I., Lepow, M. L., Gotschlich, E. C., Mauck, F. T., Bachl, F. and Randolph, M. (1973). Immunogenicity of group A and group C meningococcal polysaccharides in human infants. *J. Infect. Dis.*, **128**(6), 769

48. Gold, R., Lepow, M. L., Goldschneider, I., Draper, T. L. and Gotschlich, E. C. (1975). Clinical evaluation of group A and group C meningococcal polysaccharide vaccine in infants. *J. Clin. Invest.*, **56**, 1536
49. Gold, R., Lepow, M. L., Goldschneider, I. and Gotschlich, E. C. (1977). Immune response of human infants to polysaccharide vaccines of groups A and C *Neisseria meningitidis. J. Infect. Dis.*, **136**, S31
50. Wahdan, M. H., Rizk, F., El-Akkad, A. M., El Ghoroury, A. A., Hablas, R., Girgis, N. I., Amer, A., Boctar, W., Sippel, J. E., Gotschlich, E. C., Triau, R., Sanborn, W. R. and Cvjetanović, B. (1973). A controlled field trial of a serogroup A meningococcal polysaccharide vaccine. *Bull. Wld Hlth Org.*, **48**, 667
51. Erwa, H. H., Haseeb, M. A., Idris, A. A., Lapeyssonnie, L., Sanborn, W. R. and Sippel, J. E. (1973). A serogroup A meningococcal polysaccharide vaccine. *Bull. Wld Hlth Org.*, **49**, 301
52. Peltola, H., Mäkelä, P. H., Käyhty, H., Jousimies, H., Herva, E., Hällström, K., Sivonen, A., Renkomen, O. V., Pettay, O., Karanko, V., Ahvonen, P. and Sarna, S. (1977). Clinical efficacy of meningococcus group A capsular polysaccharide vaccine in children three months to five years of age. *N. Eng. J. Med.*, **297**(13), 686
53. Wyle, F. A., Artenstein, M. S., Brandt, B. L., Tramont, E. C., Kasper, D. L., Altieri, P. L., Berman, S. L. and Lowenthal, J. P. (1972). Immunologic response of man to group B meningococcal polysaccharide vaccines. *J. Infect. Dis.*, **126**(5), 514
54. Kasper, D. L., Winkelhake, J. L., Zollinger, W. D., Brandt, B. L. and Artenstein, M. S. (1973). Immunochemical similarity between polysaccharide antigens of *Escherichia coli* 07:K1 (L): NM and group B *Neisseria meningitidis. J. Immunol.*, **110**,(1), 262
55. Egan, W., Liu, T. Y., Dorow, D., Cohen, J. S., Robbins, J. D., Gotschlich, E. C. and Robbins, J. B. (1977). Structural studies on the sialic acid polysaccharide antigen of *Escherichia coli* strain Bos-12. *Biochem.* **16**(16), 3687
56. Gold, R. and Wyle, F. A., 1970. New classification of *Neisseria meningitidis* by means of bactericidal reactions. *Infect. Immun.*, **1**(5), 479
57. Gold, R., Winkelhake, J. L., Mars, R. S. and Artenstein, M. S. (1971). Identification of an epidemic strain of group C *Neisseria meningitidis* by bactericidal serotyping. *J. Infect. Dis.*, **124**(6), 593
58. Frasch, C. E. and Gotschlich, E. C. (1974). An outer membrane protein of *Neisseria meningitidis* group B responsible for serotype specificity. *J. Exp. Med.*, **140**, 87
59. Frasch, C. E. and Chapman, S. S. (1972). Classification of *Neisseria meningitidis* group B into distinct serotypes. I. Serological typing by a microbactericidal method. *Infect. Immun.*, **5**(1), 98
60. Frasch, C. E. and Chapman, S. S. (1972). Classification of *Neisseria meningitidis* group into distinct serotypes. II. Extraction of type-specific antigens for serotyping by precipitin techniques. *Infect. Immun.* **6**(2), 127
61. Frasch, C. E. and Chapman, S. S. (1973). Classification of *Neisseria meningitidis* group B into distinct serotypes. III. Application of a new bactericidal-inhibition technique to distribution of serotypes among cases and carriers. *J. Infect. Dis.*, **127**(2), 149
62. Frasch, C. E. and Chapman, S. S. (1972). Classification of *Neisseria meningitidis* group B into distinct serotypes. IV. Preliminary chemical studies on the nature of the serotype antigen. *Infect. Immun.*, **6**(5), 674
63. Zollinger, W. D., Kasper, D. L., Veltri, B. J. and Artenstein, M. S. (1972). Isolation and characterization of a native cell wall complex from *Neisseria meningitidis. Infect. Immun.*, **6**(5), 835
64. Zollinger, W. D., Pennington, C. L. and Artenstein, M. S. (1974). Human antibody response to three meningococcal outer membrane antigens: comparison by specific hemagglutination assays. *Infect. Immun.*, **10**(5), 975
65. Munford, R. S., Patton, C. M. and Gorman, G. W. (1975). Epidemiologic studies of serotype antigens common to groups B and C *Neisseria meningitidis. J. Infect. Dis.*, **131** (3), 286
66. Sippel, J. E. and Quan, A. (1977). Homogeneity of protein serotype antigens in *Neisseria meningitidis* group A. *Infect. Immun.*, **16**(2), 623
67. Mandrell, R. E. and Zollinger, W. D. (1977). Lipopolysaccharide serotyping of *Neisseria meningitidis* by hemagglutination inhibition. *Infect. Immun.*, **16**(2), 471

68. Farquhar, J. D., Hankins, W. A., DeSanctis, A. N. DeMeio, J. L. and Metzgar, D. P. (1977). Clinical and serological evaluation of purified polysaccharide vaccines prepared from *Neisseria meningitidis* group Y. *Proc. Soc. Exp. Biol. Med.*, **155**, 453
69. Farquhar, J. D., Hankins, W. A., DeSanctis, A. N., DeMeio, J. L. and Metzgar, D. P. (1978). Clinical and serological evaluation of meningococcal polysaccharide vaccine groups A, C, and Y. *Proc. Soc. Exp. Biol. Med.*, **157**, 79

18
Development of meningococcal vaccines

R. TRIAU

INTRODUCTION

A few years after the discovery of *Meningococcus* by Weichselbaum in 1887[1], numerous vaccines were described and tested almost everywhere in the world. Davis[2] seems to have been the first to attempt active immunization, in 1907, using meningococcal cultures heated to 60 °C. A number of other researchers followed on similar lines: Sophian and Black[3]; Chalmers and O'Farrel[4]; Riding and Corkill[5]; Neujean[6]; Blanchard[7]; Saleun and Ceccaldi[8], etc.

This work was reviewed in 1971 by Cvjetanovic[9] who found that very few of these tests met the requirements of a modern clinical trial (Table 12.1), a majority being simple field observations unacceptable as proof of efficacy of any of the vaccines tested, whose tolerability was also far from satisfactory (whole-cell vaccines).

Shortly before World War II, the discovery of sulphonamides and then of antibiotics rendered meningococcal vaccines obsolete. In fact, provided that they were used in good time, these drugs proved capable of effecting recovery in the majority of cases of cerebrospinal meningitis. Used as a prophylactic weapon they gave the impression of being able to cut short epidemics of the disease.

In 1963 the appearance of meningococci resistant to sulphonamides and to antibiotics led three research teams working in the USA, Canada and France to turn once more to new, effective and well-tolerated meningococcal vaccines. Their work has been encouraged and supported throughout by the WHO and now it is well advanced, having perfected and developed A and C polysaccharide vaccines.

Table 1 Controlled field studies of meningococcal vaccines

Authors and source	*Area and population*	*Type of vaccine and dosage*	*Type of epidemic strain*	*Type of study*	*Population inoculated*	*Control group*	*Total cases in immunized (and deaths)*	*Total cases in control group (and deaths)*	*Effectiveness of vaccine (statistical significance)*
Zrdnek, K. Feierabend, B. *Trav. Inst. Hyg. publ. Tschech.* (1931) **2**, 1	Czechoslovakian Army, Brno, Olomouc: Two studies were made	Freshly isolated local strains, agar-grown, heat-killed, phenol preserved 4000 million organisms in 1 ml. 3 doses: 0.5, 1.0 and 1.0 ml.	?	Soldiers with names A–M were vaccinated. N–Z were control	14 654 6 626 21 280	13 330 6 354 19 684	4 (1) 4 (2) 8 (3)	3 (2) 5 (1) 8 (3)	None None
Riding, D. Corkill, N. W. *J. Hyg.* (1932) **32**, 258	Sudan, Khartoum and Deims civilians, all ages.	Nine freshly isolated local strains (group B) agar-grown phenol-killed and preserved, autolysed to liberate endotoxin. 2000 million organisms in 1 ml. Only one dose of 1 cc was given	Group B	People were inoculated. at random either with CSM vaccine or TAB vaccine which served as a control	9 713	9 720	12 (5)	17 (7)	None
Russell, A. J. H. *Bull. Off. int. Hyg. Publ.* (1936) **26**, 1106	India (1) Lahore prison (2) Lahore, borstal institute (3) Delhi, prison 1934	Vaccine prepared by C. R. I. Kasauli. Three doses given: 0.5, 1.0 and 2.0 ml., 14 days apart	?	Population was divided into two approx. equal groups. One was inoculated. The other was control	(1) 1 002? (2) 766 (3) 228? 1996?	1 002? 766? 228? 1 996?	0 0 0 0	0 0 3 (1) 9 (1)	Dubious because of small number of cases
Maclean, I. H. Bevan, C. E. *Proc. roy Soc.* Med. (1939) **32**, 1	Cyprus Nicosia Limassol Paphos	Fourteen strains of group A and B blood serums agar-grown, heat-killed, 1000 million organisms in 1 ml. Dose ½ and 1 cc, 10 days apart	Group B	TAB vaccine was used as control. Vaccination was done in between two epidemic waves	6 856	5 899	7 (1)	5 (0)	None

MENINGOCOCCAL A AND C VACCINES

Since Gotschlich's[10] publication, of his production method, further modified by Ayme,[11] many scientific meetings held in America and in Europe have attempted to define and standardize the vaccines thus obtained. The complete text of 'Requirements for Meningococcal Polysaccharide Vaccine' as approved by the 27th Expert Committee on Biological Standardization is published in No. 594 of the WHO Technical Reports Series (1976).

Seriological efficacy

Serological methods for checking of meningococcal vaccine activity in man are numerous indeed. In practice, three techniques are being currently used in specialized laboratories:

(a) the technique of passive haemagglutination[12].
(b) Farr's technique modified by Gotschlich[13]
(c) assay of bactericidal antibodies[14].

With the approval of French authorities we used the data obtained in Dakar and in Lyon and they are presented here in Figures 1–3.

These serological pre- and post-vaccination titres were obtained by the Vandekerkove[12] technique of passive haemagglutination. The series com-

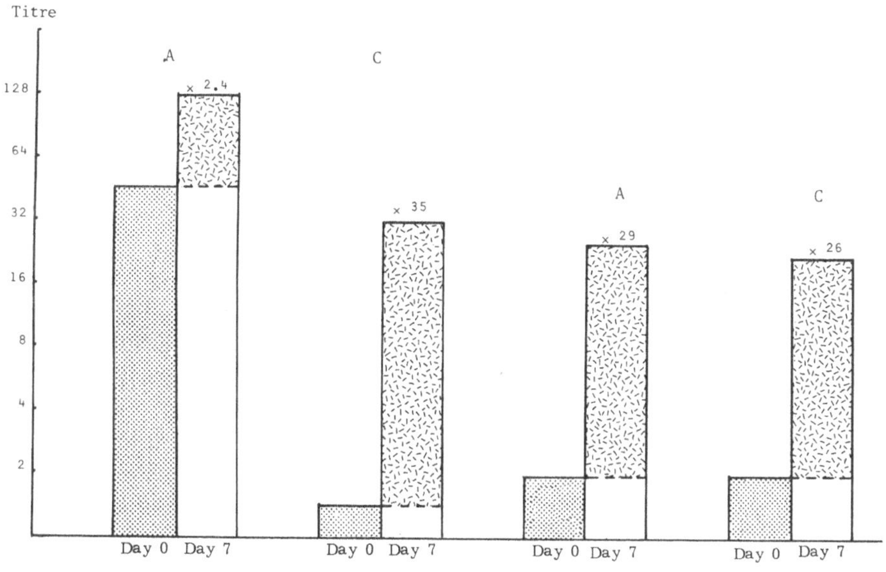

Figure 1 Relation between initial titre and homologous increasing factor 7 days after bivalent vaccination (Dakar; $n = 103$)

prised 103 children aged 9–14 years in Dakar (Professors Diop Mar and Michel Rey) and twenty-three adults in Lyon (Dr Nicolas, Dr Stellman and Miss M. C. Mynard).

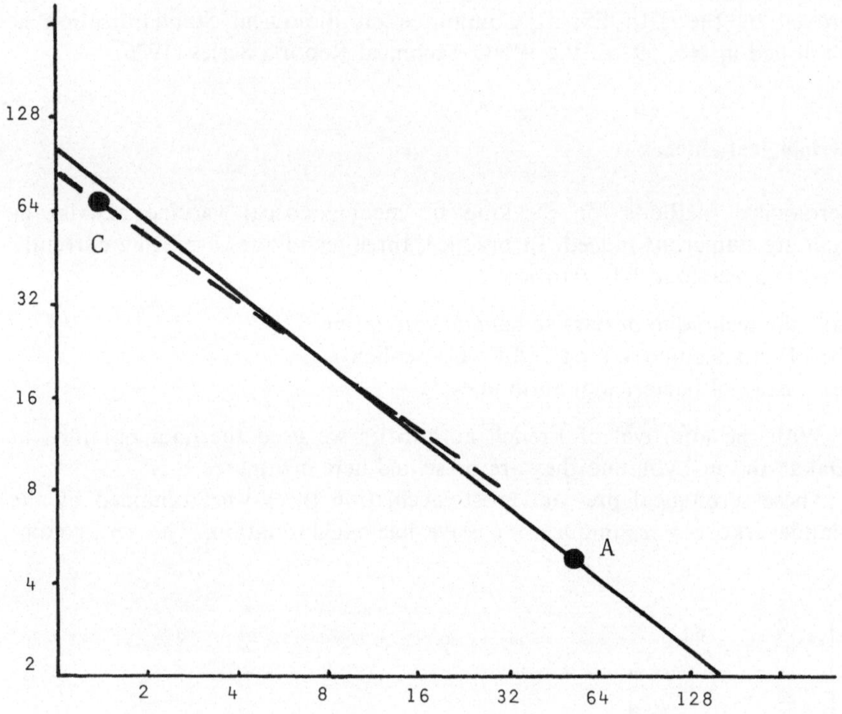

Figure 2 Relation between initial titre and homologous increasing factor 7 days after bivalent vaccination (Dakar; $n = 103$)

The homologous increases of the A and C antibody titres are closely linked to the initial antibody titres, and in order to compare the results obtained in trials carried out in epidemiologically very different countries it is necessary to analyse antibody distribution before vaccination and to account for this factor in all comparisons.

With the help of Miss M. T. Fayet we measured also the pre- and post-vaccination antibody titres by radioimmunological techniques. This was carried out in the same group of adults as above[15] (see Tables 2 and 3; Figures 4 and 5). This work, soon to be published, shows again that the lower the initial antibody level, the better the post-vaccination response. Besides, antibody curves over a period of 1 year show well sustained high titres likely to persist for many years.

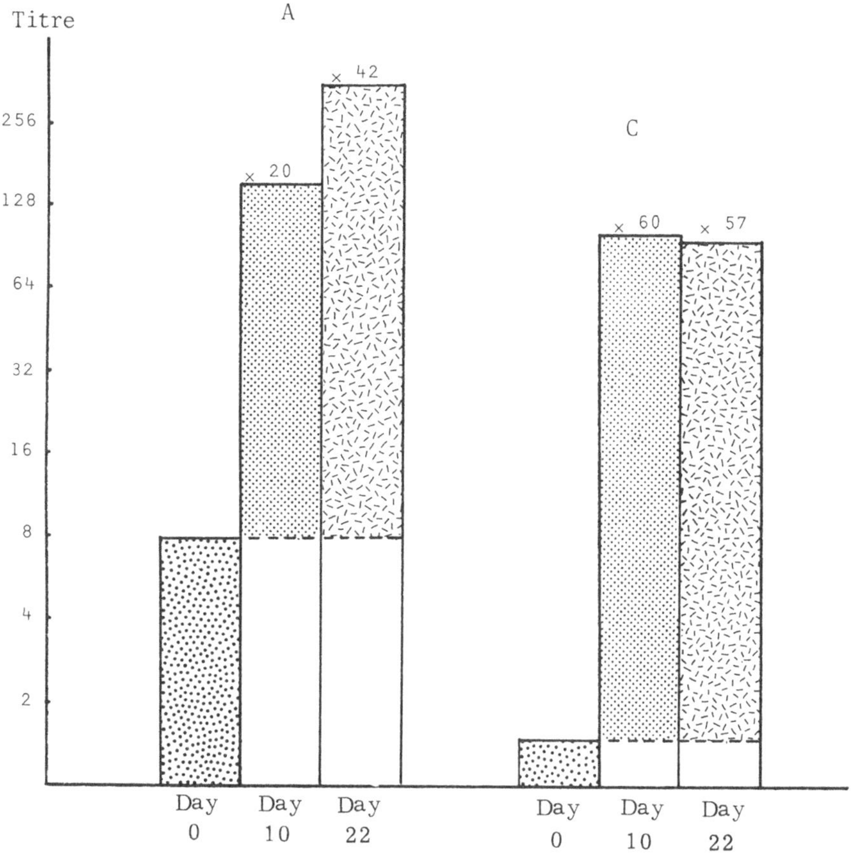

Figure 3 Relation between initial titre and homologous increasing factor 10 and 22 days after bivalent vaccination (Lyon; $n = 23$)

Table 2 Antibody to meningitis type A. (Mean of results of 7 series of samples)

Sample	*Time after vaccination*	*n*	*Mean amount (µg antibody/ml)*
1	0	21	1.68 < 2.14 < 2.72
2	10 Days	25	16.8 < 21.8 < 28.1
3	22 Days	21	27.7 < 35.2 < 44.8
4	4 months	24	27 < 34.1 < 43.4
5	6 months	24	21.3 < 27.4 < 35.3
6	10 months	20	12.4 < 15.5 < 19.4
7	12 months	20	12.1 < 15.7 < 20.4

Table 3 Antibody to meningitis type C

Patient	*Time after vaccination*	*Antibody levels* (μg/ml) ($p = 0.95$)
1	0	$0.54 < 0.79 < 1.15$
2	10 Days	$25.7 < 34.0 < 44.9$
3	22 Days	$29.7 < 41.9 < 59.1$
4	4 months	$34.1 < 46 < 62.1$
5	6 months	$28.8 < 38.9 < 52.5$
6	10 months	$26.3 < 33.1 < 41.7$
7	12 months	$17.4 < 25.4 < 37.1$

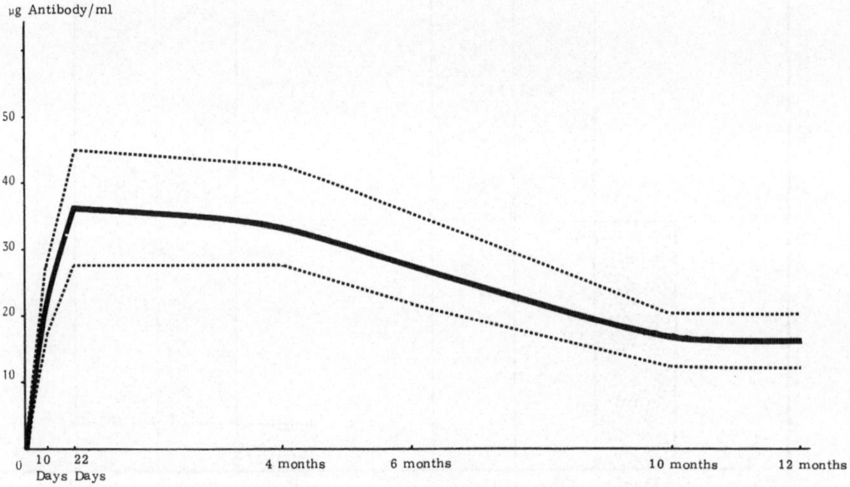

Figure 4 Antibody to meningitis type A in immunized groups

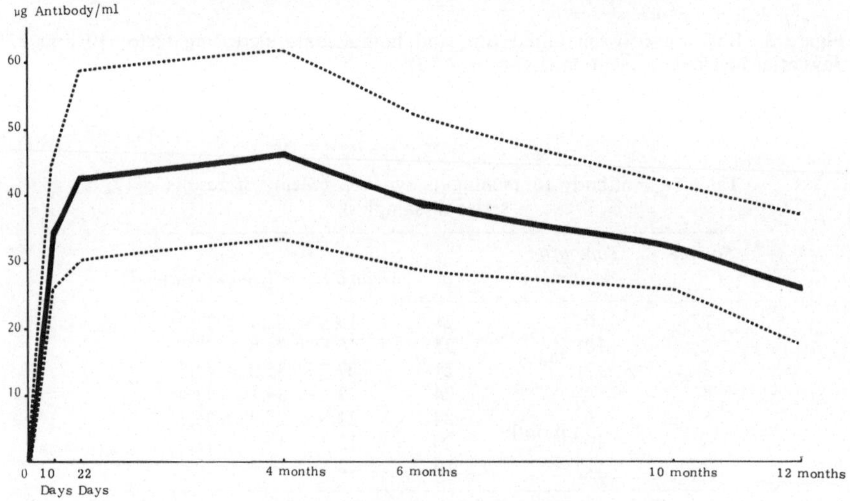

Figure 5 Antibody to meningitis type C in immunized groups

Results of field use of meningococcal polysaccharide vaccines in Brazil in 1974–75

The results of the antimeningococcal vaccination programme in Brazil are an outcome of a number of factors as follows:

1. A new policy for antimeningitis campaign: (a) the principle of striking hard and promptly; (b) the conviction that vaccination of isolated groups is ineffective.
2. A new operational method based on co-ordinated planning.
3. Adequate preparation of vaccination teams, from the technical, as well as psychological, standpoint.
4. A good logistic base.
5. A clear formulation of the aims and exact timing of the entire operation.

As the curve in Figure 6 clearly shows, after mass vaccination of 10 million people over a period of 4 days in April 1975 in Sao Paulo, the incidence of the disease fell dramatically and, as expected, the usual winter rise in the incidence was prevented.

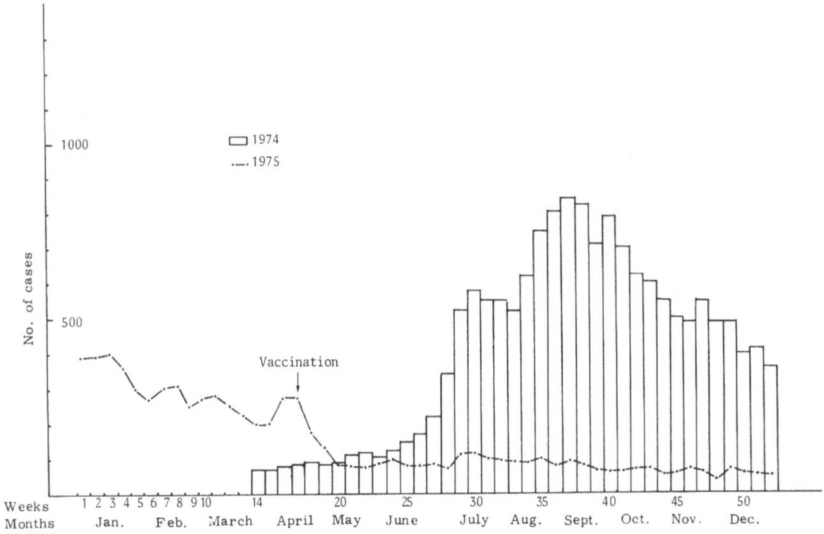

Figure 6 Meningitis cases noted in Sao Paulo during 1974–75 epidemic

The immediate efficacy of the vaccination was clearly demonstrated in certain special population groups. For instance, Figure 7 shows the incidence of the disease in babies aged 0–5 months who were not vaccinated, in comparison with those aged over 1 year who received the vaccine. The effect in the latter group is quite striking.

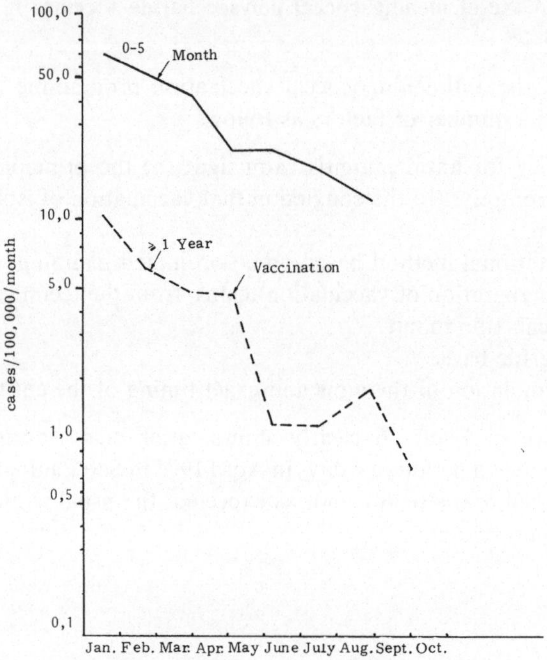

Figure 7 Cases of meningitis in Sao Paulo

Safety of meningococcal polysaccharide A and C vaccines

For many years the vaccines in question were described as satisfactorily safe by all the authors concerned. However, the vaccinated subjects were mainly schoolchildren, adolescents and adults. The occasionally reported pyrexial reactions were attributed to intercurrent infections, e.g. respiratory ('influenzal states'). Nevertheless, in our own experience in Africa (work in Senegal with Professors Diop Mar and Michel Rey) and during the vaccination programme in Brazil a number of severe pyrexial reactions, though of short duration, have been reported. Recently, the problem has been

Table 4 General reactions following meningococcal type A vaccination in 388 Finnish infants aged 3 months–5 years (percentages)

		Hours after vaccination			
		1–24 h	*25–48 h*	*49–72 h*	*72 h*
Irritability		24	6	4	2
Temperature	37.5–38.5 °C	32	12	7	6
	> 38.5 °C	2.1	0.8	1	3
Influenzal State		14	15	19	23

Table 5 Percentages of children reporting various reactions after vaccination with different lots of the Men. A and H. i. b. vaccines (calculated for the whole observation period) compared with the endotoxin content of the vaccines (measured by the *Limulus* assay and the rabbit pyrogenicity test)

	Kymi project: (Men. A lots used)					*Main project*	
	0778	*591*	*590*	*589*	*572*	*Men. A Lot 572*	*H.i.b.*
Local reactions	50	46	44	47	61	75	53
General Reactions							
without flu	27	22	22	24	24	39	26
with flu	0.8	1.9	1.5	2.0	3.1	12	13
No reactions at all	15	26	26	21	13	13	29
Number analysed	602	940	2264	1687	1413	388	365
High fever							
without flu	1.5	1.4	1.1	1.4	2.3	3.9	0.?
(> 38.5°C or > 101.3 °F	(0.5, 3.3)*	(0.9, 2.1)	(0.7, 2.1)	(0.9, 2.0)	(1.8, 2.9)	(1.8, 7.4)	(0.1, 3.0)
with flu	0.3	0.9	0.6	0.8	1.0	2.1	1.0
Number analysed	602	2673	3543	3140	6767	388	365
Limulus assay (μg endotoxin activity per 100 μg of polysaccharide)	6	6	0.6	2	14	14	0.0
Pyrogen test highest amount (ng polysaccharide per kg rabbit) giving a negative response	25	25	25	2.5	2.5	2.5	250

* 99% confidence interval

studied by Finnish authors[16], whose conclusions may be summarized as follows: the following triad of general post-vaccination symptoms may be observed in children under 6 years of age: irritability; pyrexia; malaise. Local reactions at the injection site are common, mild and short-lived.

The main significance of the Finnish study lay in that it established a degree of correlation between these reactions and the vaccine's residual endotoxin content (Table 5). This is why, at present, the manufacturers tend to increase the purity of their product by ultracentrifugation as advocated by Gotschlich and also, and this is the main point, by using polysaccharides precipitated from supernatant culture liquid in preference to whole cultures. This obviously reduces the yield but results in excellent tolerability. In the winter of 1975–76 in the mass vaccination campaign in Finland (1 400 000 subjects) use was made of meningococcal vaccines produced by one American and one French laboratory, whose endotoxin content was reduced more than 100-fold. The incidence of pyrexial reactions was thereby reduced from 1–4% to 0.4%.

As Figure 8 shows, symptoms vary in incidence with the age of the subjects.

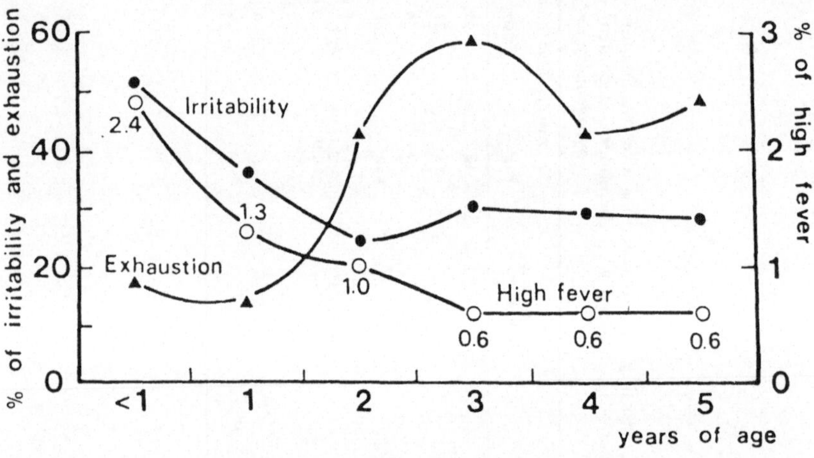

Figure 8 Post–vaccination symptoms as a function of age (Finland trial, 1976)

EFFICACY OF VACCINATION

A good polysaccharide vaccine A and/or C, that is, a vaccine of high molecular weight – over 100 000 dalton (Kd < 0.35 or 0.40 or 0.50 according to French, American or WHO norms), used in adequate doses (30–50 μg) – appears highly effective from the epidemiological standpoint as indicated above serological efficacy can best be shown by radioimmunological assay of antibodies. As Figure 9 shows, the response is positive even in 3-month-old babies, and it increases with age. Generally speaking, *it has been currently estimated that protection is provided by antibody (A or C) concentration of 2 μg/ml of serum.*

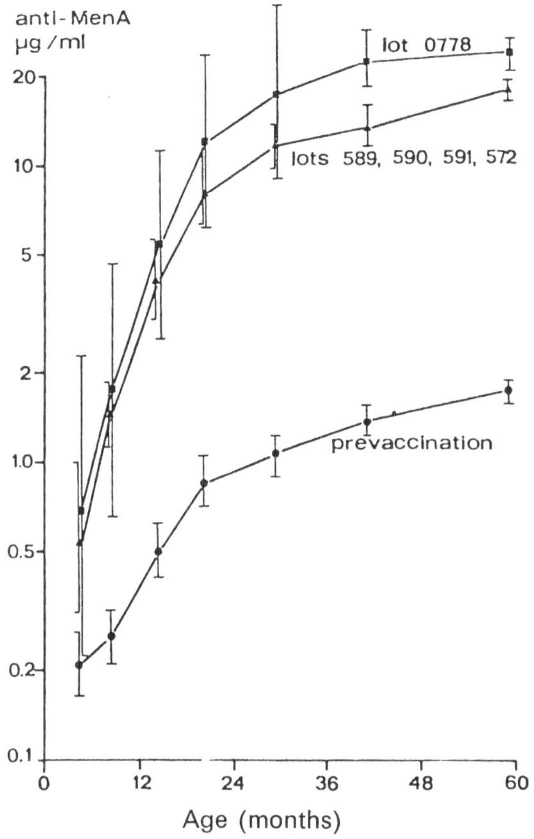

Figure 9 Post-vaccination serological responses as measured by radioimmunoassay[16]

PROSPECTS FOR MENINGOCOCCAL VACCINE B

We know that the first vaccine based on capsular polysaccharides of meningococcus which proved satisfactory in the field belonged to serogroup C. A little later, a serogroup A vaccine became a practical proposition. As regards high molecular weight polysaccharides, however, meningococcus B extracts proved, curiously enough, non-immunogenic and the problem of vaccination against meningitis caused by meningococcus B remains unsolved.

At present, the most promising in this respect seems the studies of Carl E. Frasch[14,17].

Nine serogroups of *Neisseria meningitidis* are distinguished, as follows:

A; B; C; D; X; Y; Z; 29E and W135.

This subdivision is based on distinct immunological properties of *capsular polysaccharides* of each serogroup. In addition, serotypes can be distinguished within each serogroup and these are denoted with Arabic numerals 1; 2; 3; 4; etc. This type specificity depends on the surface protein (STA). In 1967, Roberts[18] noted that antisera against two strains of meningococcus B showed neither opsonin cross-activity nor equivalent bactericidal activity. This suggested the existence of variants within strains belonging to the same serogroup. A year later, Frasch found that meningitis B convalescent sera showed marked differences in their bactericidal activity on various test strains of meningococcus B. In 1972 Frasch[14], using a new microtechnique for bactericidal activity testing was able to distinguish within serogroup B 12 serotypes as follows:

1; 2; 3; 4; 5; 6; 7; 8; 9; 10; 11; 12

On the other hand, in 1970, Gold and Wyle[19] were able to distinguish a number of serotypes within the serogroup C, but only one serotype in serogroup A.

The STA (serotype antigen) of group B is extracted at 100 °C in a slightly alkaline medium and the serotyping is done by precipitation in capillary tubes or, preferably, by the technique of double diffusion in gelose. Extraction may be also effected at +45 °C, in a medium containing lithium chloride and sodium acetate.

An important point is that serogroups B; C; Y and W135 share the same STA.

In common with other authors, Frasch noted that a majority of cases of meningitis due to serogroup B were caused by serotype 2 which is often found in the immediate social environment of the patient. Also, the bactericidal convalescent antibodies are generally active against STA2 rather than against polysaccharide B.

Serotypes 8 and 9 also seem to be associated occasionally with meningococcal infections, or cases of cerebrospinal meningitis, outside epidemics.

The nature of the prospective anti-B vaccine follows thus from the above observations: it should consist of STA2, which is likely to offer protection not only against the pathogenic meningococcus B but also against certain organisms of serogroups C; Y and W135 which share the same antigens.

Frasch prepared two vaccines based on antigens of high lipido-proteino-lipopolysaccharide molecular weight. An essential step was removal of endotoxin (the toxic lipopolysaccharide portion of the antigen). This was achieved by treatment either with Triton X-100 (vaccine 1) or sodium desoxycholate (vaccine 2), by precipitation, centrifugation or gelfiltration. The desoxycholate-treated vaccine contained less residual endotoxin than the Triton-treated one, but it was also less immunogenic when tested on guinea pigs.

We intend to test the two vaccines in the near future, first in adults (tolerability, immunogenicity, dose, etc.) and then in children, who seem capable of synthesizing anti-serotype 2 antibodies at a very young age, provided their blood does not yet contain them or at least does not contain them in high titres.

MENINGOCOCCAL CEREBROSPINAL MENINGITIS: THE CURRENT WORLD SITUATION

Cerebrospinal meningitis is an endemic–epidemic disease of world-wide distribution. In the last decade its relative importance seems to have increased

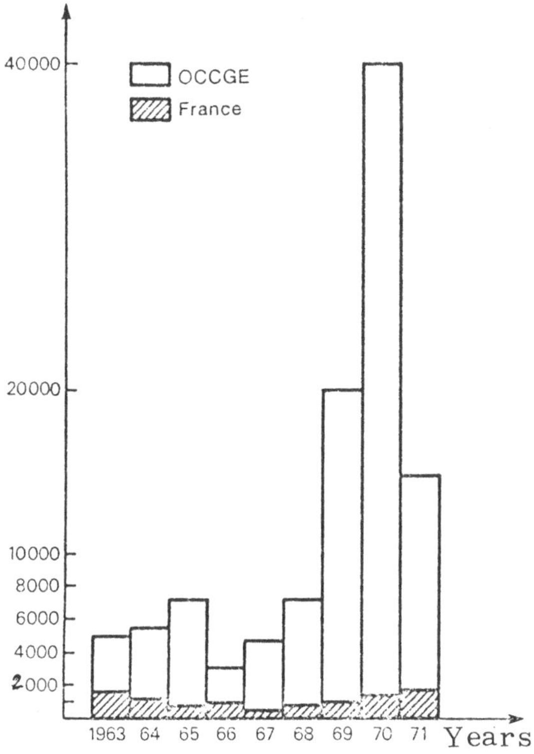

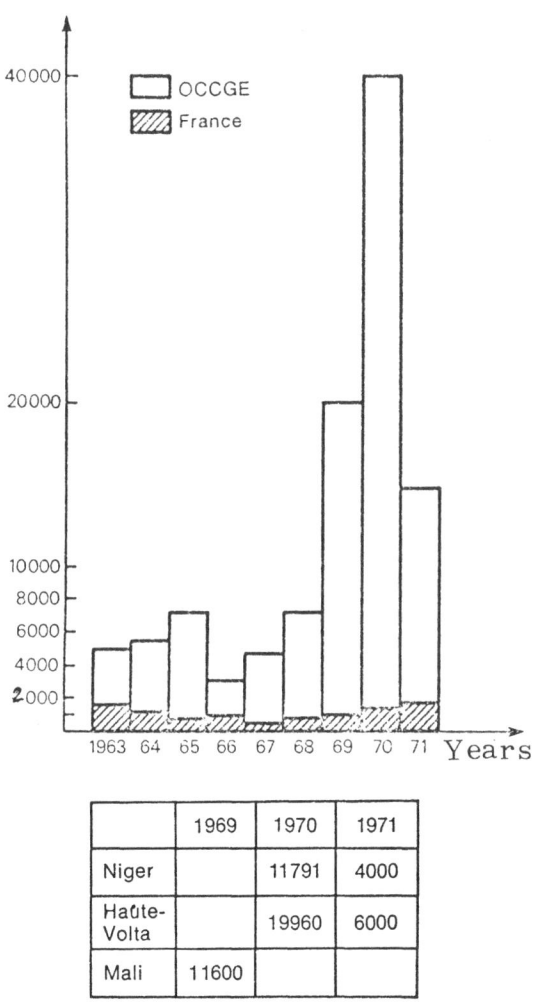

	1969	1970	1971
Niger		11791	4000
Haute-Volta		19960	6000
Mali	11600		

Figure 10 Cerebrospinal meningitis cases in France and OCCGE countries, 1967–71

in many countries. In both distant and recent past great outbreaks of cerebrospinal meningitis had occurred lasting several months to several years, when the numbers of cases were counted in tens of thousands and the numbers of victims in thousands. Very often the disease produced states of panic with political repercussions.

In Africa (Figure 10)

Cases of cerebrospinal meningitis occur everywhere, but the Sahel and the Sudan savannah north of the equator remains particularly notorious in this respect (the classica l'meningitis belt' of Lapeyssonnie). This situation seems largely due to the predominance of meningococcus A in the area. However, meningococcus C is encountered with increasing frequency.

In Europe

In France, in the last two decades, the number of cases of cerebrospinal

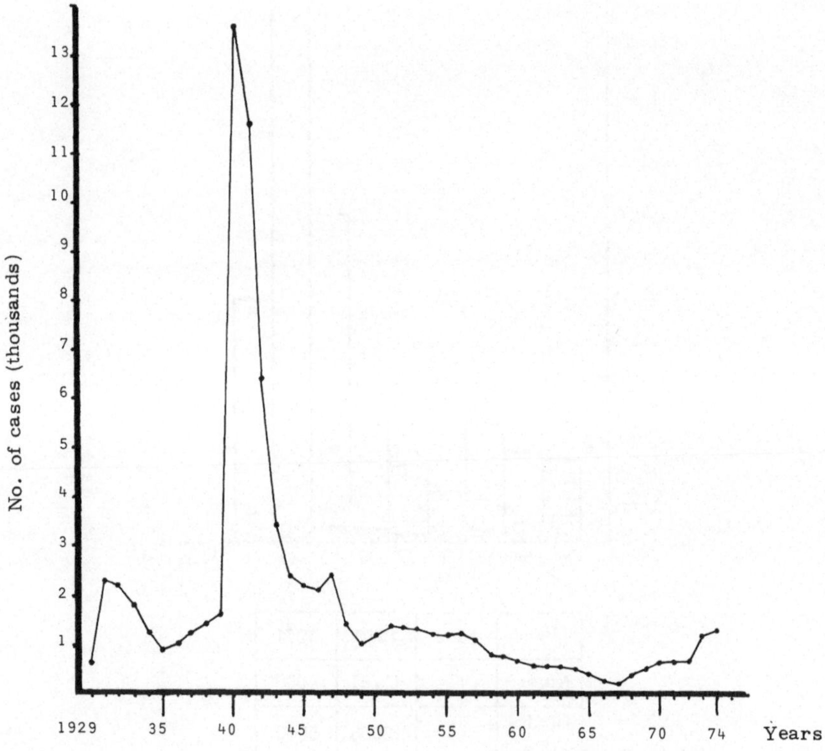

Figure 11 Meningococcal infection, England and Wales, 1929–74: Registrar General's notifications. Cases were notified as follows: 1912–49 cerebrospinal fever; 1950–68, meningococcal infection; 1970 to the present, meningococcal meningitis. Figures for 1968, 1969, and 1974 are estimates

meningitis was 500–1500 yearly. The incidence of the disease is thus low and in the range of 1–3 cases per 100 000 inhabitants per year. The mortality is usually under 10%. What is worrying, however, as regards the future is the diminishing relative incidence of the serogroup B combined with an increasing relative incidence of the epidemiogenic serogroup A.

The situation in England and Wales is similar to that obtaining in France. Figure 11 clearly shows a conspicuous rise of the incidence of the disease at the outbreak and during World War II, culminating in a figure of about 13 000 cases in one year.

In Belgium an outbreak occurred in the period 1969–1973, since when the figures have been falling.

1966 – 41 cases	1971 – 518 cases
1967 – 50 cases	1972 – 519 cases
1968 – 39 cases	1973 – 418 cases
1969 – 131 cases	1974 – 422 cases
1970 – 352 cases	

In Finland the incidence curve (Figure 12) at present shows a downward trend.

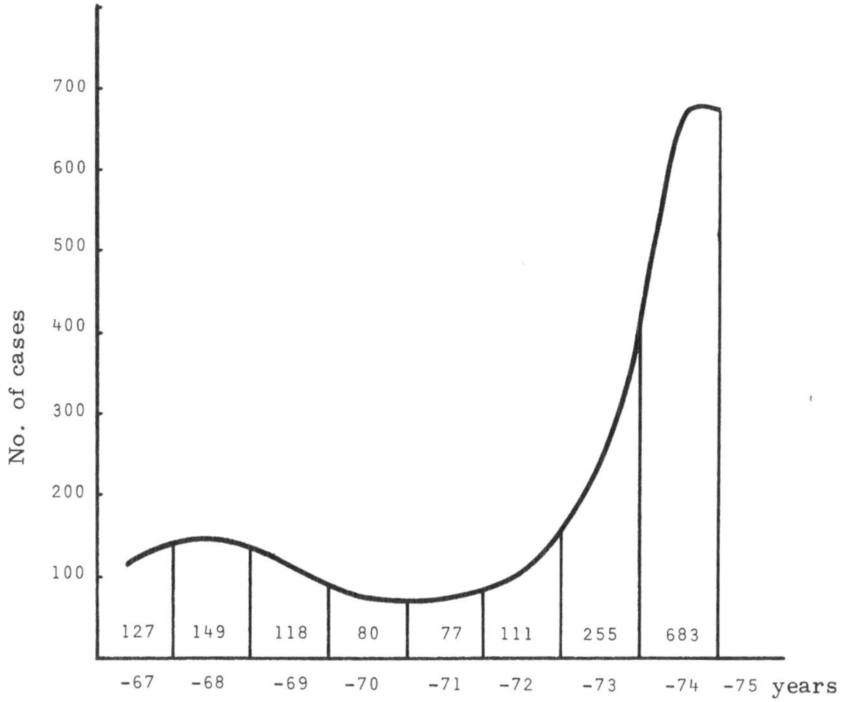

Figure 12 Cases of cerebrospinal meningitis in Finland (1967–74)

In Asia

In Turkey the incidence of cerebrospinal meningitis has been high, with 3178 cases in 1973 and 3923 cases in 1974.

In Iraq, on the other hand, and in Mongolia, meningococcal infection is strongly endemic (in 1975 in Mongolia 1800 cases were recorded, with 217 deaths).

In America

The Brazilian epidemic apart, in 1965–75 outbreaks occurred in Argentine, Paraguay, Peru, Costa Rica and Haiti. The incidence of the disease in the

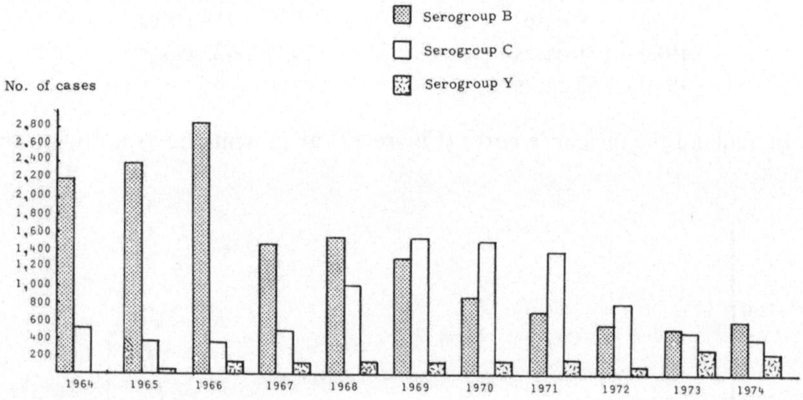

Figure 13 Estimated number of cases of disease caused in civilians by *Neisseria meningitidis* of serogroups B, C, and Y, USA, 1964–74. (Figures are based on isolates studied at the Center for Disease Control and the number of cases reported to state epidemiologists.)

USA is falling (Figure 13), with a preponderance of serogroup B and a relative rise of serogroup Y. Following the example of Brazil, Uruguay has been conducting a mass vaccination campaign.

WHEN SHOULD VACCINATION AGAINST MENINGITIS BE CARRIED OUT?

We now have thus at our disposal an excellent vaccine A and/or C, which has proved both effective and safe.

In recent years a number of countries have employed this new immunoprophylactic weapon without hesitation on a large scale:

1. In the USA: for systematic vaccination of all military personnel on their

admission into the services (Men. C). To all practical purposes the disease has been eradicated as far as the armed forces are concerned.

2. In Brazil: for vaccination of over 80 million people; a measure which put an end to the epidemic raging in this country for many years.
3. In Finland: to control an outbreak of the disease caused by meningococcus A; this was stopped by vaccination of all inhabitants aged 0–18 years (for those from 0–6 years old the dose was reduced to 30 μg).
4. In Uruguay: where 2 million young people have been immunized.
5. In Saudi Arabia: where a decision has been made to vaccinate the Mecca pilgrims every year.

In our opinion, at present it would be difficult to carry out antimeningococcal vaccination in countries where the epidemiological situation is quiescent. By the same token vaccination of the young when the epidemiological indices begin to rise should be easy. In France, for instance, we would have thought that vaccination of the young (0–20 years) is likely to be decided upon when the incidence of the disease increases from the current figure of 1–3 to 3–5 per 100 000 inhabitants.

LABORATORIES CAPABLE OF PRODUCING THE VACCINES

In South Africa:	Richardson Merrell.
In America:	
USA	Merck, Sharp & Dohme, West Point, Pa.
	Merrell National Lab., Swiftwate, Pa.
Brazil	Institute Oswaldo Cruz, Rio de Janeiro.
In Europe:	
Austria	Sandoz
France	Institute Mérieux, Lyon
Holland	Rijks Institute, Bilthoven
Hungary	Institute 'Human', Budapest
Italy	Istituto Sieroterapico, Milan
	Istituto Sclavo, Siena*
Yugoslavia	Immunological Institute, Zagreb

i.e. 11 private or state-owned laboratories.

The list will no doubt increase rapidly.

CONCLUSIONS

Subcutaneous or intradermal vaccination with meningococcal capsular polysaccharides A and C in doses of 30–50 μg provides protection against the corresponding type of endemic–epidemic cerebrospinal meningitis in at least 90% of inoculated subjects. One requirement, however, is a high molecular weight of the polysaccharide, over 100 000 and over 400 000 daltons for A and C respectively (Kd $< 0.30/0.40/0.50$). Children from the age of 3 months show very good immunological response to polysaccharide A, while vaccine C is likely to benefit only children over the age of 2 years. No doubt this problem will be re-examined with a view to reducing the age limit. The vaccines are tolerated very well indeed, and pyrexial reactions of 38.5 °C and over were recorded in less than 1% of cases in young children only.

In the light of experience gained in Egypt the immunity resulting from polysaccharide A vaccination is thought to last 3 or more years and Sudanese experience indicates that the same vaccine can put a stop to a localized outbreak within 5 days.

In 1975 mass vaccination of 80 million Brazilians with vaccine A + C put an end to a most serious epidemic, raging with particular ferocity in Sao Paulo and responsible for thousands of deaths. In this city 10 000 000 people were inoculated over a period of several days, and this operation was made possible by excellent logistic planning and by the use of pedojets. Immediately afterwards the weekly incidence curve for all types of suppurative meningitis returned to its pre-epidemic level.

Recently, many other countries have turned to mass vaccination: A + C in Uruguay, A in Finland for subjects aged 0–18 years.

Limited vaccination programmes have been undertaken in Egypt, Sudan, Saudi Arabia, Upper Volta, Mali and Mongolia.

Whereas serogroup A anti-meningococcal vaccination has been perfected, and is very effective in the fight against major epidemics likely to be caused by this organism, the problem of anti-B vaccination remains to be solved. It is possible that in the near future a type-specific protein antigen, notably serotype B_2, will prove capable of providing protection not only against the pathogenic meningococcus B but also against meningococci of serogroups C; Y and W135.

At present several European and American laboratories are capable of large-scale production of polysaccharide vaccine, in spite of the costly and difficult technology suggested by Gotschlich.

The logistics of mass vaccination of millions of people in a very short period of time presented the Brazilian government with problems which will also have to be faced in other countries embarking on a similar undertaking.

Epidemiological, serological and bacteriological surveillance of cerebrospinal meningitis, such as is already enforced in several advanced countries, is thus advisable also in others, to provide a constant supply of up-to-date data on the types of circulating meningococci, their serogroups and serotypes, as well as on their resistance or otherwise to sulphonamides and antibiotics. This will enable good use to be made of important recent developments in the field of these new and excellent antibacterial vaccines.

References

1. Weichselbaum, A. (1887). Ueber die Aetiologie der akuten Meningitis cerebro-spinalis. *Fortschr. Med.*, **5**, (19), 620
2. Davies, D. J. (1907). Studies in meningococcus infection. *J. Infect. Dis.*, **iv**, (4), 558
3. Sophian, A., Black, J. (1912). Prophylactic vaccination against epidemic meningitis. *J. Amer. Med. Assoc.*, **59**, (7), 527
   Black, J. H. (1914). Prophylactic vaccination against epidemic meningitis. A supplementary note. *J. Amer. Med. Assoc.*, **63**, 2126
4. Chalmers, A. J. and O'Farrell, W. R. (1916). Preliminary remarks upon epidemic cerebrospinal meningitis as seen in the Anglo-Egyptian Sudan. *J. Trop. Med. Hyg.*, 19, (9), 101
5. Riding, D., Corkhill, N. L. (1932). Prophylactic vaccination in epidemic meningococcal meningitis. *J. Hyg.* (*Lond.*), **32**, 258
6. Neujean, G. (1938). Etude sur l'épidémiologie, la prophylaxie et le traitement de la méningite cérébro-spinale épidémique dans le territoire de Kitega. *Ann. Soc. Belge Méd. Trop.*, **18**, 585
7. Blanchard, P. (1914). L'oeuvre sanitaire de la France en Afrique équatoriale. *Rapport officiel du Ministère des Colonies*
8. Saleun, G., Ceccaldi, J. (1936). Etude des méningocoques en Afrique équatoriale française et vaccination antiméningococcique. *Bull. Soc. Path. Exot.*, **29**, 996
9. Cvjetanovic, B. (1971). Immunization in the control of cerebrospinal meningitis. In *Proc. Symposium on Bacterial Vaccines*, pp. 281–90. (Zagreb: Yugoslav Academy of Sciences and Arts)
10. Gotschlich, E. C., Liu, T. Y., Artenstein, M. S. (1969). Human immunity to the meningococcus: preparation and immunochemical properties of the group A, group B, and group C meningococcal polysaccharides. *J. exp. Med.*, **129**, 1349
11. Ayme, G., Donikian, R., Mynard, M. C. and Lagrandeur G. (1974). Production and controls of serogroup A Neisseria Meningitidis polysaccharide vaccine. In *Table Ronde sur l'immunoprophylaxie de la méningite cérébro-spinale*, Le Mas d'Artigny, St. Paul de Vence, France, Octobre 1973, éd. Fondation Mérieux, Lyon; pp. 4
12. Vandekerkove, M., Bideau, J., Nicoli, J., Faucon, R. (1968). Reaction d'hémagglutination indirecte permettant la mise en évidence d'anticorps sériques antiméningococciques. *Ann. Inst. Pasteur*, **115**, (2), 212
13. Gotschlich, E. C., Rey, M., Triau, R., Sparks, K. J. (1972). Quantitative determination of the human immune response to immunization with meningococcal vaccines. *J. Clin. Invest.*, **51**, 89
14. Frasch, C. E. and Chapman, S. S. (1972). Classification of Neisseria meningitidis group B into distinct serotypes. I. Serological typing by a microbactericidal method. *Infect. Immun.*, **5**, (1), 98
    II. Extraction of type-specific antigens for serotyping by precipition technique. *Infect. Immun.*, **5**, (2), 127
15. Fayet, M. T., Triau, R. and Stellmann C. (1976). Mesure radio-immunologique des anticorps antiméningococciques. Soc. Frce Microbe., Réunion sur les Neisseria, Abbaye de St Maximin, 18 Septembre
16. Peltola, H., Makela, Ph., Elo, O., Pettay, O., Renkonen, O. V., Sivonen, A. (1976). Vaccination against meningococcal group A disease in Finland 1974–1975. *Scand. J. Infect. Dis.*, **8**, 169
17. Frasch, C. E., Friedman, G. L. Identification d'un serotype meningococcique associé à la maladie et commun aux méningocoques des groupes B, C, Y et 135 W. *Med. Trop.*, **37**, 155
18. Roberts, R. B. (1967). The interaction in vitro between group B meningogocci and rabbit polymorphonuclear leukocytes. *J. Exp. Med.*, **126**, 795
19. Gold, R., Wyle, F. A. (1970). New Classification of Neisseria meningitidis by means of bactericidal reactions. *Infect. Immun.*, **1**, (5), 479

19

Immunization with *Streptococcus mutans* against dental caries in rhesus monkeys

T. LEHNER, S. J. CHALLACOMBE AND JILL CALDWELL

INTRODUCTION

Well-controlled studies in germ-free rodents have clearly established that dental caries is a bacterial disease[1–3]. A number of bacteria can, in the presence of fermentable sugars, produce sufficient acid to depress the pH to that required for the solution of enamel[4]. *Streptococcus mutans* has been extensively studied, as it may be one of the most prevalent cariogenic organisms in man[5–7]. *Strep. mutans* produces glucosyltransferases (GTF) which are concerned in the synthesis of extracellular polysaccharides; the latter are thought to be responsible for adhesion of the bacterial plaque to enamel[8,9].

Investigation into the prevention of caries by vaccination requires a reproducible model in animals which have teeth, diet, caries and cariogenic organisms similar to those found in man. The rhesus monkey (*Macaca mulatta*) seems to be a suitable choice as it is the best-studied sub-human primate and develops caries in captivity[10,11], or particularly when placed on a high sucrose diet[12–14]. Dental caries has been induced with *Strep. mutans* and a human-type of carbohydrate-rich diet in the related *Macaca irus*[15,16].

A reproducible model for caries in deciduous teeth of rhesus monkeys has been established[17]. The development of caries is comparable to that found in man because caries can be induced by maintaining the animals on a human type of diet, containing about 15% sucrose. This is associated with an overgrowth of naturally occurring *Strep. mutans*. Caries develops in teeth that are morphologically similar to human teeth, and the type of caries resembles that found in deciduous and permanent teeth of children. Cervical and approximal caries develop after about 2 months and fissure caries after about 9 months of starting the carbohydrate-rich diet.

The incidence of smooth surface caries was significantly reduced by subcutaneous or submucous immunization with a heat-killed *Strep. mutans* (serotype c) in Freund's incomplete adjuvant (FIA)[18]. Protection had been correlated predominantly with the rate of development of serum complement-fixing antibodies to the hydroxylapatite fraction of culture supernatant (HACS) of *Strep. mutans*.

In a further series of rhesus monkeys immunized with a monkey-passaged *Strep. mutans* (serotype c), the rate of development and the incidence of smooth surface and fissure caries was significantly reduced[19]. Reduction in caries was again correlated with serum antibodies, suggesting that protection might be mediated by serum via crevicular fluid. The relative roles of crevicular fluid and saliva were tested by developing a differential technique across the plaque and the adjacent two fluid layers[19]. This revealed that the low caries score in the immunized animals was correlated with a low percentage of *Strep. mutans* in crevicular fluid and in the crevicular fluid–plaque zone and with an increased serum antibody titre to *Strep. mutans*. A similar relationship was not found with salivary haemagglutinating antibodies and *Strep. mutans* in saliva and the salivary–plaque zone which probably constitutes the bulk of dental plaque as tested conventionally.

The aims of this paper are to review the development of caries in *Macaca mulatta* over a period of up to 33 months and to correlate this with antibodies assayed by six different tests. Furthermore, the effects of four different vaccine preparations were compared with the appropriate controls, with reference to prevention of caries and antibody formation.

MATERIALS AND METHODS

Animals and injection schedule

Thirty-seven rhesus monkeys were caged, examined and maintained on a human type of diet as described previously[17]. All animals were young with a fully erupted deciduous dentition but without any permanent teeth. Their ages were assessed to range from 11 to 21 months[20]. The animals were distributed into seven groups (Table 1) and there was a comparable sex distribution in each group; animals in groups I, II, III, V, VI and VII were as previously described[17–19]. The immunization schedule is given in Table 1. Subcutaneous (SC) or submucous (SM) injections were administered at weeks 0, 4, 8, 12, 16 and 36 to animals in groups I, II, IV, V, VI (four animals) and VII (three animals). SC injections were given at weeks 0, 4, 8, 16 and 56 to animals in groups III, VI (four animals) and VII (four animals).

Examination of animals, collection of blood and saliva and examination for caries

The animals were examined at approximately monthly intervals and their weight and blood indices were recorded. Blood and pilocarpine-stimulated whole saliva were collected. Clinical and x-ray examinations were performed and dental caries were scored as described previously.[17]

Table 1 Schedule of injections in seven groups of rhesus monkeys

	Group						
	I	*II*	*III*	*IV*	*V*	*VI*	*VII*
Number of monkeys	4	8	3	3	4	8	7
Material injected	HSM*	HSM†	PHSM	HACS	CHT	FIA	Saline
Route of injection	2SC/2SM	4SC/4SM	SC	SC	SM	SC	SC

Injections given at weeks 0, 4, 8, 12, 16, 36 in all except group III, 4 in VI and 3 in VII which had injections at 0, 4, 8, 16, 56 weeks.

HSM* = Human *Strep. mutans*; brisk responders
HSM† = Human *Strep. mutans*; slow responders
PHSM = Passaged human *Strep. mutans*
HACS = Hydroxylapatite fraction of culture supernatant of *Strep. mutans*
FIA = Freund's incomplete adjuvant; all except Group VII had FIA in the first injection and Groups I, II, IV, V and 4 in Group VI had FIA also administered at week 36
SC = Subcutaneous
SM = Submucous

Preparation of vaccines

1. A human *Strep. mutans* (HSM) Ingbritt strain vaccine was prepared as described previously[18]. For SC immunization 1 ml of the heat-killed vaccine containing 10^9 organisms per ml was mixed with an equal volume of FIA and for intra-oral, SM immunization about 2×10^9 organisms per ml were added to 1 ml of the adjuvant.
2. Passaged human *Strep. mutans* (PHSM) was prepared by first implanting the HSM into the mouth of a rhesus monkey, then re-isolating the organisms from which the vaccine was prepared in the same way as for HSM.
3. The HACS vaccine was prepared from *Strep. mutans* (Ingbritt)[18] and 5 mg/ml containing 10 glucosyltransferase units (GTU) were injected into each animal with adjuvant (Table 1).
4. *Strep. CHT* is a non-cariogenic organism[21]. The vaccine was prepared in the same way as for HSM.

Implantation of *Strep. mutans*

No attempt was made to implant *Strep. mutans* into animals in group III, four in group VI and four in group VII. Repeated attempts to implant live HSM permanently to all the remaining animals failed[17,18]. However, naturally occurring Streptomycin-sensitive strains of monkey *Strep. mutans* (MSM serotype c) were isolated from about 4 weeks after they were started on the carbohydrate-rich diet. All animals had a large number of the MSM from week 24 onwards.

Culture of *Strep. mutans* and *sanguis*

A sequential analysis of randomly pooled plaque from the buccal and approximal surfaces of teeth was carried out at monthly intervals[19]. Samples of plaque were cultured under anaerobic conditions on TYC medium[22] and *Strep. mutans* and *sanguis* were identified by their colonial morphology, production of extracellular polysaccharide and carbohydrate fermentation reactions. The results were expressed as a percentage of colony-forming units (CFU) of *Strep. mutans* and *sanguis* in terms of the total number of Streptococci per mg of plaque grown on TYC medium. The role played by crevicular fluid and saliva were tested by sampling crevicular fluid, 'crevicular fluid–plaque' and 'salivary–plaque' zones and saliva[19]. The CFU of *Strep. mutans* and *sanguis* were determined sequentially over 6 months in the animals in group III, four in group VII and three in group VI.

Serum antibody tests

1. Complement fixation (CF) test

This test was performed in microplates, as described previously[23]. The antigens used were HACS and cell walls of HSM and of PHSM[24].

2. Haemagglutination test

Serum and salivary haemagglutinating antibodies (HA) to HACS and cell wall preparations of HSM and PHSM were carried out[23].

3. Precipitation test

A double diffusion in agar test was performed with HACS[25].

Preparation of serum IgG and IgM fractions for antibody assay

IgG fractions were prepared from four monkey sera by DEAE cellulose chromatography[26]. IgM was separated from each serum on a 1.5×30 cm column of Sephadex G-200 with 0.15 M PBS. The eluate was analysed for immunoglobulin content by double diffusion and those fractions containing only IgM were pooled and concentrated. The antibody activity of these fractions was then assayed in the CF and HA tests.

Immunoabsorption technique for the specificity of salivary IgA antibodies

Anti-IgA (Wellcome Reagents) was linked to cyanogen bromide-activated sepharose beads (Pharmacia Ltd.) and used for absorption[27]. Four samples of monkey saliva showing antibody activity against HACS were selected and

0.5 ml absorbed with the immunoabsorbent, at a ratio of 2:1 for 1 h at room temperature. After centrifugation the titre was compared with that of the control which had been absorbed with sepharose beads alone.

Antiglobulin augmentation technique for the specificity of salivary IgA antibodies

Anti-human IgA and IgG (Wellcome Reagents) were added to serially diluted saliva and then SRBC sensitized with HACS were added to each well as described previously[28]. A comparison was made between the agglutination titres of sera treated with anti-IgA and anti-IgG and those to which only saline was added.

Cell-mediated immune responses

In a further series of experiments[29] the incidence of caries and the growth of *Strep. mutans* in rhesus monkeys was studied sequentially and compared with the development of serum fluorescent antibodies (FA)[30], *in vitro* DNA synthesis of antigen-stimulated lymphocytes[31], leucocyte migration inhibition (LMI)[32] and *in vivo* skin delayed hypersensitivity (DH) to *Strep. mutans*[29].

The youngest three of a series of eight monkeys were given a subcutaneous injection of 0.5 ml of formalized *Strep. mutans* (serotype c) vaccine, in an equal volume of FIA, in volumes of 0.5 ml each into the right arm and left leg at the start of the experiment. The same amount of *Strep. mutans* alone was administered subcutaneously 30 weeks later. A sham-immunized group of three monkeys had injections of 0.5 ml of saline into the right arm and left leg. A further control group of two monkeys was used. The two control groups showed a very similar increase in caries and the number of colony-forming units (CFU) of *Strep. mutans*, so that they were combined for all statistical analyses.

Skin DH was assessed 24 weeks after the last immunization by injecting 0.05 ml of each antigen and of saline intradermally into the skin of the shaved abdominal wall. Induration was measured at 6, 24, 48 and 72 h by means of the 'Schnelltester'. The means of four measurements in two dimensions were used and the results are given by deducting the thickness at the site of injection of saline from that of the antigen at each measurement.

Lymphocytes were cultured *in vitro*[31] and stimulated with doubling dilutions of four preparations of *Strep. mutans*: (a) heat-killed; (b) Mickle disintegrated cells; (c) cell wall preparations; and (d) a culture extract containing glucosyltransferase activity[18]. Purified T-lymphocyte cultures were prepared from peripheral blood lymphocytes of eight monkeys by using nylon wool columns[33] and B lymphocytes from the spleens of three monkeys by rosetting with sheep erythrocytes coated with 19S antibody and mouse complement[34].

RESULTS

Examination of animals

All but two monkeys thrived. A steady increase in weight was recorded in all seven groups of animals. Each animal gained about 80 g/month, or 1 kg/year. The blood indices remained within normal range[35] throughout the investigation. The development of caries and antibodies are presented over a period of 21–33 months (Figures 1–8). Only mean indices and titres are given, without standard errors, so as to avoid confusion in comparing seven groups of animals.

Smooth surface (SS) caries (Figure 1)

The development and incidence of SS caries falls broadly into two divisions. In the non-protected animals (groups II, IV, V, VI and VII) caries started from week 4 to 24 and once caries was initiated a rapid increase followed,

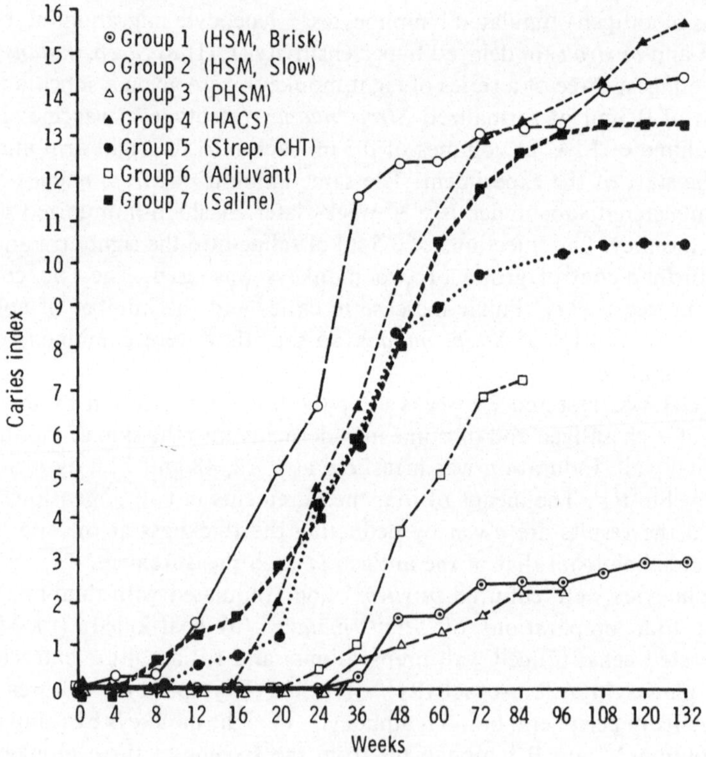

Figure 1 Mean sequential smooth surface caries indices in seven groups of rhesus monkeys

reaching a high caries index plateau of between 10 and 16 cavities per animal, between weeks 48 and 120. Group VI (FIA) should be singled out here as it showed a delay in onset of caries, although the rate of caries increased in parallel with the non-protected groups and a lower plateau of 7.6 (±2.4) cavities per animal was reached. The protected groups I and III could be clearly differentiated in that the onset of caries was delayed to week 36 and then followed a slow increase in caries, reaching a low plateau of 3.0 (±2.4) cavities per animal in group I and 2.3 (±1.4) in group III by week 84 to 120. Significant differences at the 5% to 1% levels were found between the caries indices of the HSM (group I) and PHSM (group III) animals, compared with the saline, HACS and *Strep. CHT* injected groups of animals.

Fissure caries (Figure 2)

These developed later than SS caries. In the PHSM-immunized animals (group III) fissure caries were not detected by week 96 and in group I caries started at week 84. The incidence of fissure caries in group II was similar to

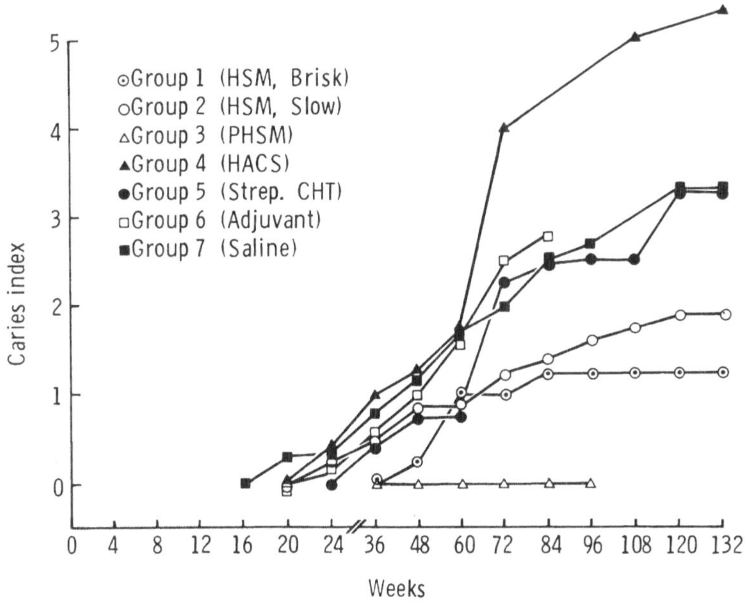

Figure 2 Mean sequential fissure caries indices in seven groups of rhesus monkeys

that of group I because by the time of onset of fissure caries the antibody titres in the two groups were similar. In the remaining groups of animals fissure caries started from week 20 to 36 and a caries index plateau was reached by about week 120 to 132, ranging from about 3 to 5. The 5% level of significance was not reached by the Student's *t* test on comparing group I and the other groups except group IV (HACS). Similar results were obtained with group III, except that in addition to HACS, *Strep. CHT* (group V) also showed a significantly higher caries index.

Serum complement-fixing antibody titre to HACS (Figure 3)

Sequential results in individual animals showed that the SC and SM routes of immunization elicited comparable antibody profiles, except that after week 48 the SC group showed less variation in titre ($\log_2$ 1 to 2) than the SM group

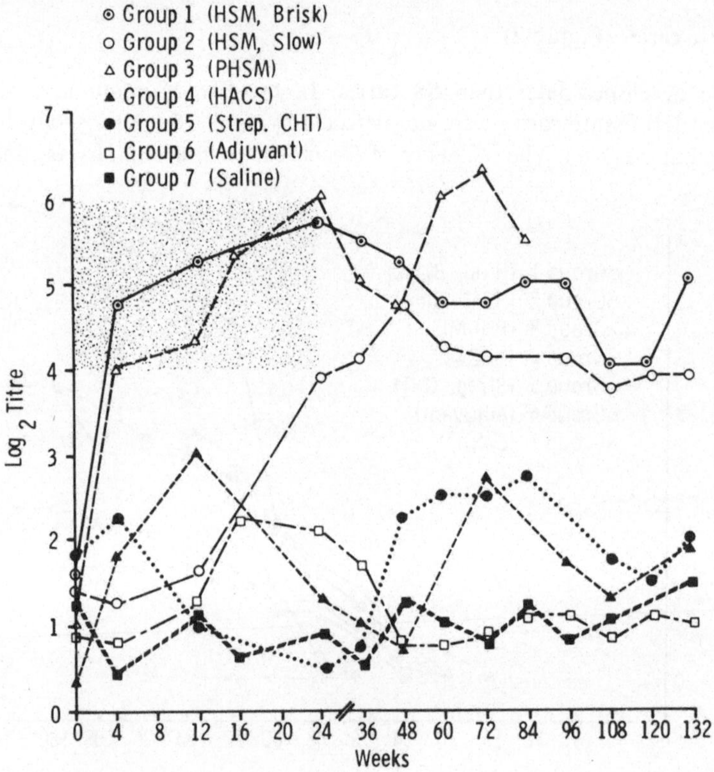

Figure 3 Mean sequential complement-fixing antibody titres to HACS in seven groups of rhesus monkeys

($\log_2$ 1 to 5) among the different animals. The most important feature, however, was the variation in the rate of increase in antibody titre between different animals. Similar differences in the development of the other antibodies led to the division into brisk (group I) and slow (group II) responders. Animals in group I yielded a brisk serum antibody response within 1 month of immunization with HSM, whereas those in group II showed a slow antibody response, taking over 5 months and four to five booster injections to reach an optimum titre. The mean CF antibody titre to HACS was $\log_2$ 4.75 ($\pm$0.5) in group I and $\log_2$ 1.25 ($\pm$0.4) in group II after 4 weeks of immunization. A mean titre of $\log_2$ 4 ($\pm$0.6) was also reached within 4 weeks by group III (Figure 3). The starting antibody titre in all groups was $<\log_2$ 2 and the mean titre in the other four groups remained below $\log_2$ 3.

Serum complement-fixing antibody titre to the cell wall preparations (Figure 4)

This also showed a rapid increase to a titre $\log_2 > 6$ in groups I and III. This level was reached in group II only after 48 weeks but sera from monkeys in group IV reached a titre of $\log_2$ 6 ($\pm$1.1) within 4 weeks. Sera from group V

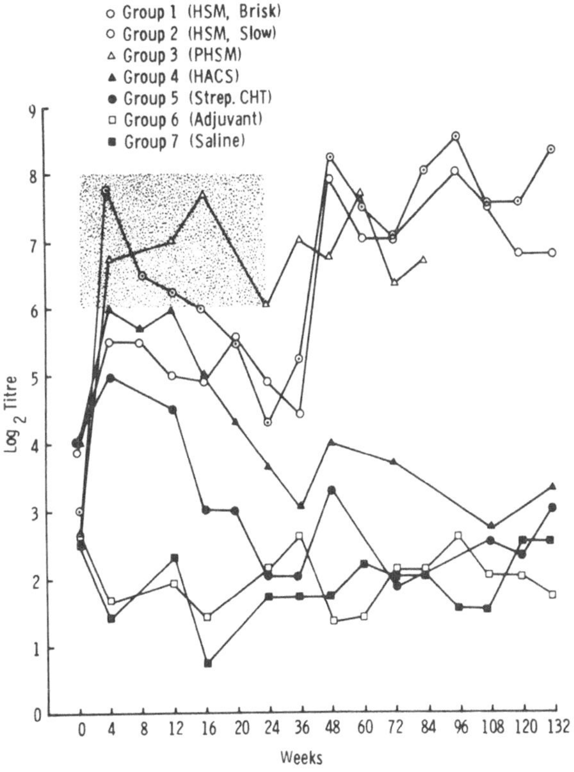

Figure 4 Mean sequential complement-fixing antibody titres to cell walls in seven groups of rhesus monkeys

also showed a high titre (up to $\log_2$ 5) within 4 weeks. The lack of clear differentiation initially between the antibody levels of the seven groups of animals may be accounted for by the high pre-immunization titre of $\log_2$ 2.5–4.0.

Haemagglutinating antibody titre to HACS (Figure 5)

This increased within 4 weeks to a titre $\log_2 > 9$ in groups I, III and IV. In the other groups the titre was $\log_2 < 9$. The pre-immunization HA titres

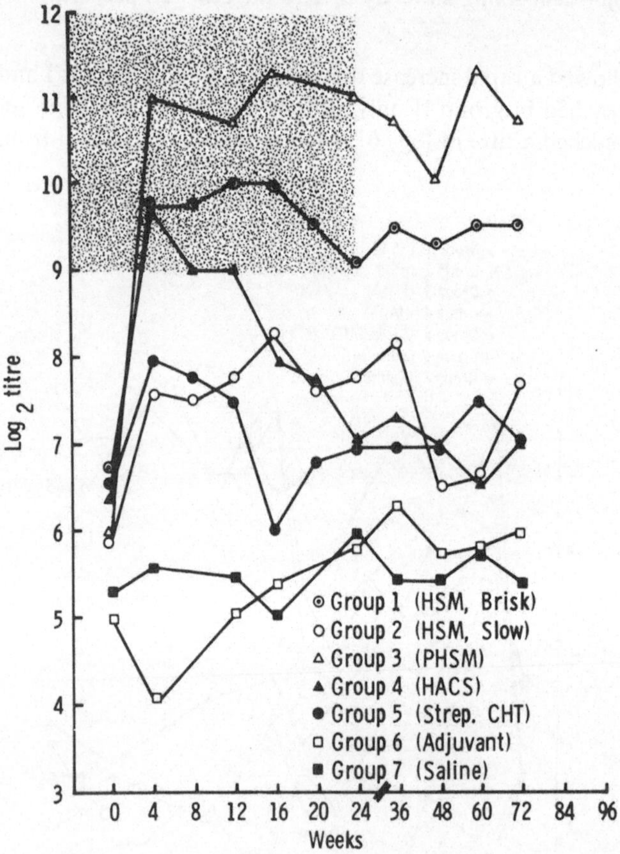

Figure 5 Mean sequential haemagglutinating antibody titres to HACS in seven groups of rhesus monkeys

were somewhat higher, ranging from $\log_2$ 5 to 7. There was no differentiation in the antibody level between the protected animals in groups I and III from the unprotected ones in group IV.

Haemagglutinating antibody titre to the cell wall preparations (Figure 6)

This increased within 4–8 weeks to a titre $\log_2 > 6$ in groups I and III. In the other groups the titre was always below $\log_2$ 5, except in group II sera which reached a mean titre of $\log_2$ 6.1 ($\pm$0.3) by week 20.

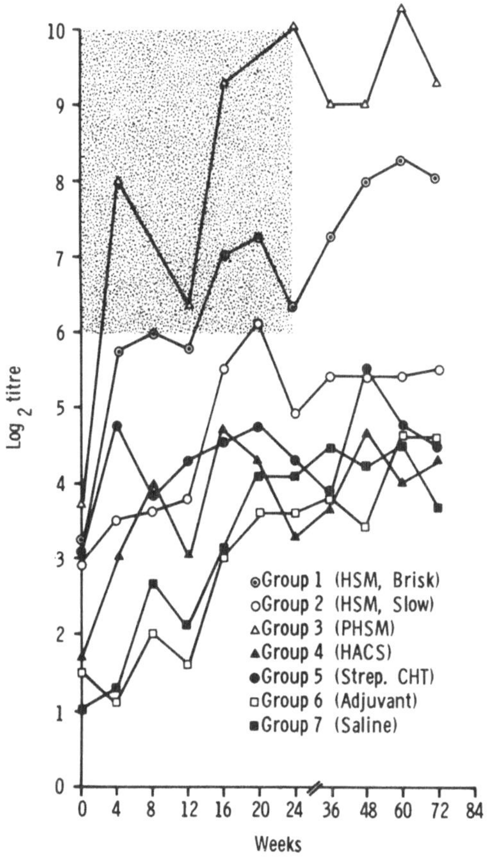

Figure 6 Mean sequential haemagglutinating antibody titres to cell walls in seven groups of rhesus monkeys

Precipitating antibodies to HACS (Figure 7)

All animals in groups I and III yielded precipitating antibodies within 12 weeks of immunization. This was also achieved by groups IV and II after 48 and 60 weeks, respectively. Precipitating antibodies were not found in the pre-immunization sera and they were not found in any sera from groups VI and VII.

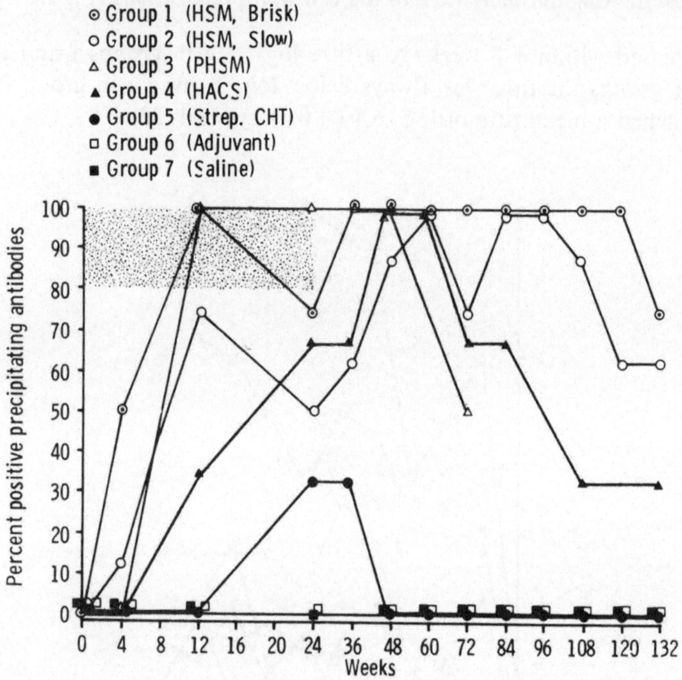

Figure 7 Sequentıal precipitatinganti bodies to HACS in seven groups of rhesus monkeys

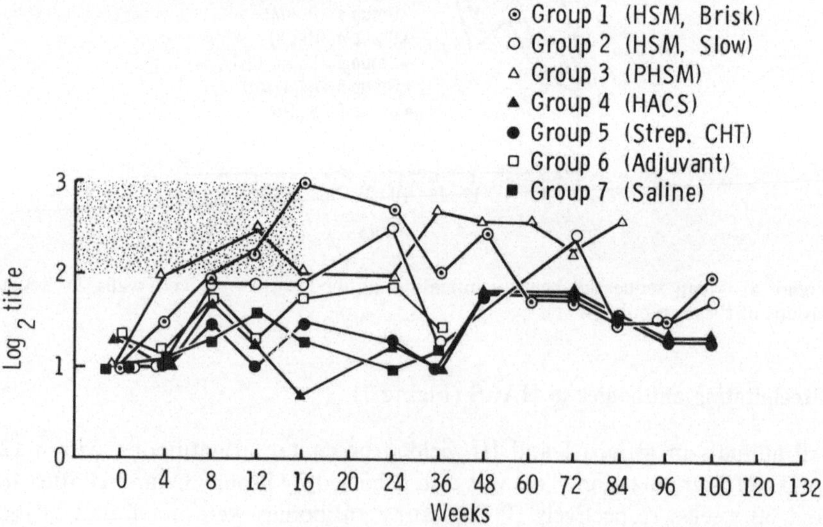

Figure 8 Mean sequential salivary haemagglutinating antibody titres to HACS in seven groups of rhesus monkeys

Salivary haemagglutinating antibody titre to HACS (Figure 8)

This showed a modest increase to a titre $\log_2 > 2$, within 4–8 weeks in groups I and III only. This level was also reached by samples of saliva from group II after 24 weeks. The pre-immunization titres were about $\log_2$ 1 and varied during the 108 weeks in the other groups only by $\log_2$ of 1.

Class of serum antibodies

CF antibodies to HACS were found in the purified IgG with little activity in the purified IgM fraction. In contrast HA to HACS were found predominantly in the IgM with some activity in the IgG fraction (Table 2). The pre-immunization CF and, therefore, predominantly IgG antibody titres to

Table 2 Antibody titre to HACS of sera separated by DEAE cellulose chromatography and gel filtration

	Whole serum	*DEAE chromatography fraction*		*Gel filtration Fraction I*
		I (IgG)	*II (IgA + IgG)*	*(IgM)*
Complement fixing antibodies	7	4	4	0
	6	6	1	0
	5	4	2	1
	5	2	1	0
Haemagglutinating antibodies	7	1	2	4
	11	2	5	3
	7	2	5	5
	9	1	5	3

HACS were 0.25–1.75 and the IgM HA titres were 5–7. Fraction II of the DEAE chromatography showed IgA and some IgG, so that the possibility cannot be excluded that the antibody titres might be due to IgG. However, the HA titres in fraction II were consistently 2–5 times higher than those in fraction I so that some IgA class of antibodies are likely to be present.

Specificity of secretory IgA antibodies

The specificity of salivary IgA class of antibodies was established by the immuno-absorption and augmentation techniques (Table 3). Absorption of saliva with anti-IgA linked to sepharose beads resulted in almost complete absorption of antibodies. The HA assay after addition of anti-IgA or anti-IgG showed augmentation of titre predominantly with anti-IgA.

Table 3 Specificity of salivary IgA antibodies studied by absorption and augmentation techniques

Log_2 titre after absorption with		*Log_2 titre after addition of:*		
Saline	*Insoluble anti-IgA*	*Saline*	*Anti-IgA*	*Anti-IgG*
2	0	2	5	3
2	0	2	6	4
3	1	3	5	3
4	1	4	4	4

Differential quantitative assessment of *Strep. mutans* and *sanguis* in four plaque zones

A significant difference was not found between the mean CFU of *Strep. mutans* in the total plaque of immunized (54 ± 15.0), saline-treated (67 ± 7.7) and adjuvant-treated (46 ± 9.4) animals. Differential sampling of the four zones, however, showed a significantly lower percentage of *Strep. mutans* in the immunized (6 ± 4.5) than in the saline control (38 ± 4.5) groups only in crevicular fluid ($t = 4.035$; $p < 0.02$) and crevicular fluid–plaque zone ($t = 2.77$; $p < 0.05$). The results for the adjuvant group were intermediate between the saline and immunized groups. A significant difference in the corresponding results with *Strep. sanguis* was not found. Indeed, there was about nine times more *Strep. sanguis* in the crevicular fluid of immunized than saline-injected animals. It is also of considerable interest that the crevicular fluid of saline-injected animals yielded about sixty times more CFU of *Strep. mutans* (38) than *Strep. sanguis* (0.6), whereas the corresponding ratio in the immunized animals was about 1:1, or 6 CFU in each group. Preliminary determinations of the percentage of *Strep. mutans* in terms of the total anaerobic bacterial growth on blood agar showed that crevicular fluid of the saline-injected group yielded about twenty-five times more *Strep. mutans* than the immunized group.

Cell-mediated immune responses

Smooth surface (SS) caries was detected in this series from week 18 and by week 54 a mean of 8.4 (±1.2) cavities per animal was found in the control group. This compared with 2.7 (±1.8) SS cavities per animal in the immunized group (Figure 9). Only three fissure caries lesions appeared by 54 weeks in the deciduous teeth of two of thefive control, and in none of the immunized monkeys.

The decrease in the incidence of dental caries is consistent with the previous results, though there were two major differences in the experimental design. A formalin-killed *Strep. mutans* organism isolated from a rhesus monkey was used, unlike the heat-killed human strain of *Strep. mutans* in the previous studies. Furthermore, unlike the six immunizing injections in the first study[18] and five injections in the second study[19], only two injections were used at an interval of 30 weeks. Indeed, it is not certain that the boosting injection was necessary as the IgG antibody titre at that stage was decreased only by one dilution step.

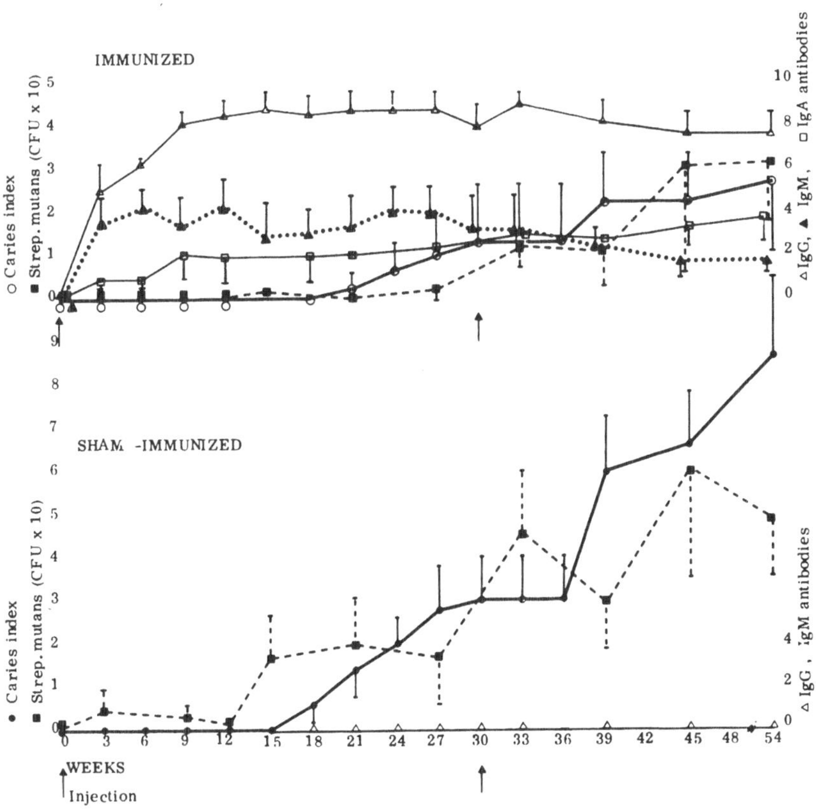

Figure 9 The effects of immunization on colonization by *Strep. mutans*, onset of caries and development of antibodies and caries

In the immunized monkeys there was a significant increase in skin DH from 1.42 (±0.17) at 6 h to 2.23 (±0.23) at 24 h ($p < 0.02$), to 2.54 (±0.45) at 48 h ($p < 0.05$) and a decrease to 2.2 (±0.45) at 72 h. The latter failed to reach the 5% level of significance as compared with the response at 6 h. The pre-immunized and sham-immunized monkeys failed to show a significant increase in induration. The results suggest a skin DH reaction which reaches maximal value at 24–48 h.

Table 4 Lymphocyte transformation induced by antigens and mitogens (Mean(±SE) of stimulation index to *Strep. mutans* antigens

Group	*No.*	*Nil.*	*Whole cells*	*Broken cells*	*Cell walls*	*Culture extract*
Control	5	1035 (±357)	1.2 (±0.2)	0.9 (±0.2)	0.7 (±0.1)	0.8 (±0.2)
Immunized	3	863 (±103)	5.9 (±1.7)	2.2 (±0.8)	2.0 (±0.05)	2.7 (±0.4)
t		0.8918	3.623	1.941	8.785*	5.245
P		ns	<0.02	>0.05	<0.01	<0.001

* Only five monkeys tested
ns = not significant

Lymphocytes from pre-immunized and sham-immunized monkeys failed to repond to any of the *Strep. mutans* preparations, so that these were combined into one control group. Significant differences between controls and immunized monkeys were found with the culture extract ($p < 0.001$), cell walls ($p < 0.01$) and whole cells ($p < 0.02$) of *Strep. mutans* respectively, though only the whole cells yielded moderate SI. The cellular responses were limited to T-lymphocytes, for 96% to 98% purified T-cells yielded significant stimulation of lymphocytes, whereas 94% enriched B-lymphocytes failed to respond.

Sequential analysis of the CFU of *Strep. mutans*[36] revealed consistently larger numbers of *Strep. mutans* in the controls than in the immunized animals (Figure 9). The results suggested that *Strep. mutans* was quantitatively related to the number of carious lesions in the control as well as the immunized groups and that both the caries index and the number of *Strep. mutans* were decreased by immunization.

DISCUSSION

Sequential analysis of the development of caries and antibodies over a period of 21–33 months has revealed that significant reduction in SS caries resulted from immunization with PHSM (group III) and with HSM in the brisk antibody responders (group I). Reduction in SS caries was not elicited in the slow responders to HSM (group II), in those immunized with HACS (group IV), or with the non-cariogenic *Strep. CHT* (group V) as compared with the sham-immunized group VII. A delay in onset of SS caries, however, was recorded in the adjuvant-injected animals (group VI). Immunization with PHSM was most effective as all animals yielded a brisk antibody response, unlike those immunized with HSM, in which only a third responded promptly. It is not possible to be certain if these differences in immune responsiveness were due to passaging *Strep. mutans* through a rhesus monkey, thereby increasing its immunogenicity, or due to strain differences between the animals. It must be assumed, however, that these animals are genetically heterogeneous.

Protection in groups I and III was correlated with the rate of development of antibodies during the critical period of initiation of caries in the first 24 weeks (boxed area in Figures 1–6). Although all serum and salivary antibodies showed some differentiation between the protected and non-protected groups, the best differential titre resulted from serum CF antibodies to HACS (Figure 3; Table 5). It should be emphasized that, of the numerous antibodies, with different specificities and classes, only a limited number may be functionally relevant. The search for specific protective antibodies is always difficult and there is not enough information to be confident about any of these antibody markers.

Table 5 The effect of four vaccine preparations on the development of caries and on six types of antibody assays

	Immunization with:				
	HSM		*PHSM*	*Strep. CHT*	
Functions	*BR (I)*	*SR (II)*	*(III)*	*(IV)*	*(V)*
Reduction in smooth surface caries	Yes	No	Yes	No	No
Reduction in fissure caries	Yes	Yes	Yes	No	No
Reduction in *Strep. mutans*	nd	nd	Yes	nd	nd
CF antibodies to HACS	>4	*	>4	⩽3	<3
CF antibodies to CW	>6	*	>6	⩽6	<6
HA antibodies to HACS	>9	<9	>9	>9	<9
HA antibodies to CW	>6	⩽6	>6	<4	<5
Precipitating antibodies to HACS	++++	++	++++	*	±
Salivary HA antibodies to HACS	>2	*	>2	<2	<2

* Titres, as in group I, were reached only after 24–48 weeks
nd = not done
CF = complement fixing
CW = cell wall
HA = haemagglutinating
Other abbreviations as in Table 1.

CF antibodies were shown on DEAE cellulose chromatography to belong predominantly to the IgG class, and virtually no CF antibodies were found in the IgM fraction prepared by G-200 gel filtration. In general, IgG antibodies to HACS (CF and precipitating) and to a lesser extent to cell walls, were better correlated with caries protection than the corresponding IgM class of antibodies. All animals showed a high pre-immunization IgM class of antibody titre both to HACS and cell walls so that a previous encounter with these or cross-reacting antigens must have occurred. Antibodies of the IgA class are also likely to be present because high titres of haemagglutinating antibodies were found in fraction II (Table 2) and an immunofluorescent method, using specific anti-IgA conjugate, confirmed serum IgA antibodies to *Strep. mutans*[37].

Immunization with HACS (group IV) failed to reduce the incidence of caries. Indeed, the highest caries indices were scored in this group. CF antibody titre to HACS, however, was low; but high titres of CF antibodies to cell walls and HA to HACS were found, as were precipitating antibodies, though rather late (Figures 1–6. Although HACS contains glucosyltransferase (GTF) activity, this does not necessarily imply that antibodies to GTF play no part in caries protection, for HACS contain up to twenty protein bands as demonstrated on polyacrylamide disc electrophoresis[38]. Immunization may have been directed towards some of the more immunogenic components of HACS than GTF and the resulting antibodies may not have been protective. The low CF antibody titres to HACS resulting from immunization with HACS suggest that, whilst HACS is antigenic, it shows poor immunogenicity. Assay of these sera using ^{14}C sucrose, however, revealed antibodies which would inhibit GTF activity[38], although a correlation between these antibodies and caries protection could not be established. The lack of effective immunization by HACS can probably be ascribed to a failure to stimulate the IgG class of protective antibodies. In addition, HACS-induced antibodies showed poor cross-reactivity with the naturally occurring MSM which was consistently isolated from dental plaque of rhesus monkeys on the human carbohydrate-rich diet.

SS caries showed parallel development in four of the five non-protected groups. Once caries started by week 20 a rapid rate of increase followed, resulting in twelve of thirteen cavities per animal by week 84. The consistency and reproducibility of caries in the deciduous dentition of rhesus monkeys was striking in view of their genetic heterogeneity. The type of caries was also similar in that about one-third of the teeth at risk had cervical caries and about one-eighth had approximal caries. Administration of adjuvant alone caused a delay in onset of SS but not fissure caries to week 24, although the rate of increase in caries thereafter was similar to the other four non-protected groups. This non-specific delay in onset of caries cannot be adequately explained, as the serum antibodies showed only a modest increase which was certainly less than the titres recorded in the protected groups. It is of interest that a significant reduction in the prevalence of caries has been reported in infants immunized with an anti-tubercle vaccine, in comparison with non-immunized controls[39]. However, in groups I and III not only was there a delay in onset of caries but also a striking reduction in caries which was maintained up to the time of shedding of the deciduous teeth.

The relationship between fissure caries, immunization and antibodies was similar to that described for SS caries, except that reduction in fissure caries reached significant levels only after 2 years. However, no fissure caries was detected in the PHSM-immunized animals by 96 weeks. A delay in onset of fissure caries in the adjuvant group was not detected. There was little difference in the prevalence of caries by 60 weeks between the brisk and slow responders immunized with HSM (groups I and II).

The differential salivary haemagglutinating antibody titres between protected and non-protected animals were poor, presumably because the titres were rather low. The relative effects of serum and salivary antibodies on the development of caries have been tested by their influence on the number of *Strep. mutans*. A differential sampling technique of plaque and the adjacent crevicular fluid and saliva revealed that the very low caries score in the immunized animals was correlated with a low percentage of *Strep. mutans* in crevicular fluid and the crevicular fluid–plaque zone and with an increased serum antibody titre to *Strep. mutans*. A similar relationship was not found with salivary haemagglutinating antibodies and *Strep. mutans* in saliva and the salivary–plaque zone, which probably constitutes the bulk of dental plaque as tested conventionally. A significant reduction in *Strep. mutans* in plaque of immunized animals was not found by others[40,41], with the exception of one out of seven groups of animals in one series[42]. It is assumed that the immune responses in crevicular fluid are mediated by serum antibodies and probably leucocytes. This will, however, have to be tested directly on crevicular fluid. The bacteriological results suggest that *Strep. mutans* colonization occurs in the immunized and control animals at about the same time (weeks 20 and 15) and precedes the onset of caries by 38 and 13 weeks, respectively. Immunization induces a significant increase in serum CF antibodies which does not seem to prevent colonization but reduces significantly the number of *Strep. mutans* in crevicular fluid. This may be responsible for the delay in onset of caries, a mean difference of 30 weeks between the immunized and control animals, and for the significantly reduced caries index.

The finding of significant skin DH as well as antibodies in immunized monkeys raised the question of whether the DH might not be a measure of T-cell helper function[43]. In order to enable analysis of linear regression to be carried out with some confidence, three additional monkeys previously immunized with *Strep. mutans* (group c) were included. A significant positive correlation ($r = 0.857$, $p < 0.001$) was found between the 48-h skin induration and the IgG fluorescent antibody titre. This is consistent with a T-cell helper function in antibody formation. As with the skin DH reaction (Figure 3), a significant positive correlation was found between the proliferative response of lymphocytes and the IgG antibodies to *Strep. mutans* ($r = 0.884$, $p < 0.001$). These results support the possibility of T-cell helper function in antibody formation, as the lymphocytes responding to *Strep. mutans* belong to the T-cell series. IgM was neither correlated with the skin DH reaction ($r = 0.0826$, $p > 0.1$) nor with the lymphoproliferative response ($r = 0.411$, $p > 0.1$). The protective mechanism against dental caries may then be dependent on the helper function of T-lymphocytes in generating IgG antibodies, as has been found in other systems[44].

Caries in the rhesus monkey seems to differ from the other animal models in that a naturally occurring *Strep. mutans* (serotype c) develops in the animals which are placed on a human type of carbohydrate-rich diet. This may be an advantage, for the development of caries mimics that found in man, and artificial implantation of organisms not normally found in the animal, or resorting to gnotobiotic conditions, are not required. On the other hand the naturally occurring MSM might differ antigenically from the immunizing organism, even if the two are of the same serotype. This might equally apply to man if a vaccine were to be used. However, serum antibodies to HSM and PHSM were absorbed both by the homologous organisms and the heterologous MSM. This was found with antibodies both of the IgG and IgM classes[37] so that the human and monkey strains of *Strep. mutans* share common antigens. In contrast, immunization with HACS, prepared from the HSM, induced poor IgG antibodies to HACS, no significant cross-reactivity with MSM and no reduction in the incidence of caries.

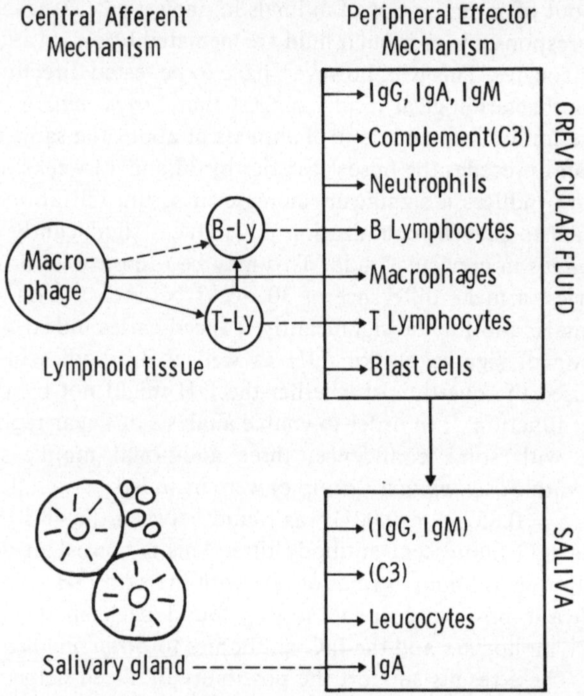

Figure 10 Cellular and humoral factors in the immunological control of caries

An attempt will be made to outline the cellular and humoral factors probably involved in the immunological control of caries (Figure 10). A central afferent mechanism is required for antigen processing, probably by macrophages, and then passing the antigens to T- or B-lymphocytes. The B-cell will proliferate to plasma cells and secrete antibodies. As IgG antibodies are T-cell-dependent and they seem to be playing an important part in caries immunity, T-cell helper function might be the limiting factor in B-cell antibody formation[44]. Both serum antibodies and sensitized lymphocytes to *Strep. mutans* have been detected in peripheral blood of man[45] and monkeys[29] so that presumably the central lymphoid tissues and the regional lymph nodes are involved.

The peripheral effector mechanism involves crevicular fluid and saliva. Plaque development on the surface of enamel might be influenced by crevicular fluid and saliva so that the tooth surface can be divided into: (a) crevicular domain, referring to the cervical and approximal sites which are exposed to crevicular fluid; and (b) salivary domain, referring to the facial, lingual and occlusal surfaces of teeth which are exposed to saliva (Figure 11). Plaque usually builds up from the gingival margin towards the occlusal surface[46,47] so that the immune components in the crevicular fluid domain may influence the type of plaque deposited. The mechanism of action of crevicular fluid is not known and is presently undergoing intensive investigation. It is evident that normal crevicular fluid contains C3, IgG, IgM, IgA and presumably antibodies, that about 90% of the leucocytes are viable[48], and that both polymorphonuclear leucocytes and monocytes contain phagocytosed bacteria. Furthermore, B-lymphocytes, some T-lymphocytes and a few blast cells are present in crevicular fluid[49], suggesting that not only antibodies but also cell-mediated immunity might reach the site where caries activity is initiated. Successful immunity to caries might be dependent on the rate of

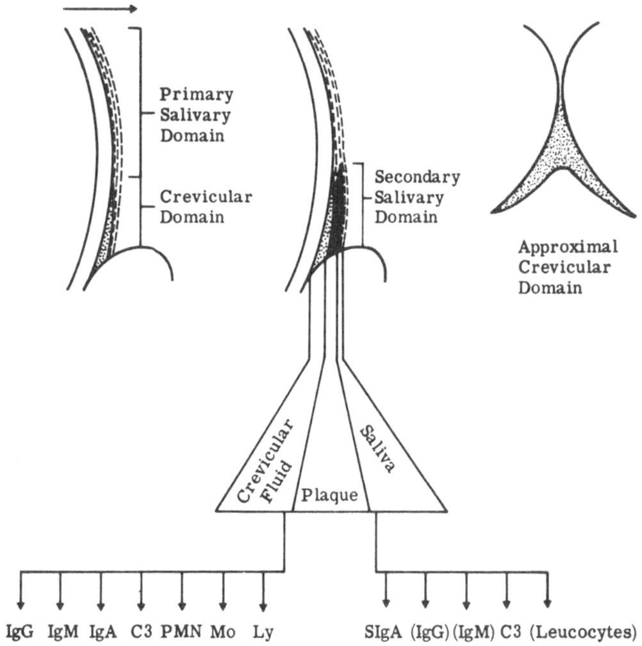

Figure 11 Three-dimensional development of plaque in relation to the crevicular and salivary domains

development of an optimum titre of antibodies, on its immunoglobulin class, antigen specificity and affinity. If any of these requirements are not fulfilled the immune mechanism may fail to function adequately, resulting in the development of caries. Antibodies may be involved in opsonizing activity of bacteria which are then phagocytosed and killed by the polymorphs and macrophages.

The salivary immune system might presumably act by secretory IgA preventing bacterial adherence to the enamel surface[50,51]. There is about 14 μg/ml of IgG, 1 μg/ml of IgM[52] and 0.5 μg/ml of C3 which is only found in 40% of whole salivas[27], so that it is doubtful if these play an active part in the salivary immune mechanism. Although a large number of leucocytes are found in whole saliva, their functional activities have not been determined after they have passed into saliva via crevicular fluid[53].

The relative merits and importance of the crevicular and salivary immune mechanisms have not been elucidated and it is likely that both may play a part in their respective domains. Nevertheless, the presence of actively phagocytic cells, IgG, complement, T- and B-lymphocytes in crevicular fluid ensures that the most powerful immune protective components are available at the site of caries initiation. The leucocytes can be replaced in about 25 min at rest, or in about 5 min on mastication[48]. The distinction between crevicular fluid and saliva is by no means clear, for most if not all crevicular fluid components enter the salivary pool where they undergo considerable dilution.

References

1. Fitzgerald, R. L. and Keyes, P. H. (1960). Demonstration of the etiological role of streptococci in experimental caries in the hamster. *J. Am. Dent. Ass.*, **61**, 9
2. Krasse, B. (1966). Human streptococci and experimental caries in hamsters. *Archs Oral Biol.*, **11**, 429
3. Gibbons, R. J., Berman, K. S., Knoettner, P. and Kapsimalis, B. (1966). Dental caries and alveolar bone loss in gnotobiotic rats infected with capsule-forming streptococci from human carious lesions. *Archs Oral Biol.*, **11**, 549
4. Krasse, B. and Carlsson, J. (1970). Various types of streptococci and experimental caries in hamsters. *Archs Oral Biol.*, **15**, 25
5. Krasse, B., Jordan, H. V., Edwardsson, S., Svensson, I. and Trell, L. (1968). The occurrence of certain 'caries-inducing' streptococci in human dental plaque materials. *Archs Oral Biol.*, **13**, 911
6. Jordan, H. V., Englander, H. R. and Lim, S. (1969). Potentially cariogenic streptococci in selected population groups in the western hemisphere. *J. Am. Dent. Ass.*, **28**, 1331
7. Littleton, N. S., Kakehashi, S. and Fitzgerald, R. J. (1970). Recovery of specific 'caries-inducing' streptococci from lesions in the teeth of children. *Archs Oral Biol.*, **15**, 461
8. Guggenheim, B. and Schroeder, H. E. (1967). Biochemical and morphological aspects of extracellular polysaccharides produced by cariogenic streptococci. *Helv. Odont. Acta*, **11**, 131
9. Gibbons, R. J. (1968). Formation and significance of bacterial polysaccharides in caries aetiology. *Caries Res.*, **2**, 164
10. Schultz, A. H. (1935). Eruption and decay of permanent teeth in primates. *Am. J. Phys. Anthropol*, **19**, 489
11. Anderson, B. G. and Arnim, S. E. (1937). The incidence of dental caries in seventy-six monkeys. *Yale J. Biol. Med.*, **9**, 443

12. Shaw, J. H., Elvehjem, C. A. and Phillips, P. H. (1945). A survey of the incidence of dental caries in the rhesus monkey. *J. Dent. Res.*, **24**, 129
13. Shaw, J. H. and Sognnaes, R. F. (1955). Developmental factors in experimental animal caries. In R. F. Sognnaes (ed.). *Advances in Experimental Caries Research*, pp. 82–106 (Washington, DC: Amer. Ass. Adv. Sci.)
14. Rinehart, J. F. and Greenberg, L. D. (1956). Vitamin B6 deficiency in the rhesus monkey with particular reference to the occurrence of atherosclerosis, dental caries and hepatic cirrhosis. *Amer. J. Clin. Nutr.*, **4**, 318
15. Bowen, W. H. (1965). A bacteriological study of experimental dental caries in monkeys. *Int. Dent. J.*, **15**, 12
16. Cohen, B. and Bowen, W. H. (1966). Dental caries in experimental monkeys. *Brit. Dent. J.*, **121**, 269
17. Lehner, T., Challacombe, S. J. and Caldwell, J. (1975). An experimental model for immunological studies of dental caries in the rhesus monkey. *Archs Oral Biol.*, **20**, 299
18. Lehner, T., Challacombe, S. J. and Caldwell, J. (1975). An immunological investigation into the prevention of caries in deciduous teeth of rhesus monkeys. *Archs Oral Biol.*, **20**, 305
19. Lehner, T., Challacombe, S. J. and Caldwell, J. (1975). Immunological and bacteriological basis for vaccination against dental caries in rhesus monkeys. *Nature*, **254**, 517
20. Hume, V. O. (1960). Estimation of monkey age by dental formula. *Ann. N. Y. Acad Sci.*, **85**, 795
21. Zinner, D. D., Jablon, J. M., Aron, A. P. and Saslaw, M. S. (1965). Experimental caries induced in animals by streptococci of human origin. *Proc. Soc. Exp. Biol. Med.*, **118**, 766
22. Stoppelaar, J. D. de, van Houte, J. and de Moor, C. E. (1967). The presence of dextran-forming bacteria resembling *Streptococcus bovis* and *Streptococcus sanguis* in human dental plaque. *Archs Oral Biol.*, **12**, 1199
23. Challacombe, S. J., Guggenheim, B. and Lehner, T. (1973). Antibodies to an extract of *Streptococcus mutans*, containing glucosyltransferase activity, related to dental caries in man. *Archs Oral Biol.*, **18**, 657
24. Challacombe, S. J. (1974). Serum complement-fixing antibodies in human dental caries. *Caries Res.*, **8**, 84
25. Ouchterlony, O. (1964). Gel diffusion techniques. In J. F. Ackroyd (ed.). *Immunological Methods*, (Oxford: Blackwell Scientific Publications)
26. Lehner, T. (1969). Characterisation of mucosal antibodies in recurrent aphthous ulceration and Behcet's syndrome. *Archs Oral Biol.*, **14**, 843
27. Williams, B. D., Challacombe, S. J., Slayney, J. M., Lachmann, P. J. and Lehner, T. (1975). C3 and immunoconglutinins in human saliva. *Clin. Exp. Immunol.*, **19**, 423
28. Challacombe, S. J. and Lehner, T. (1976). Serum and salivary antibodies to cariogenic bacteria in man. *J. Dent. Res.*, **55**, C139
29. Lehner, T., Challacombe, S. J., Wilton, J. M. A. and Caldwell, J. (1976). Cellular and humoral immune responses in vaccination against dental caries in monkeys. *Nature*, **264**, 69
30. Lehner, T. (1966). Immunofluorescence study of *Candida albicans* in candidiasis, carriers and controls. *J. Path. Bact.*, **91**, 97
31. Ivanyi, L. and Lehner, T. (1970). Stimulation of lymphocyte transformation by bacterial antigens in patients with periodental disease. *Archs Oral Biol.*, **15**, 1089
32. Federlin, K., Maini, R. N., Russell, A. S. and Dumonde, D. C. (1971). A micromethod for peripheral leucocyte migration in tuberculin sensitivity. *J. Clin. Pathol.*, **24**, 533
33. Julius, M. H., Simpson, E. and Herzenberg, L. A. (1973). A rapid method for the isolation of functional thymus-derived murine lymphocytes. *Eur. J. Immunol.*, **3**, 645
34. Bianco, C., Patrick, R. and Nussenzweig, V. (1970). A population of lymphocytes bearing a membrane receptor for antigen–antibody–complement complexes. *J. Exp. Med.*, **132**, 702
35. Krise, G. M. (1960). Haematology of the normal monkey. *Ann. N.Y. Acad. Sci.*, **85**, 803
36. Caldwell, J., Challacombe, S. J. and Lehner, T. (1977). A sequential bacteriological and serological investigation of rhesus monkeys immunized with *Streptococcus mutans* against dental caries. *J. Med. Micro.*, **10**, 213

37. Lehner, T. Serum IgA antibodies in immunisation to *Streptococcus mutans* (unpublished)
38. Russell, M. W., Challacombe, S. J. and Lehner, T. (1976). Serum glucosyltransferase-inhibiting antibodies and dental caries in rhesus monkeys immunized against *Streptococcus mutans*. *Immunology*, **30**, 619
39. Cuppini, A., Borea, G., Stefanini, F. and Capuzzi, P. (1969). Il vaccino V.D.S. e profilassi della carie dentaria: ricerche clinicostatistiche. *Mondo Odontostomat.*, **11**, 453
40. Bowen, W. H. (1969). A vaccine against dental caries. *Brit. Dent. J.*, **126**, 159
41. Tanzer, J. M., Hageage, G. J. Jr. and Larson, R. H. (1973). Variable experiences in immunization of rats against *Streptococcus mutans* – associated dental caries. *Archs Oral Biol.*, **18**, 1425
42. Taubman, M. A. and Smith, D. J. (1974). Effects of local immunization with *Streptococcus mutans* on induction of salivary immunoglobulin A antibody and experimental dental caries in rats. *Infect. Immun.*, **9**, 1079
43. Kettman, J. (1972). Delayed hypersensitivity: is the same population of thymus-derived cells responsible for cellular immunity reactions and the carrier effect? *Immun. Comm.*, **1**, 289
44. Campbell, P. A. (1972). T cells: the limiting cells in the initiation of immune responses in normal mouse spleens. *Cell. Immunol.*, **5**, 338
45. Lehner, T., Challacombe, S. J., Ivanyi, L. and Wilton, J. M. A. (1973). The relationship between serum and salivary antibodies and cell-mediated immunity in oral disease in man. In J. Mestecky and Lawton, A. R. (eds.). *The Immunoglobulin A System. Adv. Exp. Med. Biol.*, pp. 485–495 (New York and London: Plenum Press)
46. Loe, H., Theilade, E. and Jensen, S. B. (1965). Experimental gingivitis in man. *J. Periodont.*, **36**, 177
47. Ritz, H. L. (1967). Microbial population shifts in developing human dental plaque. *Archs Oral Biol.*, **12**, 1561
48. Skapski, H. and Lehner, T. (1976). A crevicular washing method for investigating immune components of crevicular fluid in man. *J. Perio. Res.*, **11**, 19
49. Wilton, J. M. A., Renggli, H. H. and Lehner, T. (1976). The isolation and identification of mononuclear cells from the gingival crevice in man. *J. Perio. Res.*, **11**, 262
50. Williams, R. C. and Gibbons, R. J. (1972). Inhibition of bacterial adherence by secretory immunoglobulin A: a mechanism of antigen disposal. *Science*, **177**, 697
51. Olson, G. A., Bleiweis, A. S. and Small, P. A. Jr. (1972). Adherence inhibition of *Streptococcus mutans*: an assay reflecting a possible role of antibody in dental caries prophylaxis. *Infect. Immun.*, **5**, 419
52. Brandtzaeg, P., Fjellanger, I. and Gjeruldsen, S. T. (1970). Human secretory immunoglobulins. I. Salivary secretions from individuals with normal or low levels of serum immunoglobulins. *Scand. J. Haematol.*, (Suppl.), **12**, 1
53. Schiött, C. R. and Löe, H. (1970). The origin and variation in number of leukocytes in the human saliva. *J. Perio. Res.*, **5**, 36

20
Vaccination against tropical parasitic diseases

A. VOLLER

The group of diseases to be considered here has been rather neglected in recent years in spite of the fact that they affect many millions of people in the Third World[1,2]. These diseases occur in areas far from the mainstream of medical research of the industrial world and the only substantial contact of the latter with these diseases has been during military operations. In addition there was little wealth in these areas to attract commercial interest in their problems. Now this is all changing: first, the moral obligations of the developed nations to assist the less fortunate have been recognized; secondly, the economic strength of many nations of the tropics has meant that their voices cannot be ignored; and thirdly, their standards of living are rising.

The World Health Organization has established a special research programme into the most important parasitic diseases – malaria, schistosomiasis, trypanosomiasis, filariasis, leishmaniasis and leprosy. One of the main objectives of this programme is to develop effective vaccines.

The major parasitic diseases have some special features which distinguish them from most other infections. They frequently infect a large part or even the whole of a population and they can persist in an infected individual for a very long time; sometimes for all his life. These features bear witness to the ability of the parasites to survive and to evade the immune responses of the host. Different parasites have different ways of doing this. These will be discussed later. This might lead one to be pessimistic about the scientific feasibility of vaccines. However, to offset this it should be noted that there is, in some instances, a fairly effective clinical immunity established by adulthood in areas where these diseases are endemic.

On the more mundane level we have to consider the practical problems posed for such vaccines. These diseases often occur in remote areas with poor communications, so that labile materials would be of little value. Medical services are frequently of a rudimentary nature and any vaccination schedule requiring multiple visits would be impracticable. Quite aside from the technical problems the financial limitations are still paramount. Expensive vaccines would do little to solve the basic disease problem since most of the people at risk are still in countries with severe economic problems. At present such vaccines could only be provided under governmental or international auspices. Possibly, at a later stage, there might be a demand at the individual level.

The specific disease problems, and the potential and progress towards their vaccines are now considered in detail.

SCHISTOSOMIASIS (Table 1)

This is a chronic disease caused by several related worms (*Schistosoma mansoni*, *S. haematobium* and *S. japonicum*) which are transmitted to man via snails in fresh water. The infected snails release forms of the parasite (cercariae) into the water and these cercariae actively penetrate the skin of people in contact with the water. After penetration the cercaria change to a new form (schistosomulum). Eventually the male and female worms pair and then migrate to the appropriate blood vessels of the viscera. The adult forms can live for many years and much of the pathology of the disease is caused by the deposition of the eggs which are laid by the female worms. These eggs can either penetrate the walls of the bladder or intestine, or get swept back and deposited in the liver causing granulomas and portal obstruction.

Table 1 Schistosomiasis: the problem

Worldwide:	Hundreds of millions infected; increasing with man-made lakes
Vector control:	By chemicals; expensive; requires high efficiency
Chemotherapy:	Does not prevent re-infection
VACCINE URGENTLY REQUIRED	

The disease affects several hundred million people at present, and is increasing as new dams are constructed in the tropics and as irrigation is extended. A great deal of effort has been put into controlling the vector snails, but this is expensive and the effect is transient unless the measures are efficiently maintained. Drugs are available for the treatment of infected individuals, but they often have unpleasant side-effects which militate against their large-scale use. Such chemotherapy does not, however, prevent reinfection. The considerations suggest that there is a real need for a vaccine against schistosomiasis.

There are pointers to the possibility of a vaccine. It is evident from experimental studies that, following an initial infection, animals can develop immunity to reinfection by schistosomes. Epidemiological studies on people in endemic areas also suggest that adults have some degree of immunity following long-term exposure. This means that viable schistosomes at some stage of their development in the human body can induce an immunological response. This has been the subject of much recent study[3].

There is evidence to suggest that in natural infections the major stimuli for the induction of immunity are the adult worms. However, these are able to escape the immunological attack, possibly by incorporating host material into their surfaces. They might then appear as 'self' and evade the immune response. This response is, however, effective in preventing superinfection[3,4,5].

The ideal schistosomiasis vaccine should prevent infection, have long activity, and be free of pathological effects. However, a vaccine which could just arrest the parasites' development or suppress the pathological consequences of infection would still be very valuable.

There appear to be two possible types of vaccine (Figure 1):

(a) *Living vaccines*
  1. With non-human schistosomes
  2. With attenuated infective or migratory forms (cercariae or schistosomulae)

(b) *Non-viable vaccines*
  These might be either whole schistosomes, extracts or secretions. Or they might be based upon purified fractions.

These two approaches will be considered separately.

Schistosomiasis vaccine

Irradiated parasites

Dead parasites (or extracts)

Live heterologous parasites

Promising in lab

To stop invasion

To reduce pathology

Promising for animal schistosomiasis

Figure 1 Possible vaccines for schistosomiasis

Live parasite vaccines

The aim of these is to provide the stimulus for immunity without the full development of the egg-laying parasite. If live heterologous schistosomes are used as the vaccine (e.g. from cattle or sheep), that may be sufficient to prevent later infection with the more pathogenic human worm. The reciprocal has been shown to be true: domestic animals exposed to the human *Schistosoma mansoni* or *S. haematobium* are partially immune to subsequent challenge with their own schistosomes[6,7]. Extensive veterinary trials will be necessary to exclude any immunopathological effects before such a vaccine could be envisaged for human use.

The use of the infective or migratory forms of the human schistosomes, irradiated to prevent their full development, seems rather promising. In the early work, irradiated cercariae were used[4] but these only remain viable for a very short time. More recently the value of the migratory phase (schistosomulum) has been appreciated. These can be irradiated, then introduced by the intramuscular, intravenous or subcutaneous routes. In the animal systems in which this type of vaccine has been investigated[8], a good level of immunity has been achieved. However, the problem of storage has never been overcome in a similar type of irradiated vaccine for 'husk' (*Dictyocaulus viviparus*) in cattle; this vaccine has now been in use for many years. To date it has been possible to store the schistosomulum vaccine for a week or two but this is scarcely sufficient for field use. The recent finding of cross-immunity between *S. mansoni* and *S. haematobium*, two human parasites, suggests that one vaccine might be effective against both[9].

Dead vaccines

Extracts, both crude and purified, of all stages of the schistosome life cycle, when injected, provoke humoral and cell-mediated responses. In some cases the antibody produced may even have a lethal effect on schistosomes *in vitro*, but these dead vaccines do not lead to immunity[10]. It seems unlikely that a non-viable vaccine will become available for schistosomiasis in the near future. Much more basic work on the antigens and their role in the immune response is needed. There is a possibility that the identification of the responsible antigen might lead to a vaccine capable of reducing the immunopathological effects of the schistosome eggs.

Opinion

It seems unlikely that a schistosome vaccine for use in man will become available in the near future, although a veterinary product seems probable. Considerable investment in personnel and financial terms would be involved in development of a human schistosome vaccine, and with little short-term prospect of success this is not likely to have commercial appeal. It is possible that the bulk of the developmental work will have to be undertaken by international and national research agencies and by foundations.

TRYPANOSOMIASIS

African (Table 2)

The diseases of man are known as Gambian and Rhodesian Sleeping Sickness and are caused by *Trypanosoma brucei gambiense* and *T. brucei rhodesiense* respectively. These trypanosomes are protozoa which are transmitted by tse-tse flies to and from man, cattle and wild game animals. It is difficult to give precise figures but many millions of people are exposed to these diseases in Africa. Because of the devastating effect of other species, *T. congolense* and *T. vivax* that infect cattle, the use of otherwise suitable land is unavailable for cattle farming. In the past, control of the disease was attempted by removal of the habitat of the tse-tse fly (e.g. brush clearing along river banks, etc.) supplemented by drug treatment of infected patients. Habitat control, however, is becoming increasingly expensive and the drugs have the disadvantage of being rather toxic, requiring long courses of treatment. Drug resistance is also a problem.

The aim of a vaccine is, ideally, to prevent infection. However, a vaccine which restricts the multiplication of the parasite in the blood or tissues and prevents involvement of the central nervous system would be of value.

There is little evidence that man or highly susceptible animals can develop an effective immunity against trypanosomiasis, although antibodies can easily be demonstrated. The parasites have a neat way of escaping the immune response by a process known as antigenic variation: as soon as antibody appears against a particular type of trypanosome it 'switches' the surface antigens to a new configuration which is not recognized by the antibody[11]. This means that any population of trypanosomes has the potential to change to many other variants. This clearly poses great problems to those developing vaccines.

Table 2 Sleeping sickness: the problem

Spreading in Africa, infects man and cattle. Number infected unknown.	
Vector control:	Expensive and difficult
Drugs:	Toxic, long treatment
Vaccines:	– Dead parasites, irradiated parasites – Effective in lab – Useless in field (too specific)

Vaccines

No vaccine has yet been used in man. In experimental animals irradiated trypanosomes have induced a high level of protective immunity[12]. Unfortunately, this immunity is only effective against the parasites of the precise type used in the immunization[13]. Obviously, under field conditions where there are many types and strains, this would be of little value. Attempts to use dead trypanosome material, either as whole parasites, crude extracts or purified antigens, have at best only produced a transient resistance[14].

Opinion

One can only reinforce the pessimistic view of Gray[15] that we are a long way from a vaccine for African trypanosomiasis. Possibly some new approach with adjuvant or non-specific boosting of immunity might be more successful, although there is no evidence for this.

TRYPANOSOMIASIS

American (Chagas Disease) (Table 3)

This disease, which is caused by *Trypanosoma cruzi*, is transmitted by triatomid bugs. In addition to man, a wide range of reservoir animals such as dogs and rodents can be infected. This disease is restricted to South America, where probably over 100 million people are exposed. In Brazil alone about 10 million people are infected.

The disease is characterized by a rather short acute phase, followed by a long chronic phase when lesions can occur in many organs including the heart, oesophagus and colon.

Control methods have been based on reducing the man–vector contact by spraying, improved building methods, etc. This is slow and costly, however. There is no drug currently available which is fully effective against the chronic stage, thus underlining the need for a vaccine.

There is good evidence of an immune response in Chagas Disease. Patients develop antibodies, and cell-mediated reactivity and acquired resistance can follow the disease. There is no indication as yet that antigenic variation can occur.

Table 3 Chagas disease: the problem

In South America	
Over 100 million exposed	
Over 10 million infected	
Vector control:	Difficult, expensive
Drugs:	No effective drugs
Vaccines:	Lab trials promising; more development needed

Vaccines[16, 17]

Dead vaccines

These can either be killed organisms or immunogenic extracts of them. The results have been very variable and confusing, but the overall impression is that these vaccines are not very effective. Recently McHardy[17] has investigated the use of dead vaccines very carefully, and he has shown that they can be effective against low challenge doses of viable organisms. The use of gentle methods for antigen extraction is expected to yield better vaccines of this type. At the present time none are suitable for human use.

Living vaccines

These are based on avirulent or attenuated organisms. X-irradiated parasites do not produce disease, but animals immunized with them are at least partially protected against subsequent viable challenge. Similarly long-cultured avirulent strains have the ability to induce protection against more virulent strains. In view of the great danger of this organism, its introduction into uninfected people, even in apparently attenuated forms, must not be lightly undertaken.

Opinion

There appears to be a possibility for a vaccine, either living or dead, for Chagas Disease. The parasite can be produced in large amounts in culture and adequate experimental animal systems are available for its evaluation. The technical problems (such as antigen extraction procedures, choice of the best adjuvant, etc.) appear to be amenable to solution if sufficient effort is devoted to them. The question of safety, both from direct effects of such a vaccine or from subsequent challenges of vaccinated people, are less easy to resolve.

MALARIA (Table 4)

Malaria is probably the most widespread disease of the tropics and affects hundreds of millions of people, especially in Africa, Asia and South America. It has been estimated that the annual mortality rate is over 1 million in Africa alone.

Malaria is caused by a group of protozoa (*Plasmodium falciparum*, *P. vivax* and *P. malariae*) which are transmitted by anopheline mosquitoes. The mosquitoes inject the 'sporozoite' stage into the blood of the human host and this quickly passes to the liver where it multiplies for a week or so. Large numbers of parasites are then released into the blood where they infect the red blood cells. Further multiplication occurs in the blood and new red blood cells are invaded by the merozoites. The disease usually has an acute phase, which can be fatal, followed by a long chronic relapsing illness.

A few years ago, the discovery of highly active long-lasting insecticides such as DDT fuelled hopes that malaria could be eradicated. However, the emergence of insecticide-resistant anophelines and the appearance of drug-resistant parasites has led to a more realistic view, in which it is accepted that malaria will be with us for many years to come.

It is a well-established fact that in malaria-endemic areas an effective immunity is established by the time that individuals reach adulthood. Unfortunately, a heavy price is paid for this adult-population immunity by a high child mortality from malaria. The function of a vaccine would be to provide at least the adult level of immunity without the mortality or morbidity accompanying the natural infection. It is possible that a vaccine might produce an immunity even more effective than that accompanying natural infection.

In natural infections immune responses are stimulated almost exclusively by the blood (erythrocytic) forms of the parasite. The sporozoites infected by the mosquito and the liver phase do not seem to be highly immunogenic normally. The prime stimulus to immunity appears to be either the mature parasite in the red cell or, more probably, the merozoite which traverses from one red blood cell to another. These are also the stages of the life cycle which are affected by the immune response. As with the other parasites we have discussed, the malarial parasites also partially evade the immune response by 'antigenic variation' in the same manner as the African trypanosomes[18].

Table 4 Malaria: the problem

People infected over 200 million	
Annual mortality over 1 million	
Current control:	Insecticides; anti-malarial drugs
Problems:	Resistance
VACCINE URGENTLY NEEDED	

Vaccines[19] (Figure 2)

There are two points in the parasites' life cycle which might be susceptible to a vaccine. The first is immediately after the mosquito bite when the sporozoites are en route to the liver, and the second is during the parasites' multiplying phase in the erythrocytes.

Sporozoite vaccines

In experimental studies on malaria in rodents and chickens injection of inactivated sporozoites resulted in protection against subsequent viable challenge. The best results were obtained using irradiated sporozoites injected intravenously.

The appeal of this system led to further work on the more relevant primate malarias and even on human volunteers. In practice, this vaccination is achieved by allowing mosquitoes to feed on a malaria-infected host. The malaria infection is then allowed to develop in the mosquitoes which are X-irradiated. The mosquitoes are then allowed to bite, thus introducing the irradiated sporozoites. Alternatively the sporozoites can be isolated and then injected. Experiments on monkeys revealed that after several immunizations they became resistant to subsequent challenge. Of particular interest is the finding that several of the human volunteers immunized in this way became resistant and were protected against all strains of the species of malaria (e.g. *P. falciparum*) used in the immunization. The protection had a duration of several months.

MALARIA VACCINE

	IRRADIATED MOSQUITO STAGES	KILLED BLOOD STAGES
Production	In mosquitoes	Culture
Effect	Transient	Long-term ?
Protection	Must be absolute	Can be partial

Figure 2 The malaria vaccine possibilities

Opinion

The results obtained to date indicate that sporozoite vaccines are theoretically possible. However, there are appalling practical difficulties for large-scale production. Even though mosquitoes can be reared by the millions, there is little immediate prospect of being able to infect them with human malaria as there is no suitable animal host or culture.

The transient nature of the immunity suggests that this type of vaccine could only be considered for short-term use; e.g. for military personnel, or tourists visiting the tropics. A particularly serious drawback is that if a single viable sporozoite does reach the liver of the vaccinated host then a normal infection will result as this type of vaccine does not inhibit multiplication of the red blood cell forms of the parasite.

Erythrocytic stage vaccines

As mentioned earlier, it is known that this is the stage of the parasite's life cycle which, under natural conditions, is the major stimulus to immunity in malaria. Long ago experimental studies indicated that mature asexual parasites, if killed and then injected with an adjuvant, induced a good level of protective immunity. This has been confirmed recently, although the presence of much erythrocytic material in such a vaccine would be a major disadvantage for its use in man.

A major step forward was made by Mitchell and colleagues[20] who were able to isolate the merozoites on their passage between erythrocytes and to use these effectively in a vaccine against a monkey malaria. These merozoites were more effective than the intra-erythrocytic parasites, and had the advantage of being free of red cell contaminants. Preliminary results in monkeys vaccinated in a similar way against the human malaria *P. falciparum* were also promising[21]. The recent development of an *in vitro* culture system for that human parasite[22] means that one of the major stumbling blocks has now been overcome, in that larger quantities of antigenic material will be available.

Opinion

The malaria merozoite vaccine is promising. Possibly the major problem at the moment is to develop an effective acceptable adjuvant to replace Freund's adjuvant which cannot reasonably be used in man. Human trials of a merozoite vaccine will present special problems, since it will only be of value if effective in children. It will be difficult to monitor the long-term effects of immunized people who are subjected to viable challenge in malarious areas. It will be especially important to determine if there are any of the immunopathological sequels which occasionally accompany malaria infections.

A very large investment will be required for any commercial undertaking to enter this field. In addition to highly specialized expertise, facilities for expensive primate experiments will be essential. Close collaboration with national health and international agencies will be required. It is the author's opinion that a malaria vaccine is feasible but that it will not make any impact on the world malaria situation within the next decade.

References

1. Rowe, D. S. (1976). The forgotten people. *World Health*, **17**
2. Dorozynski, A. (1976). The attack on tropical disease. *Nature*, **262**, 85
3. World Health Organization (1974a). Immunology of schistosomiasis. *Bull. Wld Hlth Org.*, **51**, 553
4. Smithers, S. R. (1976). Immunity to trematode infections. In S. Cohen and E. H. Sadun (eds.). *Immunology of Parasitic Infections*, pp. 298–332 (Oxford: Blackwell Scientific Publications)
5. Smithers, S. R. and Terry, R. J. (1969). Immunity in schistosomiasis. *Ann. N. Y. Acad. Sci.*, **160**, 826
6. Hussein, M. F., Safed, A. A. and Nelson, G. S. (1970). Studies on heterologous immunity in schistosomiasis. 4: Heterologous immunity in cattle. *Bull. Wld Hlth Org.*, **42**, 745
7. Massound, J. and Nelson, G. S. (1972). Studies on heterologous immunity in schistosomiasis. 6: Observations on cross-immunity to *O. turkestenicum*, *S. bovis*, *S. mansoni* and *S. haematobium* in mice, sheep and cattle in Iran. *Bull. Wld Hlth Org.*, **47**, 591
8. Taylor, M. G., James, E. R., Nelson, G. S., Bickle, Q., Dunne, D. W. and Webbe, G. (1976). Immunization of sheep against *Schistosoma matthei* using either irradiated cercariae or irradiated schistosomula. *J. Helminth.*, **50**, 1
9. Smith, M. A., Clegg, J. A. & Webbe, G. (1976). Cross immunity to *S. mansoni* and *S. haematobium* in the hamster. *Parasitol.*, **73**, 53
10. Murrell, K. D., Dean, D. A. and Stafford, E. E. (1975). 'Resistance to infection with *S. mansoni* after immunization with worm extracts or live cercariae. *Amer. J. Trop. Med. Hyg.*, **24**, 995

11. Gray, A. R. (1967). Some principles of the immunology of trypanosomiasis. *Bull. Wld Hlth Org.*, **37**, 177
12. Duxbury, R. E. and Sadun, E. H. (1969). Resistance produced in mice and rats by inoculation with irradiated *T. rhodesiense*. *J. Parasitol.*, **55**, 859
13. Duxbury, R. E., Sadun, E. H., Wellde, B. T. and Anderson, J. S. (1972). Immunization of cattle with X-irradiated African trypanosomes. *Trans. R. Soc. Trop. Med. Hyg.*, **66**, 349
14. Soltys, M. A. (1964). Immunity in trypanosomiasis. I: Immunization of animals with dead trypanosomes. *Parasitol.*, **54**, 585
15. Gray, A. R. (1976). Immunological research and the problem of immunization against African trypanosomiasis. *Trans. R. Soc. Trop. Med. Hyg.*, **70**, 119
16. Neal, R. A. and Johnson, P. (1977). Immunization against *Trypanosoma cruzi* using killed antigens and with saponin as adjuvant. *Acta Tropica*, **34**, 87
17. McHardy, W. (1977). Immunization of mice against *T. Cruzi*. *Z. Tropen. med. Parasit.*, **28**, 11
18. Brown, K. N. (1976). Resistance to malaria. In S. Cohen and E. H. Sadun, (eds). *Immunology of Parasitic Infections*, 268–291 (Oxford: Blackwell Scientific Publications)
19. World Health Organization (1975). Development in malarial immunology. *W.H.O. Technical Report*, **579**, 52
20. Mitchell, G. H., Butcher, G. A. and Cohen, S. (1975). Merozoite vaccination against *Plasmodium knowlesi* malaria. *Immunol.*, **29**, 397
21. Mitchell, G. H., Butcher, G. A., Richards, W. H. G. and Cohen, S. (1977). Merozoite vaccination of Lourocouli monkeys against falciparum malaria. *Lancet*, **i**, 1335
22. Trager, W. and Jensen, J. B. (1976). Human malaria parasites in continuous culture. *Science*, **193**, 673

21
Notes on veterinary vaccines

A. J. BEALE

In a book devoted to various specialized aspects of human vaccines a single chapter on veterinary vaccines must inevitably be incomplete and superficial.

There are three aspects to the veterinary vaccine market. First, there are vaccines primarily used to control diseases in animals that are transmissible to man. Second, there are vaccines used to control diseases in domestic pets, which is an important and expanding segment of the market. Finally, there are vaccines used to control diseases in economically important animals. These animals can be divided into those affecting production directly and those affecting acceptance of the product. For example, in many parts of the world acceptance of milk depends upon the leucocyte count rather than overt mastitis, and the meat market is influenced as much by lack of carcase blemish as by the rate of weight gain.

The development of veterinary vaccines is also of great interest to those concerned with the development of human vaccines. Thus, new technical developments can be assessed more easily by the use of vaccines in animals in the first instance.

Also there is a possibility of using the target species for experimental work and of including direct challenge tests for efficacy.

It is only possible to deal with a few of these matters. The hazards to man from animal diseases can be handled in a number of ways:

1. By control of the disease in the animals; for example, by vaccination of domestic animals against rabies, or gassing of foxes, or by vaccination followed by eradication for brucellosis.
2. By prevention of spread from animals to man; for example, by elimination of stray dogs and muzzling orders to prevent rabies, or by pasteurization of milk to prevent the spread of milk-borne diseases.
3. Finally, resort can be made to increasing the resistance of man by vaccination.

In recent years there has been an increasing awareness of the hazards to man from leptospira present in animal products. There are a number of ways of tackling the problem by means of vaccination, for example, vaccinating workers at highest risk, e.g. those in abattoirs, or vaccinating the animals not only to control a disease of economic importance, but also to prevent latent infection and the danger of spread to man. The species of leptospira involved varies from country to country, but in New Zealand for example the predominant ones are *Leptospira pomona* and *L. hardjo*. Vaccines against these species can be prepared, but until recently these have required the use of serum in the medium to get adequate growth. This has precluded the use of vaccines in man and also the use of intensive schedules in animals that are likely to be effective in preventing carriage or clearing up latent infections. Using a completely synthetic medium, workers at the Wellcome Research Laboratories have recently succeeded in growing all leptospira species, and the results of trials in hamsters show that these vaccines made in serum-free medium are of excellent potency where good challenge strains exist. Moreover, high titres of agglutinating antibodies are produced to both antigens in cattle. It is too early to be sure that these titres will reduce carriage of organisms. When these experiments are concluded satisfactorily, then not only will the disease be prevented in animals, but the danger of spread to man will be reduced. Moreover, a safe and effective vaccine would be available for man should the need arise.

Foot rot in sheep is a serious and painful disease with adverse effects on the condition of sheep and therefore their value as production animals. The disease is an infection of the hoof bed and somewhat surprisingly it was found that parenteral vaccination gave rise to protection against the disease, provided the antibody levels were high enough. The problem is to produce large quantities of antigen. This resolves itself into two parts: identifying the important antigen and then devising conditions for the bulk growth of organisms that yield a lot of this antigen. Experience in this philosophy and attendant technology came first in the development of vaccines against the clostridial diseases of sheep and cattle. These are now prepared in 1000-litre tanks under optimal conditions for antigen production. Sometimes the antigen has to be concentrated and purified and new techniques (for example, immunopurification for tetanus toxin) have proved particularly valuable. This enables a single step to achieve greater degrees of purity than was previously obtained by a multistep process. This large-scale processing and manufacturing capacity is important in making the benefits of immunization available on a large scale.

Another vaccine where production technology has played a decisive role is foot-and-mouth disease. This is the single most important disease of cattle, and the market for the vaccine is the single largest feature in veterinary vaccines. The best substrate for virus production are cells grown in suspension, for example the baby hamster kidney cell line BJK clone 21. This can be grown in large tanks up to 5000 litres and probably more. The problems of harvesting cells, washing them free of media and infecting them have been solved by the use of special filter presses which hold the cells. They can then be easily washed and infected. Similar technology could easily be applied to the production of other viral antigens which can be purified andin activated.

One of the greatest challenges left for those engaged in vaccine research is protection against the diseases of surface mucous membranes, especially the alimentary and respiratory tracts. A considerable amount has been learned about the important aetiological agents, but more needs to be learned. It is a feature of these diseases in animals that there is massive infection and with many agents, so that sorting out the important ones and defining the role of different agents is essential. Sometimes, however, a vaccine may need to be effective against only one component in the aetiology; for example, in foot rot the disease is due to the combined action of *Fusiformis necrophorus* and *F. nodosus*, but a vaccine composed of only *F. nodosus* is effective. This is because the disease requires the action of both organisms.

Protection against respiratory and especially alimentary tract infections can be conferred by immunization of the mothers. For pigs, for example, *Escherichia coli* is an important cause of neonatal scours due to strains containing K88 antigen which enables them to adhere to the gut and produce toxin. If vaccines rich in K88 are given to the dams, this protects piglets when they are exposed to direct challenge, or when they are exposed on farms. There are other causes: scours and rotaviruses and the virus of transmissible gastroenteritis are two important examples in pigs. There are different problems in stimulating immunity in the gut or respiratory tracts of older animals. The relative importance of different aspects of the immune system is still subject to active debate. It is clear that in many systems the liver-circulating antibody gives a rough guide to local immunity, but that this breaks down under certain conditions. Thus, immunity from living 'flu vaccine, or previous influenza, is superior to that produced by killed 'flu vaccines. Similarly, the gut immunity from killed poliovaccine is inferior to that produced by living vaccine, even when the antibody titres produced by killed vaccine are much higher.

The mechanism of immunity at the surface of the gut has received much attention, as has research into the best means of stimulating such immunity. The work of Gowans and others (Husband[1]), has traced the circulation of the IgA-containing cells from the Peyers patches back via the lymphatics to the thoracic duct and back again to the lamina propria of the intestinal wall. A secondary immune response in this system has been established, also the localization of the response preferentially to areas exposed directly to antigen. Pierce and Gowans (quoted by Husband[1]) have shown tha t IgA antibody can be stimulated by parenteral followed by local boosting, or by local administration. The best means of exploiting this new knowledge are under active investigation.

Control of respiratory virus infections of animals and man remains a challenge because we neither understand the immune mechanisms satisfactorily nor have we elucidated the aetiological agents. Thus, although many viruses have been implicated in the aetiology of bovine respiratory disease, efforts to transmit the disease experimentally to satisfy Koch's postulations have been unavailing. In order to supplement such studies we have, in collaboration with workers at the Agricultural Research Council's station at Compton, shown that a vaccine against parainfluenza type 3 virus prevents virus multiplication but has no effect on respiratory disease in a field study. Indeed the field study levels show parainfluenza type 3 as of little importance.

One other area deserves mention: this is the control of diseases to herpes virus infections. In general, killed vaccines against these diseases have been unsatisfactory. Living vaccines, for example, against the respiratory pathogens infectious bovine rhinotracheitis or infectious laryngotracheitis of fowls, or against the lymphomatous tumours of chickens called Mareks disease, have been notably successful. They have, however, served to highlight the problems of latency and possible malignant change associated with these viruses. Efforts to prepare killed vaccines against Mareks disease show considerable promise, and open up important prospects for the control of diseases of importance in both men and animals, using killed herpes virus vaccines.

Reference

1. Husband, A. J., Monié, H. J. and Gowans, J. L. (1977). The natural history of the cells producing IgA in the gut. *CIBA Foundation Symposium* **46**, (New Series), 29–42

22
Standardization and control of allergen extracts

W. D. BRIGHTON

In the UK two kinds of allergen extract materials are available for use in humans. The first kind is provocation material, used for skin tests and nasal and bronchial inhalation challenge tests. The second kind is composed of those extracts used for hyposensitizing vaccines. Both are injected beneath the skin and both therefore come within the purview of the Medicines Act 1968. This means that both are subject to control by the UK Licensing Authority.

Under the terms of the Biological Standards Act 1975 one of the duties of the National Institute for Biological Standards and Control is to produce standard materials for use in biological assays, and the other is to control vaccines.

Before control can be applied it is necessary to have control regulations which state the methods to be used. Draft proposals for inclusion in the 'Compendium of requirements for biological medical products for human use' have now been written and circulated to the manufacturers in the UK and to the Association of British Pharmaceutical Industries. No doubt there will be further discussions about the proposals and these may be modified in view of the discussions, but in the UK the stage has been reached where control of allergen extracts is imminent.

PRESENT POSITION

After many problems over the supply of antisera and labelled antiglobulin a collaborative trial of an *in vitro* method for comparing potency of allergen extracts was started earlier this year in thirteen laboratories, some in this country, some in Europe and some in the USA. The results are not yet all to hand, but those that have been returned are good, and I think that it will be possible in the near future to recommend a standardized RAST method for comparing extract potency.

In this work I am most grateful for the cooperation and active participation of the manufacturers, and for discussions with them as to acceptable limits of tolerance of the results of the potency assays. When this standardized method of laboratory assay is used it will become doubly important to produce standard preparations of each of the materials to be tested, as the results will be obtained by comparison with the standard; the evidence that we have obtained suggests that acceptable variation in potency would be between 25% and 400% of the potency of the standard.

If this tolerance level is adopted as a legal requirement it is also then required that the standard itself has an acceptable potency, both *in vitro* and *in vivo*, and the latter must be determined by clinical workers. In the UK we have adopted a system of collaborative trials in which clinicians assay by a statistically controlled skin test in sensitive patients in parallel with laboratory tests by the standard RAST. The first trial was that of three different extracts of Cocksfoot pollen. There was good agreement between the skin test assay and the two variations of RAST that were used, and the tests showed a 30-fold difference in potency of the three extracts, though the comparison between the skin test assay and histamine released from sensitized monkey skin *in vitro* was so poor as to be unusable; we have therefore not proceeded with this any further.

As a result of this trial the 1st British Standard of Cocksfoot pollen extract was created from a batch of material kindly prepared by Bencard (Clarendon Road, Worthing, Sussex), lyophilized and submitted to accelerated degradation tests to determine its storage stability. After 6 months the ampoules stored at 56 °C have lost about 70% of their initial potency, those at 44 °C about 20% at 37 °C there is an insignificant loss and at 22 °C, 4 °C, −20 °C, −70 °C and −150 °C the titres are indistinguishable from those of the original, as shown in Table 1.

Table 1 Loss of activity of 1st British standard Cocksfoot pollen extract in 6 months

Temperature (°C)	*Remaining activity* (%)
56	30
44	80
37	98
22	100
4	100
−20	100
−70	100
−150	100

We have confidence therefore that suitable preparations, suitably lyophilized and stored, can be used for long-term standards of pollen without significant degradation.

The second of these collaborative trials is under way at the present time. This time, nine extracts of *Aspergillus fumigatus* have been obtained, some from commercial manufacturers, some from university workers and other sources. The trial is being conducted by four clinicians with different patient populations, and ten laboratories. Preliminary results show a 7000-fold variation in potency of the nine preparations.

Because of the possible very wide variation in the potency of these extracts we thought it prudent to carry out a preliminary survey of the extracts before the main part of the trial. The final assessment must wait until all the results have been received, but again, I am confident that we shall be able to select a preparation and method of production which will enable a standard to be produced within the next few months.

Without a formal collaborative trial we have also been involved in much work with extracts of *Candida albicans*. We were persuaded to make a batch of cytoplasmic proteins, and this was made available to thirty-four workers for their study and comment. As a result of this activity the following decisions have been made:

1. A suitable strain for standard preparations is NCPF 3153.
2. Four preparations are required:
   (a) Cytoplasmic proteins
   (b) Mannan
   (c) Live culture for *Candida* killing
   (d) Whole extract (proteins + mannan)

These preparations have now been made, and are being lyophilized and labelled at the present time.

Table 2 Standards from *Candida albicans* strain NCPF 3153

1. 1st Standard preparation of cytoplasmic proteins. Mannan was removed by affinity chromatography on Concanavalin A columns. Lyophilized.
Uses: Type IV hypersensitivity testing. Lymphocyte transformation. MIF. Serology.

2. 1st Standard preparation of purified mannan. Free from proteins. Made by the copper precipitation method of Peat, Whelan & Edwards. Lyophilized.
Uses: Type I hypersensitivity testing. Serology.

3. 1st Standard preparation of live cells of strain NCPF 3153. Lyophilized.
Use: Candida killing test (Lehrer & Cline).

4. 1st Reference preparation of whole soluble extract. Contains proteins, glycoproteins and mannan. Lyophilized.
Uses: Lymphocyte transformation. Serology. Electrophoresis.

In addition to these activities which have been conducted within the UK, there have been close contact with members of the International Union of

Immunological Societies, Allergen procurement group and Serum procurement group to provide a pool of internationally accepted reagents. The decision was taken at the WHO/IUIS Symposium in Copenhagen (1975) that the ten most needed standards internationally were as shown in Table 3.

Table 3 Ten most-needed standards

Cocksfoot	Birch
Timothy	*Altenaria*
Rye	House dust
Ragweed	Honey-bee venom
White Oak	Cat dander

With the exception of the honey-bee venom and house dust, batches of these materials have now been obtained. In the UK, manufacturers are required to submit samples and protocols for each batch they make. It is therefore possible for us to estimate, if we accept that the manufacturers actually use and sell their materials, the frequency with which each specification is used by clinicians in this country. Under the provisions of the Biological Standards Act it cannot be revealed what individual manufacturers supply, but the estimates show that the most-used extracts in the UK, taken as a whole, are those shown in Table 4.

Table 4 Most frequently used hyposensitizing vaccines

Mixed grass pollen
House dust mite (*Dermataphagoides pteronyssinus*)
House dust without mites
Aspergillus fumigatus
Cat dander
Dog dander
Horse dander
Birch pollen
Altenaria
Honey-bee venom (*Apis mellifera*)
Mugwort pollen (*Artemesia vulgaris*)
Plantain pollen (*Plantago spps*)
Mixed flower pollen
Candida albicans
Nettle pollen (*Urtica diocia*)
Alder pollen (*Alnus glutinose*)
London plane pollen

Unfortunately, not all of the pools of matching sera that we had hoped to collect have yet materialized. By cooperation with clinical colleagues enough serum has been obtained to make an IgE anti-grass-pollen standard, and almost enough to make an IgE anti-cat-fur standard, and enough has been purchased for an IgE anti-tree-pollen standard and an anti-*D. pteronyssinus* standard. After lyophilization these sera must be subjected to collaborative assay, and then they can be used for control purposes.

There is one aspect of standardization which I have not yet covered. The methods of assay that I have discussed hitherto have been to measure the overall, combined potency of the many components included in present-day extracts. I now wish to tell you of some work that we have been able to do in close association with Dr Jonathan Brostoff.

My colleague Dr Michael Topping has recently refined and developed the technique of isoelectric focusing in polyacrylamide gel to isolate from the gel slices sufficient quantities of material to make it possible to do *in vivo* assays. This developed technique has been applied to the problem of determining what the standard should contain. The question to be answered was whether or not standards should consist of purified single components, and whether a search like that for antigen E of Ragweed was necessary for each allergen extract.

The 1st British Standard Cocksfoot Pollen extract has a complex composition with about twenty-eight components. The problem really is which of these components is biologically active. We therefore made preparations of thirty fractions of sliced polyacrylamide gels and tested them for biological activity by skin passive transfer tests in rats and monkeys, using human sera in the monkeys and homologous sera in the rats. Appropriate control tests with blank gels were included.

As a result of these tests it could be seen that there was no reaction to the blank gel extracts, but there were reactions to some of the fractions of the Cocksfoot gels, particularly to the fractions 15–17, fractions 1–3 and 21–23.

After we were reasonably sure that no untoward reactions would develop from use of these extracts in humans, ten patients, sensitive to the standard Cocksfoot extracts, and two not sensitive, were tested with all thirty fractions. There was a wide variation in individual activity against the different fractions in sensitive individuals, and the insensitive patients did not react at all.

This work was originally undertaken as a much shorter way than those used in the USA for Ragweed and antigen E to identify and prepare in a pure form the active constituents of a pollen. We believe now that certainly for the pollen extracts used in skin testing, and most probably for other complex skin testing extracts the concept of a single antigen for testing all patients is no longer tenable. We believe that the standard must contain all the immunologically active components, but with non-specifically reacting materials removed. We suggest that we have demonstrated a method by which, with co-operation between clinician and standardizer, the correct standard can fairly readily be selected.

A combination of skin and serum testing with fractionated materials has shown considerable variation in the response of different individuals to different fractions. We hope that, if a full clinical investigation of each patient is made by these means, it may prove to be possible to prepare hyposensitizing extracts that are more discriminating and more successful than those in use at present.

Much work remains to be done, and a major impediment is the number of extracts that have to be examined. However, if our present close collaboration both with clinicians and manufacturers can be maintained, and also if sufficient serum is forthcoming, I believe that we can achieve not only a useful set of standards, but also practicable methods of control.

References

1. Medicines Act 1968. Elizabeth II, Chap. 67
2. Biological Standards Act 1975. Elizabeth II, Chap 4
3. WHO/IUIS Symposium: (1975). 'Standardization of Allergens'. *J. Biol. Stand.*, **3**, 121

Index

adjuvants 49, 65, 213
allergen extract vaccines 315–321
  composition of cocksfoot extract 319
  most frequently used 318
  potency assays 316, 317
  standards 316, 317
    ten most-needed 318
antibody 2
  caries 278, 279
  hepatitis 157–161, 163–167
  meningococcal 248, 259, 260
  production related to age 25
  rubella 108–110
    persistence 109
antigen 4, 7, 8
  hepatitis 156, 157, 172–174
  herpesvirus 180, 181
  meningococcal 249
Australia antigen 156, 157

bacterial vaccines
  use in paediatrics 23–25
  see also streptococcal, pneumococcal, meningococcal and influenza vaccines
BCG vaccine 25
  see also tuberculosis

caries
  animal model 275, 276
  antibody 278, 279, 282–288, 290–294
  cell-mediated immunity 279, 288–290, 293, 294
  fissure 281, 282, 292
  smooth surface 280, 281, 292
  vaccine
    effect 291–296
    preparation 277
Chagas disease 304, 305
chickenpox *see* varicella
cholera
  antigens 225–227
  economic considerations 232, 233
  epidemiology 223, 224
  immunity 227–229
  pathogenesis 225
  serologic responses 227
  vaccine 229–231
    future prospects 231, 232
cost–benefit 16, 67, 68, 77, 93, 94, 113, 232, 233
cowpox 2
cytomegalovirus 26, 27, 179
  see also herpesvirus

Dane particle 157
dental caries *see* caries
diphtheria–pertussis–tetanus vaccine 19–21, 43, 119
  see also quadruple vaccine
DTP *see* diphtheria-pertussis-tetanus vaccine

epidemiology 15, 16, 59, 223, 224, 246
Epstein–Barr virus *see* herpesvirus

foot rot 312, 313

German measles vaccine *see* rubella vaccine
Guillain-Barré syndrome 83
  see also swine influenza
hepatitis
  antibody 157–161, 163–167
  antigen 156, 157, 172–174
  risk groups 171
  vaccine 155–169, 171–177
    efficacy 158–161, 171
    polypeptide 173, 174
    potency 157, 158
    safety 174, 175
    subunit 172, 173
    synthetic 175
  virus 155, 157, 163

herd immunity
  polio 128–136

herd immunity *continued*
  rubella 112, 113
herpesvirus
  antigen 180, 181
  vaccine 179–210
    in Marek's disease 179, 180
    in neoplastic disease 180
    veterinary 314
  viral components 181–183
    structure of EHV-1 183–198
    stabilization 198–200
    see also virion *and* nucleocapsid

influenza vaccines 63–69
  cost–benefit analysis 67, 68
  effectiveness 63
  influenza high-risk groups 65, 66
  manufacture 68, 69
  potency 63,
  purity 64
  swine *see* swine influenza
  types of 64, 65
  vaccination policy 67
  veterinary 313

malaria vaccine 305–308
  erythrocytic 307, 308
  sporozoite 306, 307
manufacture 7–11, 68, 69, 106
  quality control 9–11, 247
Marek's disease 179, 180, 314
measles vaccine
  benefit–cost analysis 60
  combination with other vaccines 59
  epidemiology 59
  inactivated 55, 56
  indications 60
  live 57–59
    conversion 57
    reactions 58
  use in paediatrics 22, 23
memory, immunological 125, 127
meningitis, cerebrospinal 267–270
meningococcal vaccine 245–253, 255–273
  antibody 248, 259, 260
  efficacy 247–249, 257–260, 264, 265
  historical development 255, 256
  indications 270, 271
  potency 247
  production laboratories 271
  prospective vaccine 266
  purity 247, 257
  reactions 262–264
  use in field 256, 261, 262
meningococci
  antigen 249
  epidemiology 246
  serogroups 245, 248, 266
mortality
  effect of vaccine developments on 11–15, 17
  following influenza outbreaks 76
  pneumonia 237
mumps vaccine 23
Mycobacterium tuberculosis 211
  vaccine 212, 213, 218, 219
  see also tuberculosis *and* pertussis

Neisseria meningitidis 245, 246
  serogroups 266
neoplastic disease vaccine 180
nephrotic syndrome, pneumococcal vaccine in 240, 242
nucleocapsid
  EHV-1
    disruption 192, 202
    effect of formamide on 193, 196–198
    morphology 192
    trypsinization 193–195

otitis media, pneumococcal vaccine in 240

parasitic disease vaccine 299–309
  malaria 305–308
  schistosomiasis 300–302
    killed 302
    live 301, 302
  trypanosomiasis
    African 303, 304
    American 304, 305
pertussis vaccine 29–54
  controversy 48–50
  effect 42
  reactions 43–48
  standardization 42, 43
  trials 42
  use in paediatrics 20, 21
    reactions 21
  see also whooping cough
pneumococcal vaccines 212, 218, 219, 237–243
  antibody levels after vaccination 241, 242
  reactions 238
  use
    in chronic nephrotic syndrome 240, 242
    in otitis media 240
    in sickle-cell anaemia 240
polio vaccine 117–150
  administration route 136
  antibody 124–127
  failures 124
  herd effect 128–136
  killed 21, 22, 120
    immune response to 120
  live 21, 22, 117, 118
    inactivation 145–148
    potency 117, 119

polio vaccine *continued*
reversion 22, 117, 137, 141
memory, immunological 125, 127
use in paediatrics 21, 22
vaccination program, effect of 136–145
vaccinology 148, 149

quadruple vaccine 43, 46, 120
see also diphtheria–pertussis–tetanus vaccine

rabies vaccine 87–101
avian embryo 88, 89
diploid cell 92
Fermi 88
nervous tissue 87, 88
polyvalent 96, 97
post-exposure vaccine 95, 96
reactions 88, 92
Semple 88
subunit vaccine 95
tissue culture
human 91–94
veterinary 90, 91
wildlife 97
reactions 43–48, 58, 75–77, 88, 92, 238, 262–264
respiratory virus vaccines
use in paediatrics 25, 26
veterinary 314
ribosomal vaccines 211–222
RNA
double-stranded 211
stimulation of immune system 213
rubella vaccine 23
administration in pregnancy 111
conversion 108
cost–benefit 113
efficacy 111
historical development 103–105
intranasal administration 110

Salmonella typhimurium vaccine 213–217, 219
live 216
schistosomiasis *see* parasitic disease vaccine
sickle-cell anaemia, pneumococcal vaccine in 240
sleeping sickness 303
smallpox 2, 3, 14, 15
streptococcal vaccine 217, 218
caries 275
swine influenza, New York immunization program 71–86
cost 77
Guillain-Barré syndrome 83
organization 71–74
problems 77–85
vaccine reactions 75–77

tetanus vaccine 20
see also diphtheria–pertussis–tetanus vaccine
trypanosomiasis *see* parasitic disease vaccine
tuberculosis 25, 212

vaccines
caries 275–298
historical background 1–5
hyposensitizing allergen extract 315–321
new developments 7–17
paediatric 19–27
pneumococcal 212, 218, 219, 237–243
reactions *see* reactions
ribosomal 211–222
veterinary 311–314
see also measles, mumps, whooping cough, influenza, rabies, rubella, hepatitis, herpesvirus, cholera
vaccinology 148, 149
varicella 26, 179
see also herpesvirus
veterinary vaccines 311–314
Escherichia coli 313
foot rot 312, 313
herpesvirus 314
leptospirosis 312
Marek's disease 179, 180, 314
respiratory 314
virion 9
EHV-1 183–191, 200–202

whooping cough 29–31
mortality 34–42, 50–53
notification 31–34
see also pertussis vaccine